JANUA LINGUARUM

STUDIA MEMORIAE
NICOLAI VAN WIJK DEDICATA

edenda curat

C. H. VAN SCHOONEVELD

Indiana University

Series Maior, 28

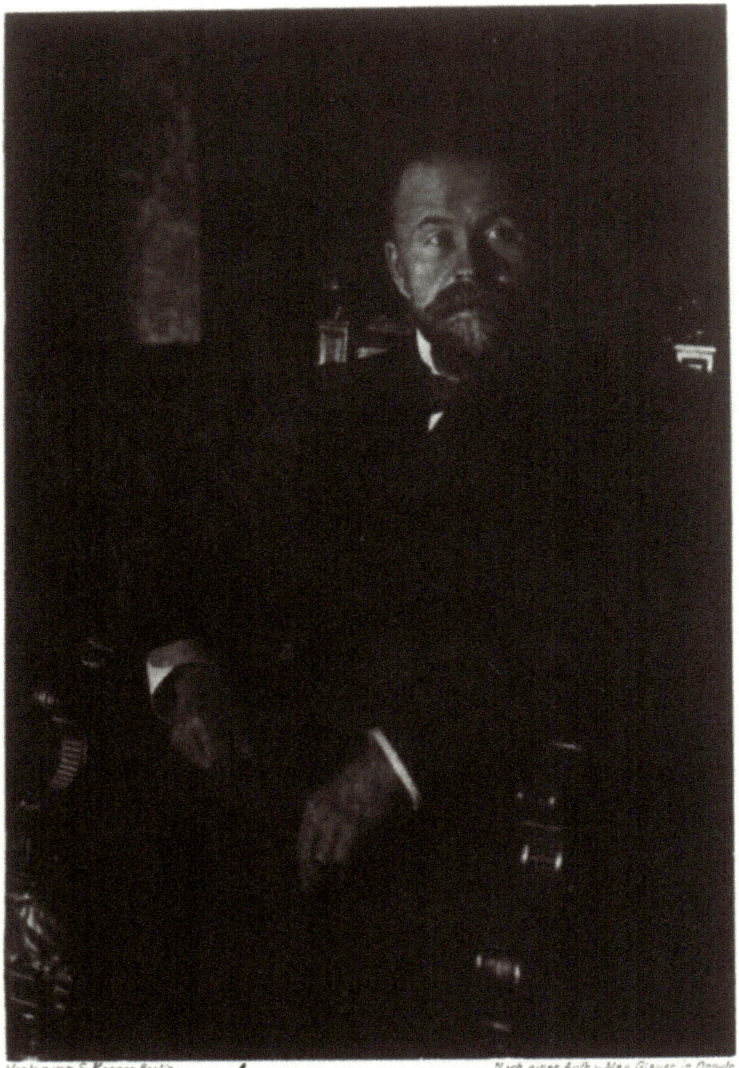

Verlag von S. Karger Berlin. Nach einer Aufn. v. Max Glauer in Oppeln

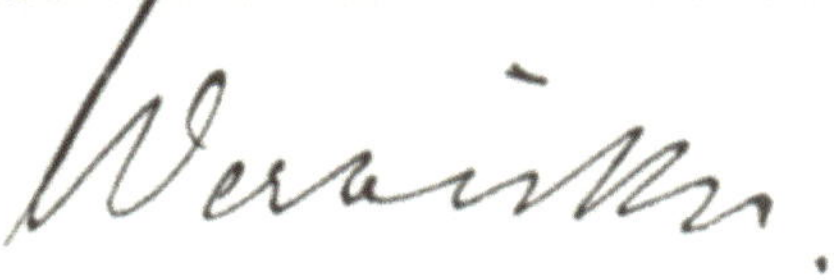

CARL WERNICKE
1848–1905

Wernicke's Works on Aphasia
A Sourcebook and Review

Early Sources in Aphasia and Related Disorders
Volume 1

Gertrude H. Eggert, Ph.D.

Chief, Speech Pathology Service
Veteran's Administration Lakeside Hospital,
Chicago

Mouton Publishers
The Hague · Paris · New York

ISBN 90-279-7985-5

Printed in the Netherlands

To
MY MOTHER
and the memory of
MY FATHER

In the course of years I have yet much to learn, but also much I have accepted as true from others has proved inaccurate. I believe that this double-edged discovery spares no one who holds an earnest striving, and that one need not thereby be wholly disenchanted.

If man would not be a mere counting-machine or registrar, he remains exposed to error. But should he, therefore, hold the counting-machine as his ideal? May that thought hold as little sway in my riper years, as it has in the past.*

CARL WERNICKE
Breslau, 1892

FOREWORD

In 1967, when in the process of selecting a topic for her doctoral dissertation at Northwestern University, Dr. Eggert expressed an interest in doing a translation and interpretation of Carl Wernicke's works on aphasia. I strongly encouraged her to undertake this project for two reasons. There was a great need for such a work to be accomplished and beyond this, Dr. Eggert had excellent qualifications for doing it. Not only did she have the knowledge of German so obviously necessary, but she also had a strong academic and clinical background in the field of aphasia as a speech pathologist. Her decision to do this research, rather than to do a more limited experimental study more typical of thesis research in applied sciences, is amply justified by this volume; and I believe that with it, Dr. Eggert has made a singularly significant contribution.

Perhaps the greatest value of Dr. Eggert's work is that it brings to English-speaking aphasiologists the work of a genius whose contributions have not, until recently, been sufficiently appreciated nor understood. Though his concepts did receive considerable attention during his lifetime, Carl Wernicke's influence on the field of aphasia did not remain constant. The biased assault of Henry Head, in 1926, on Wernicke, his contemporaries, and his students – Head derisively labeled them as "diagram makers" – was successful enough to produce more than a quarter century of indifference and neglect towards these highly important contributions. Head's success in drawing attention away from Wernickean interpretations of language and aphasia was in no small way abetted by the unfortunate tendency towards linguistic parochialism among English speakers. Thus, more often than not English summaries and criticisms replaced Wernicke's work itself as the chief source of information. Neglect would have been bad enough; but to the extent that Wernicke's ideas were not neglected, they were often grossly misinterpreted.

Happily, Wernicke's contributions have been brought to the fore anew. This renaissance has been due in large part to the brilliant work of Myers, Sperry, and others at the California Institute of Technology on "split-brain" phenomena, and to the equally brilliant work of Dr. Norman Geschwind on the application of Wernicke's theories on brain function to disconnexion syndromes in animals and man.

The present volume now affords the opportunity to peruse Wernicke's works in English, an opportunity that should be relished by anyone with a scholarly interest in aphasia who has not had access to this material or who does not read the German language competently. The reader will discover that much of what Wernicke wrote in the late nineteenth and early twentieth centuries has a distinctly modern aura; indeed, his concepts are highly congruent with much contemporary thought on brain function in relation to language and to language pathology. At the same time, it is quite clear that Wernicke often could not transcend the limited neurological and psychological knowledge of his time. As a result, certain of his concepts are out-dated and, on occasion, absolutely incorrect. A significant aspect of this volume is the analysis and discussion of Wernicke's works by Dr. Eggert, which helps to place these concepts in a historical perspective so that we may appreciate the man's accomplishments and also recognize his limitations and failures.

With Carl Wernicke's monumental contribution, as Dr. Geschwind has emphasized, we truly enter into the modern era of thought on aphasia. This volume thus opens the door to the beginnings of this era for neurologists, speech and language pathologists, psychologists, linguists, and to others seeking an understanding of the cerebral mechanisms on which are based language functions and dysfunctions.

November 3, 1976

GERALD J. CANTER, Ph. D.
Professor of Speech Pathology
Northwestern University

ACKNOWLEDGEMENTS

This investigation was supported in part by a Public Health Grant, S0, 05420, from the National Institutes of Neurological Diseases and Stroke.

By a happy coincidence the appearance of this volume follows in the wake of the one-hundredth anniversary of Wernicke's discovery of sensory aphasia. It is hoped that this discussion and the translation of his works may serve to mark this event and to encourage a reassessment of his contributions. This volume is the first of a series of critical reviews and translations of early works on aphasia and related disorders.

The major portion of this work was undertaken as a doctoral study at Northwestern University. The translation of Wernicke's 1906 monograph on aphasia and Chapters V and VI have been added later. With the exception of a recent translation of the 1874 work and an early (1908) translation of the 1906 work, this is the first appearance of Wernicke's writings on aphasia in English.

I am particularly indebted to my colleague, friend, and former professor, Dr. Gerald Canter, who strongly encouraged this undertaking and who generously provided helpful direction and suggestions throughout the study. I would also like to express my appreciation for the helpful criticism of members of the Northwestern University faculty, Dr. R. Koenigsknecht, Dr. Donald Olson, and particularly, Dr. Harold Westlake, whose contributions to neurological speech disorders has stimulated an interest in that area among so many of his students.

The studies of the late nineteenth and early twentieth century workers in neurology and aphasia have provided the major source material for the discussion section of this volume.

Of contemporary workers in this area, Dr. Norman Geschwind has been particularly instrumental in redirecting attention to the significance of Wernicke's works, and I would like to acknowledge his important contributions to this area.

Special gratitude is due my family and particularly, my mother, for providing continuing support during the preparation of this study.

Finally, an analysis of the early work within a contemporary framework would not have been possible without the opportunity for clinical study of a broad population of aphasia patients. I am grateful for the opportunity for such study and the professional exchange with colleagues from a variety of disciplines at a number of medical facilities – The University of Minnesota Hospitals, Milwaukee County Hospital, Louisiana State Medical School, Wayne State Medical School and the VA Lakeside Hospital in Chicago.

Chicago, Illinois
November, 1976

G. H. E.

TABLE OF CONTENTS

PART TWO

A Translation of Carl Wernicke's Major Works on Aphasia

LIST OF FIGURES

PART ONE

A DISCUSSION OF CARL WERNICKE'S CONTRIBUTIONS TO APHASIA

I.

INTRODUCTION

The study of a science or discipline is enhanced and becomes intelligible through a perceptive understanding of its past. Such a historical perspective provides some kind of coherent framework for evaluation of current theory and development.

The study of aphasia has its roots in nineteenth century neurology. New insights in assessing contemporary trends may be gained by a review of ideas bred in that earlier era, a vigorous and productive epoch in the history of aphasia research.

Interest in this period has recently been revived by Geschwind and others. One aspect of current research has focused on implications of corpus callosal connections in cerebral function and interhemispheric relations. These concepts, however, are in fact not new but may be considered as extensions of the connectionistic theory generated in the work of Carl Wernicke and his followers, the Breslau-Halle school of aphasia. Indeed, Liepmann, Lissauer, Storch, Heilbronner, Dejerine, Pick and other contemporaries of Wernicke carried out the first studies of disconnection syndromes some sixty years ago.

Unfortunately, the lack of primary sources in English, describing the work of these men, leaves many workers in neurology, speech pathology and other disciplines with a cloudy and often distorted picture of their contributions. The secondary sources available tend to be sketchy in information and frequently biased in interpretation. Moreover, the lack of primary sources may at times result in loss or neglect of pertinent information, as is true of the early callosal studies, thus delaying progress in certain areas.

Carl Wernicke launched this era in the history of aphasia in 1874 with his publication, *Der aphasische Symptomencomplex: Eine psychologische Studie auf anatomischer Basis.* This monograph was to become a model for later research and is regarded as a classic in aphasia literature. Wernicke's other works in this area provide a rich source of information for the student interested in tracing the history of aphasia through the eyes of the man whose work was of unique significance in forging the direction of that history.

Wernicke is remembered primarily as the discoverer of sensory aphasia. However, the real substance of his contribution lies not merely in his identification and localization of that clinical entity but in his formulation of a theory of psychic life of which language behavior formed a part. His formula which related behavioral findings to anatomic and pathological data permitted the evolvement of an aphasia model and the development of a scientific approach to the study of aphasia.

In historical retrospect, the Wernicke era emerges as perhaps the most productive and significant period in the history of aphasia. Head's (1926) review has been utilized as the major English reference for the literature of this period. Unfortunately, a study of the original sources leads to a serious questioning of the accuracy of Head's assessment. The value of his work as an objective critique is weakened by its strong holistic bias and its rather superficial treatment of the earlier works. This bias is reflected in his dismissal of Wernicke as well as many of his British and French contemporaries under the label of "diagram-makers." Their contributions were summarized in a chapter entitled "Chaos."

Wernicke's original monograph, *Der aphasische Symptomencomplex,* and his later writings on aphasia constitute significant primary sources in the area of aphasia and historically provide a unique contribution to our early professional literature.

The study which follows includes a translation of Wernicke's major writings on aphasia and attempts to explore the impact of his works on later historical trends and the significance of his ideas to current concepts of aphasia.

This discussion does not intend to provide still another critique of localization and holistic points of view, a subject which has been the target of much analysis and debate in the history of aphasia. It is felt that history has revealed the validity of both approaches in the study of higher mental processes. Furthermore, it is well recognized that the achievements of the nineteenth-century workers reflect and are restricted by the limits of the scientific and medical knowledge of that time, and this review shall not attempt to focus on such obvious limitations.

This discussion shall rather attempt to present an exposition of Wernicke's contribution to aphasia and an examination of its effect on later developments in aphasia.

Moreover, it is the hope that this discussion together with a presentation of the original writings may invite a new appraisal of nineteenth century concepts of aphasia as reflected in the works of one of its chief representatives.

Finally, it is hoped that the mode of presentation chosen, which has attempted to facilitate the availability of the original works, may point up the importance of the use of primary sources in the study of aphasia.

II

BIOGRAPHICAL REVIEW

EARLY LIFE

Carl Wernicke was born on May 15, 1848 in a village in upper Silesia, close to the Galician border. After attending the public schools in this small town, his education was continued at the academies of Oppeln and Breslau. Details of his early life are scanty. Some of the events of his early home life were confided to Liepmann, who was his closest assistant and colleague. The memorial accounts and early summaries by his assistants and colleagues have provided the chief sources of information for this discussion (Bonhoeffer, 1905), (Heilbronner, 1905), (Kleist, 1905, 1959), (Liepmann, 1905, 1911, 1922), (Siemerling, 1905), (Ziehen, 1905). Later reviews of his life and works have been sketched by Buesz (1955), Gruhle (1948), Goldstein, (1953), Hildebrandt (1921), Schroeder (1939), and most recently, Geschwind (1966).

Wernicke grew up in a family of modest means. The father, a secretary to a town official, is described by Liepmann as a taciturn, reserved man who did not openly show affection to his wife and children. The mother, pictured as a devout, soft-hearted woman, was strongly interested in Wernicke's education and hopeful that he would study for the ministry.

Shortly before Wernicke's admission to the University of Breslau, his father died. In view of the family's limited means, his guardian advised that young Wernicke take an apprenticeship and train to become a locksmith. However, the mother's strong determination that his education be continued prevailed. Although he chose medicine instead of theology, she somehow found the means to support his studies. Her death, however, occurred shortly before his state examinations, and she did not live to see the realization of her struggles.

At Breslau, Wernicke studied medicine under Haidenhain, Meddledorph, Spiegelbert, and Lebert. His college days were apparently happy, and he enjoyed the reputation of being "a good fellow".

Some indecision regarding a field of specialty marked the completion of Wernicke's studies. At first he considered the possibility of entering private practice in Görlitz. However, the skill and personality of Foerster, the ophthalmologist, led to a decision to spend a six-month assistantship in the Eye clinic at the University of Breslau. Foerster was sensitive to Wernicke's unique potential and remained his life-time friend and patron.

Following this short experience, Wernicke entered service in the Franco-Prussian War of 1870 and assisted the surgeon Fischer in treating the wounded on the battle field.
This experience also had an influential effect on Wernicke, and he briefly considered surgery as a possible speciality. The direction of his future interests, however, took a decisive turn when he returned to Breslau to accept an assistantship in the Psychiatric Institute of the Allerheiligen Hospital under Heinrich Neumann. It is quite evident that the seeds of his later interest in psychiatry and higher mental processes were laid in these early years at Breslau. His fellow assistants during that period included the neuropathologist Carl Friedländer and the neurohistologist Weigert, who remained his life-long friends. During his assistantship at Breslau, Neumann allowed Wernicke to spend a six-month period of study with Meynert in Vienna.

This renowned neuroanatomist was to have a profound and lasting influence on Wernicke's development. It is quite likely that this experience supplied an immediate channeling of his interests into the area of neuroanatomy and directed his early interest to the problem of aphasia. The appearance of his first major work on aphasia shortly after may well reflect the significance of the Vienna visit. The publication of *Der aphasische Symptomencomplex* in 1874 focused strong and somewhat surprised attention of the neurological community on the young twenty-six year old assistant. This significant event marked the close of the first period of Wernicke's medical training and his early years at Breslau.

THE BERLIN YEARS

Wernicke was next drawn to Berlin, the nucleus of the German medical world. Here in 1875 he accepted an assistantship under the urbane and gifted Westphal. The psychiatric polyclinic at the Berlin Charité Hospital offered a wealth of opportunity for the study of neurological and psychiatric disorders. In Berlin his talents were soon recognized and in Liepmann's words, he was considered a "rising star". In 1876 he completed his 'Habilitation', a level of achievement in German medical training which permitted assistants to become junior members of the medical faculty and to charge lecture fees. However, this promising beginning came to an abrupt end. Wernicke became involved in a conflict with the hospital administration in regard to some private matter, the nature of which is not clear. Apparently his obstinacy in the matter intensified the antagonism of the authorities, and as a result his assistantship was terminated. Unfortunately this event, which led to the permanent enmity of Althoff, the powerful Ministerial Director who held power to veto applications for medical faculty advancement, was to haunt Wernicke for the remainder of his career.

The break with the Charité hospital in Berlin occurred in March of 1878. Wernicke was now without university connections and research facilities. For a period of seven years he was forced to make a living in the private practice of neurology. Although this was a lean period financially and limited in opportunity for clinical study and research, it was productive in professional publication. The characteristic talent which Wernicke used to exploit his misfortunes is strongly evident here.

The freedom from academic duties permitted him time and energy to work on his *Lehrbuch der Gehirnkrankheiten* [Textbook of Brain diseases], an impressive work which promoted and solidified the distinction won by his first work on aphasia. His early interest in neuroanatomy and neurology continued to be a dominant influence in his thinking during this period. However, the seeds of his interest in psychiatry, planted in the Breslau years, were still active under the surface, as is reflected in publication of his essay, "Ueber das Bewusstsein" [In Regard to Consciousness] in 1879.

Wernicke's reaction to this rather bleak Berlin period has been described by Liepmann: "In spite of misfortune he energetically lost himself in his scientific writing and nourished himself in a large circle of friends made up of artists and writers" (1922)*. The latter included the poet Sudermann, the sculptor Hilger, and the writers Ludwig Pietsch and Steinen. One wonders if the influence of Westphal, Wernicke's cosmopolitan chief at the Charité, was perhaps instrumental in his introduction into this circle.

The possibility of an academic affiliation to permit continuation of his scientific work was repeatedly frustrated. A possible position at the Psychiatric Institute at Dalldorf miscarried as a result of Virchow's protest and Althoff's influence. The latter was still angry about the Charité incident.

THE RETURN TO BRESLAU

Finally, in 1885, an offer to succeed Neumann at the University of Breslau gained Wernicke a return to academic life. His old friend and supporter, the ophthalmologist Foerster, was largely responsible for this opportunity. In 1890 he was promoted to the position of Ordinarius and became chairman of the Department of Neurology and Psychiatry. At long last Wernicke had a clinic of his own, students, a wealth of clinical material, and even a modest laboratory. Liepmann says of this time, "He could now put into practice the interest in psychiatry which had long been active under the surface".* The lar-

* Quotations designated by * have been translated from the original German sources by the author.

ger clinical population available to him provided unlimited opportunity for the study of focal neurological symptoms, an area which had been a strong interest in the past. The Breslau stay was to last for almost twenty years. Although much of Wernicke's activity during this period centered on the study of mental illness, his interpretation of psychic symptoms continued to carry the stamp of his early concentration and interest in neuroanatomy and neuropathology. Indeed, his later formulation of psychic theory was an extension of the model evolved in these earlier years.

This was a fruitful and productive time in Wernicke's life, one which saw the early formulation, elaboration, and testing of his psychic theory, a period for the accumulation of clinical data, and a time marked by the association of gifted colleagues and assistants. Among these are counted distinguished names in the history of neurology – Liepmann, his most intimate assistant and colleague, Lissauer, whose promising work was cut short during his assistantship, Heilbronner, Foerster, Kleist, and Goldstein.

It was also a productive period in study and research in aphasia. These years saw Lichtheim's extension of the Wernicke aphasia schema which was to stimulate and popularize the use of complicated schemas in Germany, France, and England. It provided the soil in which were bred the works of Liepmann on apraxia, Lissauer on visual agnosia, Heilbronner on asymbolia, and Storch on psycho-physiological aspects of aphasia. Wernicke himself produced the classic work on tactile agnosia during this time.

Although the opportunities offered in Breslau provided a release from the earlier frustrating period with its lack of university affiliation, this small provincial academic setting was hardly the ideal or ultimate goal for a man of Wernicke's achievements and potential. Three choice university positions fell vacant in Germany at this time. Niessl von Mayendorf (1925) reports that Wernicke was selected to become chairman of the Department of Neurology and Psychiatry at Vienna, which had been formerly held by Meynert and recently vacated by Krafft-Ebing. Before the offer was officially presented, however, a false rumor of Wernicke's refusal was circulated in a number of Viennese newspapers, and the offer never materialized. Furthermore, during this time, the influence of his old foe Altmann is reported by Liepmann to have checked an opportunity to become director of the Neurological Clinic at Berlin. Another possible opportunity in Munich was lost in favor of Kraeplin. Wernicke's last years at Breslau were filled with frustration. The Psychiatric Clinic at the university was under municipal administration which at this time severed connections with the Institute. The state was reluctant to supply funds for the building of a new Clinic. Wernicke, who simultaneously held a position at the city hospital, was still permitted the use of clinical material and the opportunity to lecture at this Institute. However, even this privilege was later withdrawn. For a year Wernicke was without university affiliation and had access only to a municipal neurological polyclinic. As a result he lost his assistants, among them Liepmann, who went to Dalldorf.

Again, Wernicke turned misfortune to advantage and devoted the year to his famous work on psychiatry, *Grundriss der Psychiatrie* [Foundations of Psychiatry]. He later confessed that without this year of freedom from official duties this work would likely not have been possible.

Although his privileges at the municipal institute were later restored, Wernicke was disenchanted with the entire frustrating situation at Breslau. An offer in 1904 to direct the Clinic of Psychiatry and Neurology at the University of Halle was accepted as a welcome solution.

THE HALLE PERIOD

Many of the specific and intimate details of Wernicke's brief years at Halle, cut short by his death, have been supplied by Kleist, one of his youngest assistants. At the University of Halle he was successor to Ziehen, who had received the offer to Berlin which had been denied Wernicke by Althoff's animosity.

The kind of effect Wernicke had on his assistants is evident in the words written by Kleist many years later. "When I first wrote his memorial some thirteen days after his passing, I was still filled with his presence and shattered by his death" (1959).* Kleist's description of his first encounter with Wernicke provides a glimpse of him at a medical meeting in October, 1903. "My companion pointed to a darkly-clothed, serious man strolling about during a break in the sessions. He said only, 'That is Wernicke;' but the manner and respect with which the words were spoken showed that this was no ordinary man" (1959).*

Kleist has also described the preparation of the young assistants for their new chief at Halle. This took the form of reading his *Grundriss* late into the night and absorbing his new concepts on mental illness.

Among the distinguished guests who attended Wernicke's inaugural ceremony was Hitzig. Ten years earlier, he had been the originator of the free, open-type psychiatric clinic at Halle, which emphasized new techniques in the treatment of mental patients.

This year was also marked by the meticulous collection of data on mental illness which was applied to the testing of Wernicke's psychic theory, now in its final stages of development, and by further exploration into the areas of neurohistology and neurosurgery. Data from these latter studies was designed to further test and advance his hypotheses on the problems of mental illness.

The achievements and stimulation of this period were reflected in changes in Wernicke. Kleist reports that he appeared happier, freer, and "more mellow", enjoying the stimulation which the new opportunities at Halle offered. His efforts were now devoted almost entirely to the study of psychiatric problems, although he encouraged and followed with interest the studies of his assistants in the area of neurology and particularly aphasia and related disorders.

During the Halle period, Wernicke appeared renewed by the stimulation of his studies and students, content in his family life and a circle of close friends and colleagues, and in recreation which included mountain climbing, gymnastics, and cycling.

This new contentment met an abrupt end on June 15, 1905, when a cycling accident claimed his life. Pfeifer, the young surgical colleague from his clinic was his companion on the death-trip. Cycling along a narrow road in the Thüringer forest, they met a timber cart and in the course of the narrow passing Wernicke fell under the cart, the rear wheel crushing his chest. Later advances in thoracic surgery which might have saved his life were not yet available. He lived for two painful days but until the last would not permit his wife to be called, to spare her the anguish of his suffering.

Wernicke was 57 and in the midst of new discoveries when the accident occurred. The immediate shock and sorrow of his colleagues and associates is readily evident in their memorial accounts. Such reviews, however, also presaged the impact of his work on the future. This hope and forecast of his future influence may be summarized in Liepmann's (1905) closing eulogy:

> The man is gone from us. But his teaching will continue to reap fruit as one of the most vital forces and most productive influences in the continuing development of our science.*

III.

CARL WERNICKE: SKETCHES

WERNICKE: THE WRITER

Wernicke left a considerable body of writing which represents a summary of his contributions in the areas of aphasia, neuroanatomy, clinical neurology, and psychiatry. These works reflect his central absorption with the problem of the relationship between neuroanatomy, physiology, and psychic behavior.

His first as well as his last important work concerned the problem of aphasia. Few writers open their careers with the dramatic acclaim met by the 1874 *Aphasia Symptom-Complex,* which presented the discovery of sensory aphasia and contained Wernicke's first formulation of his aphasia doctrine. This was followed by a brief paper on aphasia and anarthria in 1882 and a longer essay, "Ueber die motorische Sprachbahn und das Verhältnis der Aphasie zur Anarthie" [The Motor Speech Path and the Relation of Aphasia to Anarthia] in 1884. His second important monograph on this subject, " Einige neuere Arbeiten ueber Aphasie" [Recent Works on Aphasia] appeared in 1885. Wernicke returned to this topic once again shortly before his death in his "Deutsche Klinik" *Aphasische Symptomencomplex* which was posthumously published in 1906 and later appeared in English translation (Church: 1908). This discussion was preceded in 1903 by a paper on agraphia which had been stimulated by his observation of an isolated form of this disorder during this period. These works will be reviewed in greater detail in the chapters which follow.

The bulk of Wernicke's writings was devoted to the areas of neuroanatomy, neuropathology, and clinical neurology. An early evidence of the effect of his visit to Meynert may be seen in two papers published shortly after the Vienna trip, "Das Urwindungssystem des menschlichen Gehirns" [The Primordial Gyral-System of the Human Brain] and "Erkrankung der inneren Kapsel" [Diseases of the Internal Capsule]. The first paper attempted to relate certain features of the primate brain to those of the human in its early stages of embryonic development. In this study he directed attention to the appearance of the "primordial gyral-arc." which was noted to enclose the entire speech area, including motor and sensory areas together with the supramarginal and angular gyri. Ziehen (1905) commented that Wernicke was first to recognize the three major sulci and their relationship to the total plan of the brain. This reveals Wernicke's characteristic approach to problems, in which the total structure of the design was scanned and subordinate details placed in their proper relationship to the complete picture.

The major fruit of the Berlin period and Wernicke's most significant contribution to the area of clinical neurology may be found in his textbook on neurological disorders, *Lehrbuch der Gehirnkrankheiten* [Textbook of Brain Diseases], which appeared in 1881-82. This three-volume work was a major accomplishment for a man who was still in his early thirties. It contained an anatomic-physiologic review based largely on Meynert's works, a classification of brain diseases, and a discussion of the general pathology of focal cerebral involvement. This publication, which championed the localization approach, is described by Liepmann as "not merely a compilation of facts and a review of the literature, but the presentation of a unique theory of the same" (1905).* Ziehen later commented that, in this work, "Wernicke opened wide the door to the study of brain anatomy. . . Meynert's renowned work was too brief and too obscure" (1905).* The *Lehrbuch* was regarded as the major textbook in neurology until the appearance of Von Monakow's work in the late 1890's.

One year later Wernicke undertook a translation of Duchenne's study on the physiology of movement. This task reflected his interest in the mechanisms of normal and disturbed muscle function. Not only did his translation serve to focus attention on this important French work, but as Liepmann has reflected, may likely have provided the stimulus for Wernicke's later studies on residual hemiplegia.

In 1893 another significant publication appeared. This was Wernicke's *Gesammelte Aufsätze und kritische Referate zur Pathologie die Nervensystems* (Collected Essays and Critical Reviews in Neuropathology). This compilation contained reprints of his works on aphasia, a few early essays in the area of psychiatry, a number of original papers on neuroanatomy and clinical neurology, and concluded with a series of critiques of current French and German studies on cerebral localization and neuropathology. This work was dedicated to the memory of Friedländer, his earlier fellow-assistant at Breslau. In this work and in his textbook can be found reports of his original discoveries including a study of hemiopic pupillary reactions, the clinical picture of polioencephalitis hemorrhagicca superior (Wernicke's disease), the tracing of the pyramidal tract to the spinal cord, and a description of residual hemiplegia.

Together with Freidländer, Wernicke published the first detailed clinicopathological study of cortical deafness in 1883. His case study and discussion of tactile agnosia, "Zwei Fälle von Rindenlasion" (Two Case Reviews of Cortical Lesions), is also considered classic.

Wernicke's early interest in psychiatry was evident in a number of short essays produced during his Berlin years. These include two papers on consciousness published in 1879. They were followed later by shorter publications in the area of psychiatry, including a paper on the relationship of aphasia to mental illness which appeared in 1890.

Although Wernicke's later writings were largely devoted to this area, his continuing interest in neuroanatomy is revealed in his *Atlas des Gehirns* [Atlas of the Brain], which was published in 1897-1903. This ambitious work, produced in three sections, was put into the hands of his assistants, H. Sachs, Mann, Schroeder, and Foerster. Liepmann has observed that this publication was first to present a review of cerebral anatomy which included enlarged and unretouched photographs of serial sections of the human brain.

The last years at Breslau were marked by the appearance in 1899-1900 of Wernicke's three-volume *Krankenvorstellungen aus der psychiatrischen Klinik in Breslau* [Clinical Studies from the Breslau Pyschiatric Clinic], a compilation of case reviews which provided the basis for his *Grundriss der Psychiatrie* [Foundations of Psychiatry]. This latter work represented an attempt to relate neuroanatomic, pathologic, and neurophysiologic principles to psychic function and approached the problem of psychiatric disorders from a neurologic standpoint. It contained three parts, an introductory section on psychophysiologic aspects of mental processes, a second on paranoid disorders, and a final section on the acute pyschoses. Although Wernicke's interpretation and classification in the area of mental illnesses did not survive, this work continued to be valued for its wealth of clinical observation and insight. Jasper, for example, representing an entirely different orientation, commented years later that Wernicke had created "one of the outstanding works in psychiatry. . . which no psychiatrist. . . can afford to neglect" (Liepmann, 1922).*

Wernicke's neurologic interpretation of psychic processes has been referred to by Liepmann as "the bridge which leads from the diseased psyche to the brain." He went on to observe:

> To have been first to cast the mold of such a span shall remain the immortal legacy of Wernicke. Who can predict whether all of its shafts and girders will hold? It would go beyond the strength of one man to achieve such a huge task at a single blow. But if in the course of time, sections of the structure are replaced, even if the final appearance is far different from the original plan, yet this shall be the bridge by which coming generations shall reach the opposite shore (Liepmann, 1905).*

WERNICKE: THE MAN

Scattered glimpses of Wernicke as a person can be detected in the memorial accounts of his colleagues and assistants referred to above. These reviews show that Wernicke's interests were not limited to his work. He enjoyed nature and recreation, music, culture, his home and family, as well as the comradeship of a circle of intimate colleagues and friends.

The trait which was his chief characteristic as a scientist was also true of him as a person. He was tenacious and unflinching in pursuing his goals and refusal to compromise. In his personal dealings he tended to be somewhat brusque and direct. He did not curry favor nor was he influenced by the impression of others. If he believed an action to be correct, the criticism as well as the applause of others went unnoticed, while he held steadily to his course. In his personal affairs as in his work, he instinctively struck at the heart of an issue and dealt with it deftly and directly. Liepmann has commented that he was not a man of many words but often effectively employed an ironic, humorous reply.

The hardships and frustrations of his early life and career were met with a kind of stoicism softened by a streak of humor and lack of bitterness. Periods of frustration such as the Berlin years were turned to advantage and he lost himself in his writing and cultural interests. The reserve and sharp aspects of Wernicke's personality were balanced by a streak of the "good fellow" as described by Liepmann. He enjoyed the companionship of a circle of intimate friends, a bottle of good wine, and late evening discussions on topics which he with some amusement referred to as "the deeper questions of life."

Kleist reports that at times his students and assistants were invited to his home where he gave the impression of being the devoted housefather and husband." Little information is available about Wernicke's wife who is described as "much younger than he, pleasant, and somewhat submissive" (Kleist, 1959). Wernicke had three children, two daughters and a son. After the day's work he could often be seen going out into the country-side with a child on each hand.

Although Wernicke was not physically robust, he enthusiastically took part in many different sports such as mountain climbing, cycling, skating and hiking. At one time he climbed the Matterhorn. Music was among his interests, and later on in life he took up piano playing. Evenings were frequently spent accompanying a trio or playing duets with Kaufmann, a member of his clinic staff. Later on in life, he took up the study of higher mathematics which he felt would be useful in his work.

Von Koschützky, a Berlin journalist, who numbered among Wernicke's close friends, has offered some sketchy glimpses of Wernicke's religious and philosophical feelings (Kleist, 1959). Occasionally he followed theological works and was particularly interested in the writings of Harnack, a popular theologian of the day. At one time when the two friends were hiking in the Glatzer mountains, discussing the chief goals in life, Wernicke made the comment, "There is only one proper motive in work and that is. . ." and standing still he groped for the unfamiliar words. . . 'Seek ye first the kingdom of God and all the rest shall follow'." (Kleist, 1959).*

At another time Foerster, his old friend and patron, observed that somewhere in the universe there must be a point where the final riddle of life is resolved." To this Wernicke is said to have answered, "No, I absolutely feel no need to comprehend everything which lies beyond my understanding... and do not feel compelled to wander in the realm of the transcendental" (Kleist, 1959).*

Von Koschütsky has commented that the unbending, tenacious aspects of Wernicke's nature was also the source of his success as a scientist. This trait appears again and again in the accounts of his colleagues. If someone did not appeal to him, he did not try to hide it. In Liepmann's words, "He could be a determined foe, but also a warm, true friend... He went his way and would not humble himself, bowing to the left or right, or up or down, but carried himself with the proud awareness of one who has been entrusted with an important mission in life" (Liepmann, 1905).* It was this relentless striving, this singleness of purpose, which holds the key to Wernicke as a man and as a scientist.

WERNICKE: THE TEACHER

Wernicke attracted a creative group of assistants and students during his years at Breslau and Halle. This group, the Breslau-Halle school of aphasia, was perhaps his most enduring legacy to the history of neurology. Liepmann, Heilbronner, Storch, Bonhoeffer, Sachs, Foerster, Kleist and Goldstein were among its members. The necrologies and reviews of Liepmann (1905; 1922), Heilbronner (1905), and Kleist (1905; 1959) have given us a fairly clear glimpse of Wernicke the teacher and clinic chief. The traditional teaching tools of didactic instruction, clinical observation and examination, conferences, laboratory work, and research made up the clinical program.

One dominating influence pervaded the learning atmosphere – the search to unlock the mechanisms underlying higher mental processes and formulation of a theory of psychiatric disease. This motive supplied the source of energy and enthusiasm for chief and students alike. However, this search demanded mastery of the traditional subjects of neuroanatomy, clinical neurology, and neuropathology which were the necessary tools for such exploration.

The clinical atmosphere is described as a workshop where new ideas were created and tested. The assistants were treated as co-workers and contributors to these new concepts. Wernicke taught by lecture, case-conference, and clinical examination. His lectures are described as concise, delivered with authority, but barren of showmanship or rhetoric. He had the gift of getting at the core of a problem and summarizing it in a few pithy and terse observations. With the exception of Meynert and Kahlbaum, the ideas of others were rarely mentioned. This was not so much a sign of immodesty on Wernicke's part as a reflection of his dissatisfaction with the solution of many of his contemporaries to problems which he considered significant in psychiatry. What he gave his students, therefore, as Liepmann observed, was "uniquely his own."

Wernicke's skill as a clinical examiner is repeatedly mentioned in the accounts of his assistants and colleagues. He is described as a careful and thorough investigator. His background in muscle function, stimulated by Duchenne's work, and his thorough study of focal neurological symptoms in combination with a keen hypothesis-testing approach made such clinic visits a rich learning experience for his students. Liepmann has described the routine followed in the patient examination. The task of observation and recording of symptoms was divided between various assistants. While Wernicke carried out the questioning and testing, Storch recorded all verbal behavior, and Liepmann took notes on the patient's facial expression, gestures, and manual performance. This was followed by a discussion period in which the clinical picture was reconstructed and an interpretation made of the observations reported. These comments were then recorded in "The Golden Book," a compilation of case histories which provided the basis for Wernicke's textbook on psychiatry. This tireless and exhaustive approach to clinical evaluation, characteristic of Wernicke, reveals that he worked not only deductively but empirically, carefully testing his theories with clinical evidence. At times the thoroughness and length of such examinations were the despair of his assistants. This approach led to the establishment of new clinical pictures and uncovered additional symptoms which could not be accommodated under old classification systems. Wernicke's strong emphasis on the importance of detailed clinical study is revealed in an incident reported by Heilbronner. In response to a visitor's request to see the Breslau Clinic Library, Wernicke pointed to the case-history files piled about and said, "That is my library".

Wernicke systematically broadened his clinic faculty with members from related disciplines. His diagnostic conferences were attended by such distinguished guests as Hitzig, whom he greatly admired, as well as Von Bramann, the brain surgeon. Such conferences provided an arena for lively discussion and debate, largely stimulated by these two. During this period several new staff members received appointments at Halle. Among these was Edmund Forster, who had worked with Nissl. Wernicke was well aware of the significance of the area of histology in resolving problems of mental illness and followed with interest, for example, the work of Altzheimer in this area. The study of neurochemistry and its role in brain disease was assigned to Max Kaufmann, who had studied under Zunst. This expansion of faculty reflected Wernicke's growing absorption in the problem of etiology in mental illness in the last years of life. Before this, the areas of neuroanatomical localization and symptomatology had largely absorbed his attention. Kleist has commented that this new direction of research at Halle might well have led to significant changes in Wernicke's theory of psychiatric illness. Moreover, he reports that Wernicke was already aware during the last year of his life that certain sections of his *Grundriss* would require modification.

The assistants were given a great deal of independence and freedom to explore their own areas of interest. Liepmann's work on apraxia, for example, was encouraged by Wernicke who took great pride in the results of this classic study which were published shortly before his death. The senior assistants were made section chiefs and held their own evening case conferences, which were attended by students and visting staff from the city. Wernicke had high expectations, and assistants who did not measure up or whose interests and goals did not coincide with those of the clinic program were not retained. This was facetiously referred to as "the self-purge of the clinic".

Wernicke's blunt and unpretentious ways were reflected in his way of handling his assistants. Liepmann comments that he neither "led them by the nose nor treated them pedantically" (1905). They were considered colleagues working together in an important venture. He rarely gave suggestions, but his own example, as Liepmann has remarked, was "difficult to resist." At one time when an assistant tried to justify an inaccurate diagnosis with many words, Wernicke said simply, "Dear colleague, one of us is wrong" (Kleist, 1959). He often commented on his good fortune in having assistants of such high caliber. However, as Heilbronner has observed, this was a reflection of his skill as teacher and mentor.

The Breslau-Halle school was to become the source of diverse streams in the history of aphasia, as Geschwind (1966) has recently pointed out. This is evident in the different paths taken by his students and assistants. Liepmann, Hans Sachs, and particularly Kleist reflected a strong localizationist approach while Storch, Heilbronner, and Goldstein became involved in the broader psycho-physiologic aspects of the disorder, the latter in fact, to become the chief exponent of the holistic school of aphasia. Yet in all, including Goldstein, the "Wernicke stamp" of careful attention to neuropathology and anatomy was never successfully erased. The apparent paradox that the Wernickean theory was sufficiently broad to permit development in both holistic and localizationist directions may be resolved by a closer study of Wernicke's approach to higher mental processes. His reputation as a strict localizer is contradicted by his observation in 1874 that "primary functions alone can be referred to specific brain areas" (1874, p. 118). Heilbronner was first to point to the merging of the two approaches in Wernicke's works, the neuroanatomical and the psychological, so succinctly revealed in the subtitle of his original work "A Psychological Study on an Anatomic Basis." The combination of these two elements, the anatomic and the psychological, may well account for the vitality and durability of his contribution.

A picture of Wernicke, the teacher, may be summed up in Kleist's (1905) eulogy:

To us his last assistants remains the memory of a renowned yet modest man, a model who entrusted us with far-reaching confidence and independence, a teacher who discovered in each a certain talent. . . To have been his students shall remain our pride as long as we live.*

WERNICKE: THE EXPLORER-THEORIST

It is difficult to study one dimension of an individual's life in isolation. This is certainly true of Wernicke in whom a number of roles were closely bound and realized with remarkable effectiveness. One can see in him the neuroanatomist, the dedicated clinical neurologist and psychiatrist, a venerated clinic chief and teacher, a contented husband and father, and finally a man who enjoyed recreation and the cultural aspects of life.

Which of these was Wernicke first of all? A brief scanning of his life may provide an answer. One central struggle pervaded his work and consumed his energy, the need to resolve the enigma of psychic life and its disturbances. From this perspective Wernicke emerges first of all as "Der Forscher," the explorer-theorist in quest of a theory of psychic life. His earlier pursuits then stand out, not as mere transitions or shifts of interest, but as part of a well-ordered and logically-planned design. The seeds of this central question were likely sown in the early Breslau years under Neumann, to become more clearly defined under Meynert, whose neuroanatomic theories provided the basic tools and direction of the resolution of this problem. His later work in clinical neurology sharpened his skill in the observation of symptomatology and offered an opportunity to apply his background in neuroanatomy and neuropathology to the interpretation of such symptoms. These activities then supplied the basic tools for construction of his theory and were not ends in themselves.

Wernicke's characteristic bent was to scan and extract the huge themes in life. This is clearly evident in the routine management of his clinic, in his mode of teaching, and in his approach to scientific problems. This characteristic is reflected in his approach to the formulation of a theory of aphasia. It may seem strange that the discoverer of sensory aphasia did not immediately attempt to confirm these early tenuous findings by further pathologic studies. This neglect, however, is typical of Wernicke. He was content to raise the major issues of a problem, formulate the basic questions, and to sketch possible formulas which might lead to their resolution. The elaboration and detailing of issues which did not relate to his major interest were left to others.

Wernicke then emerges as a theorist first of all. This characteristic was balanced by the ability to utilize careful testing and verification of data in his primary area of interest, the study of higher processes and psychiatric disorders. This major goal, the unraveling of the problems of such higher psychic processes, was pursued decisively and with uncompromising determination.

Wernicke's work and life were then dominated by one driving force which moved relentlessly forward toward a single goal. Along the way, however, this mainstream was fed by side-channels which prepared the soil for a productive yield in related areas – as his contributions to neuroanatomy, clinical neurology, and the study of aphasia are strong testaments.

IV.

THE WERNICKE SCHEMA OF APHASIA

INTRODUCTION

The thirty-five year period extending from the mid 1870's through the first decade of this century might rightly be called the "Wernicke era" in the history of aphasia. As this review shall attempt to point out, the impetus for the major developments of this period had its sources in the Breslau-Halle school of aphasia.

This era may be studied by tracing the evolution of the Wernicke theory of language and his aphasia model, which represented the preliminary step in his formulation of a schema of higher mental processes, his ultimate goal. The development of this model may be followed through three stages or periods which are somewhat arbitrarily defined. The first period was opened by the 1874 *Aphasia Symptom-Complex,* in which the early outlines of his theory were sketched. The middle or second period, extending from 1885 into the late 1800's, featured an expansion and further development of the schema. The final period was climaxed by his third and last important monograph on aphasia, published posthumously in 1906, which contains a recapitulation of his earlier views in the light of later findings of his contemporaries.

In the chapters which follow we shall attempt to sketch the major landmarks characteristic of these three periods in the development of the Wernicke aphasia model, selecting and concentrating particularly on concepts and ideas which were innovative or which opened new areas of approach to a study of the disorder.

WERNICKE'S EARLY APHASIA PERIOD 1874-1885

The discovery of sensory aphasia in 1874 aroused an immediate surge of interest in this clinical entity. Such an effect was not surprising since these findings signaled an important advance in the understanding of aphasia. Two brief descriptions of the loss of comprehension in certain cases of aphasia, by Bastian (1869) and by Schmidt (1871), preceded the 1874 findings. However, these papers did not stress the complete clinical symptomatology characteristic of this entity, nor did they include a confirmation of its localization by pathological studies.

The immediate impact of the discovery of sensory aphasia tended to overshadow the deeper significance of the 1874 work. Wernicke's real intent in this study lay in the presentation of a theory of aphasia approached from a psycho-neuroanatomic perspective. Heilbronner (1905) was first to point to the significance of the monograph's subtitle, "A Psychological Study on an Anatomic Basis," which revealed Wernicke's focal emphasis on the interrelationship between psychologic aspects of language behavior and its neuroanatomical substrate. Although the discovery of sensory aphasia and a new language center provided one of the cornerstones of the theory formulated in this monograph and was an indispensable component in its total structure, a presentation of these new findings was not Wernicke's basic purpose in the 1874 work.

The mode of organization of the monograph exposes its broader intent and sets it apart from the usual clinico-pathological studies of the day. The characteristic pattern of such publications commonly featured an introductory section with a review of a specific clinical picture which was followed by a discussion of the pathological findings and concluded occasionally by a brief commentary. This pattern, however, as a study of the translation reveals, was ignored by the youthful author of the *Aphasia Symptom Complex.* His review of clinico-pathological findings rather follows and is used to support the exposition of his aphasia theory to which in fact more than half of the monograph is devoted.

Wernicke's early aphasia model, as described in the 1874 work, represented his preliminary formulation of a theory of aphasia which later studies proved to be essentially complete in its major tenets. This work raised and attempted to answer questions which were to occupy the thinking of neurologists interested in aphasia during the next decades. In fact, such issues continue to be significant in the study of aphasia as well as other areas of communication today. These problems include exploration of the processes involved in language development, the mechanisms implicated in sensory-motor speech programming, the acquisition of reading and writing skills, the relationship of cerebral localization to disturbances in language and related processes, the problem of a feedback or monitoring system in speech production, and the study of the relationship of higher processes such as concept formation to language behavior. The 1874 work, as well as Wernicke's later writings, attempted to clarify some of the issues involved in these problems and in some instances to advance possible solutions. This work popularized the use of diagrams or schemas which attempted to pictorially illustrate possible

* Wernicke's 1874 work was probably largely stimulated during his Vienna visit by Meynert's paper "Ein Fall von Sprachstörung" *Wien Med. Jahrbücher*, VI, 1866 in which he refers to a total of 5 cases of speech disturbance with involvement of the island area.

mechanisms in language function and aphasia disorders.

During this early period Wernicke also directed his attention to the neuroanatomical basis underlying the differentiation of anarthia and motor aphasia. This led to his publication of "The Motor Speech Path and the Relationship of Aphasia to Anarthia," which was his other major work on aphasia during this period. Wernicke's early interest in higher mental processes and psychiatry was reflected in the publication of two short essays on the subject of consciousness at this time. The latter part of this period was marked by a number of shorter papers in the areas of neuroanatomy, neuropathology, and clinical neurology.

A review of Wernicke's works reveals two concepts as central to his theory of aphasia: (a) the Meynert doctrine of association fibers and specialized cortical centers, and (b) the theory of memory imagery. The discussion which follows shall attempt a review of these two concepts and their relationship to the Wernicke schema.

The Neuroanatomical Basis of the Wernicke System

The 1874 monograph opens with Wernicke's acknowledgment of his debt to Meynert, his former teacher at the University of Vienna. He quite frankly states that the work essentially reflects an application of Meynert's neuroanatomic approach to the study of aphasia. Acclaim is also given to Broca's localization of a motor speech area, which provided Wernicke with one of the primary cornerstones for construction of his aphasia model.

Let us now briefly sketch the major tenets of the neuroanatomic foundation presented in the original 1874 work. The core ingredients of the Meynert doctrine included a differentiation of the cerebral cortex into posterior sensory and anterior motor regions and the presence of fiber tracts linking these areas with each other. These concepts have been discussed in detail by Meynert in his work, *Psychiatrie,* which was published in 1884 and translated into English by B. Sachs one year later. An understanding of Meynert's neuroanatomic constructs is basic to understanding Wernicke's theory of aphasia.

The Projection Fiber System

Meynert divided the fiber tracts of the brain into two major systems, the projection and association pathways. In his description of the projection tracts he says:

> The cleavage system of each convolution presents radiating fibers... These radiating fibers, originating in the cortex, end in some peripheral gray substance near the nuclei of the cranial nerves... I propose to call these fibers, which begin but do not end in the cortex, projection fibers... We may argue that the cerebral cortex is the surface upon which the entire body is projected by means of these nerves. (1885, pp. 37, 38, 39).

Meynert differentiated two types of such projection paths, the centripetal tracts carrying sensory information to the cortex and the centrifugal, conveying motor impulses to the periphery. This projection system, furthermore, was divided into three orders or levels. The first level included fibers coursing between the cortex and subcortical ganglia, a second between the thalamus and the central gray matter of the brain stem, and a third order between the latter and the sensory or motor end-organs.

The Association Fiber System

Meynert described the second great fiber system, the association tracts, as bundles which in contrast to the projection paths"... begin and end in the cortex" (1885, p. 38). Shorter fibers designated as "arciform fibers" and the "fibrae propriae" made up the connection between the individual gyri (p. 39). Longer tracts coursed between various cortical areas. The major intracortical association fasciculi cited by Meynert included the medullary substance of the cingulum and the arcuate and uncinate fasciculi. The corpus callosum was regarded as a form of fibrae propriae which formed the connecting bond between the two hemispheres.

The Motor and Sensory Regions

Let us now turn our attention to the two regions which were connected with each other and the peripheral nervous system by means of these two fiber systems. A differentiation of the sensory and motor features of these two areas was fundamental to Wernicke's theory of aphasia. In the 1874 monograph, attention was focused primarily on the sensory region and its relationship to language.

Meynert used the mollusk as a model to describe the sensory and motor features of certain cortical areas:

> The prosencephalic cortex possesses centripetally conducting processes, the sensory fibers of the nervous system which may be considered its tentacles, and motor fibers which are its claws. The remainder of the body with its sensitive surfaces, its muscles and skeleton, ... serves to sustain these tentacles and claws which enable the forebrain to receive images of the external world and to react upon the latter... A single functional energy only... is inherent in the brain cell, and that is 'sensitiveness' (1885, pp. 138, 139).

Meynert's sensory-motor dichotomy of cortical areas was based on three sources of information: histology, pathology, and comparative anatomy.

The presence of hemiplegia in some cases of destruction of the "prosencephalic ganglia, particularly the lenticular nucleus," was cited by Meynert as an example of his use of pathological data for support of such cerebral differentiation, since these nuclei were known to be connected to the anterior cortical area. In contrast, the posterior cortical region was hypothesized to be sensory in function, since disorders of sensation had been observed in association with lesions of nuclei containing fiber radiations from the posterior areas.

Meynert's use of data from comparative anatomy to support his sensory-motor dichotomy may be illustrated by his comparison of olfactory lobe development in man with that of animals primarily dependent upon olfaction for obtaining food. He noted that the development of this lobe in such lower animals was much greater than that in man. Moreover, development of the fornix, which was believed to be associated with olfaction, was insignificant in man in relation to the rest of the brain. In lower animals, in contrast, the fornix demonstrated extensive development.

Furthermore, Meynert drew attention to the marked proliferation of areas of the human brain surrounding the Sylvian fossa which he hypothesized to be related to psychic processes. He emphasized particularly the extensive development of the claustrum in man which he felt had specific significance in language function.

In regard to the relationship of the island-region for speech processes Meynert stated:

> I have found that the disturbances of psychic speech which are classed under aphasia and its allied conditions depend upon lesions of the claustrum, and in general. . . upon lesions in the wall of the Sylvian fissure (1885, p. 142).

This short review has attempted to outline the major features of the Meynert doctrine of fiber associations and his sensory-motor cortical dichotomy. In addition to Meynert's influence, three other experimeters were significant in forging the doctrine of localization during this period. The studies of Fritsch and Hitzig (1870; 1874) confirming the motor function of the anterior cerebral areas coincided with Wernicke's first work on aphasia. In an addendum to this publication Wernicke applauded such research, observing that such findings "prove that the anatomic and physiologic studies directed toward achieving a deeper understanding of the brain go hand in hand" (1874, p. 69). The ablation studies of Munk (1876-79) describing psychic blindness and deafness also provided frequent sources of reference in Wernicke's textbook on neurological disorders. It is possible that these latter studies reinforced Wernicke's interest in the problems of reading and writing disorders, already evident in his first work on aphasia.

The Speech Area

Let us now turn our attention briefly to Wernicke's concept of the sensory-motor speech region which was the focus of his 1875 study, "Das Urwindungsystem des menschlichen Gehirns" [The Primordial Gyral-System of the Human Brain.]

Influenced perhaps by Meynert's example, Wernicke found the area of comparative anatomy a productive approach to study of this particular cerebral region. In the work referred to he noted the striking similarity between certain structural features of animal brains and those demonstrated at various stages of embryonic development in the human. Such studies, he felt, emphasized the underlying unitary nature of the speech region. Wernicke described this area as a "rainbow-shaped arc" formed by a single large gyrus enclosing the Sylvian fossa. The anterior portion of this arc was formed by the opercular regions of the frontal lobe, while the complexly-structured supramarginal and angular gyri of the parietal lobe represented its posterior aspect. The island and surrounding temporal lobe area made up the core of this region. The peculiar structural feature formed by this blending of the frontal, temporal, and segments of the posterior area into one apparent functional unit was designated as the "first primordial-gyrus." Wernicke felt that this feature of the embryonic brain supplied an anatomic basis for the unitary nature of the speech region in which the motor and sensory areas were brought into a close anatomical and functional relationship.

The island and the surrounding temporal lobe areas formed the hub of this region. At the time of the 1874 work the precise termination of the auditory nerve was still indefinite. Meynert had traced the nerve to the claustrum, which he regarded as its end-point. This supported the probable relationship of this particular cerebral area to auditory function. In *The Aphasia Symptom Complex* Wernicke described his own dissections of the arcuate fibers which he believed to course through the island-region. Such fibers were assumed to provide the connecting link between the motor and sensory speech areas. In his final work on aphasia published in 1906 Wernicke pointed to the significance of two association bundles, the uncinate fasciculus, extending from the third frontal gyrus to the temporal area penetrating the claustrum, and the arcuate bundle which connected Broca's area to the sensory speech region. Wernicke regarded this latter tract as the major bond between the two speech centers.

Let us now turn briefly to one other problem which occupied Wernicke's attention regarding the speech region during this early period, namely the question of the presence of a separate motor speech path. This problem was discussed in a lengthy paper published in 1884, "The Motor Speech Path." At that time Wernicke postulated the existence of a bundle of motor speech fibers, separate from the rest of the pyramidal tract, the disruption of which was assumed to result in motor aphasia. This idea was later rejected by Wernicke on the basis of Von Monakow's anatomical studies.

This review has attempted to highlight the major neuroanatomical concepts current in the early Wernicke era which furnished the foundation for his model of aphasia. However a second ingredient was necessary for formulation of this model. The theory of memory imagery constituted the second important cornerstone in this theory.

The Wernicke Theory of Memory Imagery

Wernicke's concept of memory imagery occupied a central position in his schema of psychic life. Perception ("primary identification"), comprehension ("secondary identification"), concept formation, and finally, the concept of consciousness itself constituted the essential steps in his hierarchy of psychic function.

The Meynert doctrine of cortical centers and association paths provided the skeleton or framework of such a theory while the notion of memory imagery offered a mechanism by which higher mental processes might occur.

The most detailed discussion of Wernicke's overall interpretation of memory can be found in the introductory chapters of his *Grundriss der Psychiatrie.* His interpretation of the processes involved in production of motor speech imagery was largely based on Meynert's work (1885).

In his "*Grundriss*" Wernicke defines memory as "a special feature of the nervous system characterized by permanent modifications of nerve tissue as the result of stimulation" (1900, p. 21).* This process was felt to involve transfer of the stimulation from the peripheral sensory projection endings to cell circuits in which such permanent changes occurred. The perception of a specific object was assumed to be accompanied by its own particular pattern of cortical excitation.

The "spindle association cells" (apparently referring to the sixth layer of cortical cells) together with the association fibers were believed to constitute the anatomical substrate of memory imagery. This assumption is reflected in Wernicke's statement:

> In the cortex there are ganglion cells invested with the feature of potential permanent modification of transient stimuli, of which persisting residuals remain, which we describe as memory images. (1900, p. 32).*

Wernicke, however, does not assign individual memory images to single cells. a view which has inaccurately been attributed to him by some critics, but rather to cell-circuits or constellations of cells and their association fibers. This notion is evident in his statement:

> By means of a very unique organization of these stimulated cells an image arises which we can project into a specific space.. . . I agree with Sachs and Goldscheider that memory represents a functional connection of the simultaneously perceived elements mediated by the association paths (1900, pp. 23, 25).*

Wernicke did not attempt to explain or hypothesize in any detail the specific mechanisms by which this modification might occur. It was his feeling that sufficient information for an adequate interpretation of this process was not yet available. Repetition of the same combinations of sensory stimulation was believed to result in a reduction of the resistance normally present in the association fibers and in an increase in the response to arousal of memory associations.

The stability of all associations of such memory imagery is maintained by repetition of the same or similar stimuli. . . . The simultaneous and contiguous occurrence of a number of sensory impressions results in the permanent association of such memory associations (1900, p. 25).*

Wernicke applied a Helmholtz resonance type of mechanism to his interpretation of memory revival.

If the same pattern of stimulated elements recurs, the memory image is aroused by cell elements involved in perception, since only the pertinent combinations of cells are 'tuned in' to such perceptual patterns (1900, p. 25).*

Motor Speech Imagery

Wernicke based his concepts of motor speech imagery[1] on the interpretation of Meynert (1885) and earlier workers such as Brücke and Lotze. Brücke and Lotze had differentiated the development of motor patterns into two stages, primary and secondary. Meynert applied these concepts to the speech process.

Let us briefly examine the principles underlying this idea of motor imagery. The primary reflex movements were believed to be initiated by subcortical centers. Production of such reflex movements as eye-closure, for example, in response to painful stimulation of the eye with a sharp instrument, was believed to be accompanied by the deposition of three memory images in the cortex, a visual image of the instrument used, a somatic impression of touch and pain, and an "innervatory" or motor-kinesthetic image which was associated with the motor act of closing the eyelid. Applied to the motor production of speech, this latter image was called the "motor speech image" or "motor speech-representation," and was assumed to have its representation in the motor cortex. These three cortical images maintained a close relationship by means of the association tracts and fibers.

[1] The German word used by Wernicke to refer to motor speech images, "Sprachbewegungsvorstellung", might be literally translated as "speech movement representation." A shorter term, "motor speech image" shall be used here in and the translations which follow.

Secondary motor movements consisted of consciously-produced repetitions of the primary or reflex actions and were believed to be initiated by activation of any one of these three memory images associated with production of the original act. The visual image of the sharp instrument itself, for example, might be adequate to bring about the motor act of eye-closure in absence of stimulation of the eye by the instrument.

The third and highest level of motor control was characterized by true voluntary control of the motor pattern. Unlike the secondary stage, the action which occurred at this level was not a mere repetition of the reflex movement which had initially followed arousal of one of the images. Rather, it might be represented by an inhibition or repression of such reflex action or by the substitution of a more appropriate movement or action.

Meynert's application of this principle to motor speech movements assumed that voluntary motor speech patterns evolved from earlier-established reflex speech movements. The motor speech-representation or images, i.e., motor-kinesthetic sensations accompanying the action, were believed to be laid down in the motor cortex as a sequel to early reflex speech production. Such motor speech images were assumed to be held in close association with the acoustic, visual, and tactile impressions accompanying such early events.

Meynert explained the early association of motor and acoustic components of speech production on the basis of the close anatomic arrangement of the auditory nucleus and the nuclei of the cranial nerves involved in speech production. This close anatomic relationship supplied the neuroanatomic substrate for reflex speech production. Stimulation of the auditory nerve, for example, would be followed by simultaneous excitation of the movements involved in the production of sound. A cyclic process would therefore be established. The motor activity of the production of sound was followed by further auditory stimulation and a repetition of the pattern. In this process, acoustic and motor-kinesthetic images were assumed to be laid down in the cortex in association with visual and tactile impressions accompanying the early reflex motor speech production. Meynert described the process involved in the development of the "secondary" motor mechanism of speech as "an endless number of coordinating acts in the forebrain" resulting in a conscious and "methodical imitation of the syllables heard" (1885, p. 209). One might note, parenthetically, that this concept, which was also held by Broadbent (1872; 1879), is of interest in the light of recent studies of hearing in the neonate which reveal that the infant in the early postnatal period responds only to speech sounds, ignoring non-speech auditory stimuli (Eisenberg, 1970). Wernicke's reference to this principle of primary and secondary motor speech processes in the 1874 work suggests that, although he did not accept all facets of the Meynert theory of the development of motor speech-images as definitely established, he did support the basic principle of the acquisition of voluntary speech as a sequel to the production of reflexly-produced combinations of syllables initially produced by mimicry.

Sensory Imagery

Wernicke divided the processing of incoming sensory stimuli into two stages. The first stage, "primary identification", referred to the recognition of incoming information in one sensory sphere by means of the arousal of the respective memory images. For example, an auditory stimulus such as the word "orange" would first arouse the acoustic imagery alone. Although such sound stimuli would be accurately perceived acoustically, as might be reflected in mechanical echoing of the word, at this stage such input would be devoid of meaning. "Secondary identification", the second stage in this process, was assumed to involve the association between the specific sensory imagery evoked and the related concept. This would then include arousal of all other sensory images related to the word, i.e., the visual, tactile, olfactory, and gustatory images associated with the object together with all other related associations. In this way the spoken word could be comprehended only by association of the aroused acoustic imagery with the related concept. Primary identification of course could not exist in isolation in the normal brain.

Higher levels of concept formation were regarded as products of complex associations involving varied constellations and combinations of memory images. The totality of such complex combinations made up the content of consciousness. Wernicke recognized three types of consciousness: 1) consciousness of the outer world, i.e. the totality of memory images related to the external objects in the environment; 2) consciousness of one's body, referring to somatic sensory imagery, and 3) consciousness of one's personality, which represented a synthesis of the first two types and involved the interrelationship of the personality to the corporeal self and the total environment.

Language was regarded as the medium by which abstract concepts are developed. This is reflected in Wernicke's statement:

> Articulate speech is the chief medium by which a specific organization of concepts occurs. It facilitates all complex and unique connections not only between the concepts of concrete objects but also between the events and actions which occur at the same time (1900, p. 70). . . .. It provides an abbreviated symbol for special complex associations, abstract concepts which in part are first acquired by means of speech. . . The logical sequence of elements of the sentence structure leads to the gradual development of guiding principles by which thought occurs (1900, p. 71).*
>
> . . . Although the word may be associated with an entire series of concepts, the decisive factor is not the association with the word but the interrelationship of this series of concepts with each other (1900, p. 72).*

Moreover, Wernicke observed that thought and speech were not identical.

"Speech is merely the means of learning, the taskmaster, by which concepts continue to maintain a characteristic interrelationship and organization" (p. 72).*

Wernicke summarized his interpretation of higher psychic processes in his final schema illustrated in Figure 23, p. 216. The purpose of this diagram, he readily admitted, served merely to provide an abbreviated mode for synthesizing such mechanisms and therefore represented a gross over-simplification of the complex processes involved in mental function.

In this schema, the area (s) referred to all modalities of sensory input, while (m) represented verbal as well as all other motor modes of output. The letter (B) designated the concept center which was assumed to involve the entire cortex. The ideational or goal-planning aspects of mental function were designated by (Z) which referred to the mechanisms underlying the integration and processing of all information in terms of past experience. The point (A) referred to the discharge-point for activation of all motor, verbal, and thought processes. Wernicke stated that the theoretic path (A) - (Z) represented all the varied association bonds traversed in the individual's mental activity.

This schema therefore may be regarded as Wernicke's compact mode of summarizing and synthesizing his concepts of higher psychic function and as an integration of his notions of various forms of imagery, concept formation, and consciousness within a neuroanatomic framework.

WERNICKE'S MIDDLE PERIOD 1885-1890

Introduction

The publication of the monograph, "Recent Works on Aphasia" in 1885 launched the second or middle period in the development of Wernicke's theory of aphasia. This forty-page review, little-known in contrast to his two larger works on aphasia, signaled a return to the subject after essentially a decade of silence.

The first years of this period were also marked by the return to Breslau and academic life following seven years in the private practice of neurology in Berlin. The later Berlin years, frustrating in their poverty of clinical opportunity, had nevertheless permitted a time for reflection and writing which was climaxed in his three-volume textbook on neurology, an important product of that period.

The Breslau years initiated a change of pace, fresh challenge, and new opportunity. The university and municipal clinics offered facilities for scientific research and a wealth of clinical material for the further study and delineation of clinical entities and symptomatology. During this period, under Wernicke's direction, the Breslau Clinic was to become the scene of significant advances in the area of aphasia and related disorders as reflected in the work of Liepmann, Lissauer, Storch, and Heilbronner.

Wernicke's influence in fact can be detected in many of the advances in the history of aphasia of this period. The discovery of sensory aphasia was followed by a surge of clinicopathological studies confirming the dramatic but tenuous 1874 findings. Greater attention and emphasis were devoted to testing techniques, the recording of clinical observations, and the development of new modes of eliciting language symptoms. This trend was reflected in the inclusion of special sections on diagnostic approaches and methods in various aphasia monographs of the day. Moreover, the Wernicke pictorial device of diagramming language models stimulated an explosion of such schemas. Although the majority of such diagrams were imitations or variations of the Wernicke-Lichtheim schema, they reflected the new interest in formulation of language and aphasia models and helped to focus interest on interpretation of speech processes in terms of possible psychic-anatomical mechanisms and the associationistic psychological concepts current at that time. Such diagrams were later regarded with a certain contempt because of their obvious over-simplifications of very complex processes. However, Wernicke intended such models or schemas to serve merely as a short-hand device to clarify possible theoretical mechanisms. This is clear from his statement:

> We must keep in mind that each schema, including our own, has value only as a mode of instruction and interpretation and loses its significance as soon as an easier or more accurate grouping of the data is found (1900, pp. 214-215).*

The various trends emerging during the middle aphasia period represent small but definite steps in the history of aphasia theory. The origin of many of these developments may be traced to the influence of the 1874 work and Wernicke's writings of this period. The most significant mark of this middle period, however, lay in the expansion of the Wernicke aphasia model and the emergence of a new classification system of aphasia.

The extension of this model was stimulated by Lichtheim's (1884-85) significant contributions which very likely motivated Wernicke's further attention to the subject in his monograph, "Recent Works on Aphasia."

Two new and unique concepts evolved during this period, that of the word-concept and that of transcortical language function. These ideas were of critical importance to Wernicke's interpretation of language mechanisms and his aphasia classification system. The following discussion shall attempt to explore the relationship of these concepts to the aphasia schema.

The Fundamental Components of the Wernicke Schema

The Word-Concept

Wernicke himself originated the notion of a "word-concept" and interpreted it as a union of the specific acoustic and motor features of the word and therefore a combination of acoustic and motor speech imagery. This union was achieved in early childhood and found its anatomic substrate in the arcuate fibers connecting the motor and auditory speech areas. Later, in his final work on aphasia in 1906, Wernicke used the term "word-concept" interchangeably with the French expression of "inner speech", although this latter was eventually to have broader and more complex implications than it had at that time. In his 1906 monograph he states, "The closely-bound association of the acoustic and motor imagery of the individual word has been designated by French authorities as "inner speech". However, the French interpretation, which had largely been the creation of Charcot and was later detailed by his student Ballet (1888), differed from that of Wernicke. Charcot's interpretation of this notion was based on his classification of specific visual, acoustic, and motor imagery types. This interpretation was also supported by Bastian in his explanation of various clinical pictures of aphasia.

The Wernicke word-concept was a primitive forerunner of the later complex notion of inner language. At this time, it was an incompletely formulated idea. Wernicke, for example, did not attempt to elaborate on the possible mechanisms by which it operated. Thiele (1928) has pointed out that the union of acoustic and motor imagery making up the word-concept should be regarded as a serial association of such elements and needed to be understood within the context of the association psychology of that day.

The concept of inner language aroused a great deal of interest and became a rather controversial issue in the post-Wernicke years among workers in the areas of aphasia, linguistics, and psychology. Freud, Storch, Moeli, and Goldscheider, for example, explored various facets of this idea in relation to aphasia. In France, Ballet, Egger, and Saint-Paul, building on Charcot's earlier interpretations, contributed to a further expansion and understanding of this notion. Perhaps the most complete development of the concept of inner language and its relation to aphasia was realized several decades later in the works of Goldstein and Pick. The latter recognized the significance of Wernicke's word-concept and applied it to an interpretation of the aphasia symptom of agrammatism.

A review of the evolution of various interpretations of the concept of inner language would be beyond our purposes here. However, it is of interest that this idea had its origins in Wernicke's notion of a word-concept. The latter occupied an important place in his aphasia model. Its function can best be understood in relation to the concept of transcortical processes.

Transcortical Language Function

Transcortical language function is the second important new idea in development of the Wernicke aphasia theory advanced during the middle period.

Disturbance of such function was first predicted by Lichtheim (1884-85) and later labeled by Wernicke as transcortical aphasia. The seeds of this idea were first evident in his discussion on concept formation and in his review of certain case studies in the 1874 monograph. A brief sketch of Wernicke's theory of aphasia may facilitate an understanding of this concept.

The final Wernicke aphasia schema may be described as a three-tiered hierarchical model of language function with three levels of language processes: subcortical, cortical, and transcortical.

The subcortical processes of auditory transmission from the ear to the sensory speech area and the discharge of motor impulses from Broca's area to the speech musculature constituted the first or lowest level of the hierarchy. Disruption of the white matter immediately beneath the motor and sensory cortical centers would result respectively in subcortical motor aphasia (pure word-mutism) and subcortical sensory aphasia (pure word-deafness). The second or middle level of the schema was represented by the motor and sensory speech areas. The close union of the motor and acoustic imagery formed the word-concept or inner speech. Damage at this level would characteristically result in a motor or sensory aphasia. Impairment of the word-concept was typically associated with such disruption at the cortical level. Conduction aphasia, a syndrome characterized by difficulty in mimicry, paraphasic but fluent speech, and intact auditory comprehension was believed to be caused by interruption of the arcuate fibers. The summit of the hierarchy was represented by conceptualization, the complex of visual, auditory, tactile, gustatory and olfactory associations. More abstract levels of thought involved still more complicated patterns of association. Impairment at this highest level in several sensory spheres might result in dementia. If the destruction were limited to specific sensory areas, isolated agnosias could be predicted.

Both Wernicke (1886) and Lichtheim (1885) emphasized that localization of such a "concept center" to a specific cortical site was not possible, and that such higher processes in reality involved the entire cortex. Later critics tended to neglect this broader interpretation and charged Wernicke and his contemporaries with attempts to localize higher processes such as conceptualization to a single "center."

The transcortical tracts were believed to form the anatomic substrate of association processes involved in higher mental functions. Such pathways provided the neural circuitry between the various sensory areas and linked motor with sensory areas. Wernicke described the specific function of the transcortical tracts as the association of motor and sensory imagery with the higher processes of concept formation. This description, it is felt, was meant to be theoretic and schematic rather than strictly anatomical. Comprehension of the spoken word could occur only by association between the auditory speech area and the "concept center." The spoken word was without meaning until the appropriate concept or group of concepts were aroused by the acoustic imagery. The constellations of concepts, so revived, in turn activated the appropriate motor speech imagery and thereby the word-concept, leading to final motor output of the word. The particular significance of the word-concept within the total framework of the model becomes evident in the emergence of various aphasia syndromes, dependent upon the level of disruption in the hierarchy.

Involvement at the highest level resulting in damage to concept formation has already been discussed. Such damage would result in dementia or isolated agnosias. Disruption at the middle level was characteristically followed by a motor, sensory, or mixed cortical aphasia. Damage to the transcortical tracts might cause loss of association between the word-concept and the object concept. If such damage involved sensory transcortical tracts, integrity of conceptualization might be anticipated as well as auditory perception itself. However, comprehension of the word would not be possible because of impairment in arousal of the concept by the auditory imagery. Such a situation would be reflected in parrot-like mimicry with absence of comprehension of the spoken word. Reading and writing would be essentially intact but would be typically carried out mechanically, with lack of comprehension or awareness of content, as a result of dissociation between auditory centers and the areas involved in conceptualization. Disruption of the transcortical motor tracts, which were believed to connect concepts with motor speech imagery, might result in loss or poverty of verbal expression because activation of speech by such higher centers would be absent. In such a transcortical motor aphasia, according to Wernicke's interpretation, auditory comprehension would typically be functional as would be reading, writing, and speech mimicry.

The subcortical aphasias were assumed to reflect involvement at the lowest level of the tier, disrupting specific sections of the white matter immediately below cortical centers providing connections between such and the peripheral sensory and motor organs. Thus, pure word-deafness or subcortical sensory aphasia in Wernicke's terminology was marked by adequate hearing sensitivity but impairment in auditory comprehension, in association with essentially intact oral expression, reading, and writing. The characteristic symptoms of its corollary, pure word-mutism, or subcortical motor aphasia, included disturbance in speech production, similar to that found in cortical motor aphasia, together with good auditory comprehension and integrity of writing and reading comprehension. Disturbance of inner language or the word-concept was typical of the cortical aphasias. This function, however, remained intact in the subcortical and transcortical syndromes. These clinical pictures have been described in detail in Wernicke's major work of this middle period, "Recent Works on Aphasia."

The subject of transcortical language function and transcortical aphasia became the target of much discussion and criticism during this period. Many rejected the existence of this form of aphasia because of the infrequency of occurrence of discrete damage to such tracts which were so widely dispersed over the brain. Wernicke's characteristic response to such criticism was that "pure forms are always rare." Some authorities attributed the occurrence of such syndromes to partial involvement of different centers or to combinations of such damage. Others felt that they merely represented different stages in the recovery process. Heubner (1889) reported a fairly detailed clinico-pathological study of transcortical sensory aphasia in which Wernicke's area was essentially isolated from the rest of the brain by a softening process, leaving the area itself, however, intact. The clinical symptoms coincided with the Wernicke-Lichtheim description. Recent studies reported by Kabelyanskaya and Viting (1968) Segarra and Quadfasel et al. (1961) have confirmed the existence of a transcortical form of sensory aphasia.

However, in spite of the dissenting views regarding this form of aphasia, the concept of transcortical language function was at least of value from a heuristic standpoint. It stimulated exploration and consideration of the relationship of language to higher processes and focused attention on the possible mechanisms involved in the production of various aphasia syndromes. It therefore permitted the development of important extensions of the aphasia model. The search for cases presenting the predicted clinical pictures led to more detailed study of specific symptoms or symptom-complexes and encouraged the development of test procedures to elicit various aspects of language behavior. This concept then was fruitful in contributing to further expansion of the study of aphasia and aphasia theory. The notion of transcortical processes was later applied by Wernicke to the problems of mental illness and provided the foundation for an elaboration of the aphasia model to his schema of psychic processes.

Figures 1 to 4 present the author's expanded version of Wernicke's language and aphasia models based on the latter's pertinent aphasia and psychiatric writings. Wernicke pointed to four aspects of language development; reflex crying and vocalization, mimicry, early volitional speech, and later volitional speech acquisition as shown in Figure 1.

The first diagram in Figure 1 depicts the stage of reflex speech vocalization. Although Wernicke acknowledged that the specific mechanisms and localization of reflex sound production were not known, he held that such production resulted in the deposit of an acoustic speech image in the temporal lobe and a motor-kinesthetic speech image in Broca's motor speech area.

The second stage, that of speech mimicry, (Figure 1), was marked by the development of Wernicke's "word-concept". The auditory stimulus, the spoken word, was transmitted via sub-cortical tracts to the sensory speech area, leaving behind an acoustic speech image. The impulse was then transmitted via the arcuate fibers, the link connecting motor and sensory speech areas to Broca's motor speech area. The frequent repetition of this process in childhood led to an intimate union of the motor-kinesthetic and acoustic speech images. This union was called the "word-concept" and might be viewed as a forerunner of the contemporary notion of a sensory-motor speech programmer. It was involved in the patterning of sounds and syllables in the appropriate sequences and was responsible for the automatic aspects of speech production. The "word-concept" of a word or utterance was merely the external "envelope" of the word and was devoid of meaning or any semantic content.

In the early stage of volitional speech development (Figure 1) initiation of the speech impulse took place at the concept level. During this initial period of thought activity which preceded the actual utterance, all concepts related to the idea to be conveyed were aroused and consolidated via the association tracts and were "discharged" at the "conceptual discharge site". This was followed by an "ideational goal planning stage" in which a general schema of what was to be spoken was formulated. The impulse was then transmitted to the acoustic sensory speech area where the acoustic speech images were aroused followed by the transmission over the arcuate tract to Broca's area. In this process the "word-concept" was called up, resulting in the appropriate motor acoustic patterning of the utterance. The speech corrector, in the form of acoustic imagery functioned as an unconscious monitor assuring arousal of the correct speech images. The motor discharge of the word then took place from Broca's area.

Volitional speech production later on in life (Figure 1) when motor speech aspects became more firmly established and automatic in nature, followed essentially the same course, with the exception that instead of the transmission of the speech impulse from areas involved in conceptualization (which essentially involved the entire cortex) to the acoustic sensory speech area, the impulse traveled directly to Broca's center. However, because Broca's area was part of the word-concept which represented a union of motor and acoustic speech images, the sensory speech area was still indirectly involved.

Figure 2 depicts Wernicke's two-stage schema of auditory comprehension. The auditory stimulus, the spoken word, is transmitted to the sensory speech center in the temporal lobe. Here the word is perceived but not comprehended. Wernicke referred to this stage as "primary identification" (word-sound-identification in the 1906 work). The acoustic speech images then aroused the related concepts in stage two of the process, at which point the word was fully comprehended. This stage was labeled "secondary identification" (or "word-meaning-comprehension" in the 1906 work) by Wernicke.

Figure 3 depicts the author's version of the Wernicke speech model. The aphasia model is presented in Figure 4 and an outline of his classification system in Figure 5.

Damage to the motor (Broca's) area would result in a motor aphasia with the typical picture of paucity of speech, slowed, effortful, laborious output, perseveration, and use of recurrent utterances together with relatively intact auditory comprehension. Damage to the sensory area would cause a sensory aphasia marked by impairment in auditory comprehension, a copious, confused output, literal and verbal paraphasia, word-finding difficulty, alexia and agraphia. Conduction aphasia might result from disruption of the tract connecting motor and sensory areas, the arcuate fasciculus. Typical symptoms of this aphasia form included intact auditory comprehension, fluent but paraphasic speech output, and difficulty in verbal mimicry. Alexia and agrophia might be present.

Damage to the white matter beneath the sensory speech area, together with disruption of the corpus callosum would lead to a subcortical sensory aphasia, also known as pure word-deafness. Subcortical damage to Broca's area with destruction of the adjoining callosal fibers would be followed by a subcortical motor aphasia (pure word mutism), characterized by impaired motor speech expression but intact reading and writing. Damage to the transcortical tracts which connected motor and sensory speech centers with areas involved in conceptualization would result in transcortical motor and transcortical sensory aphasia, respectively. The former would typically be marked by loss of auditory comprehension, in association with a forced echolalic type of mimicry of any words the patient might hear. The symptom-picture of transcortical motor aphasia would characteristically include poverty of speech output, an inertia in activation of thought processes and impairment in initiating the speech act together with essentially normal verbal mimicry. In his writings Wernicke also provided models and classification systems of the alexias and agraphias as has been depicted in Figure 5. His classification of the latter paralleled those of the aphasias and reflected his anatomic subcortical, cortical, and transcortical hierarchy. Wernicke's aphasia model, first submitted in his classic work and elaborated in his later writings, gained quick popularity and the discovery of sensory aphasia and formulation of this theory of aphasia, as history has demonstrated, won him lasting fame.

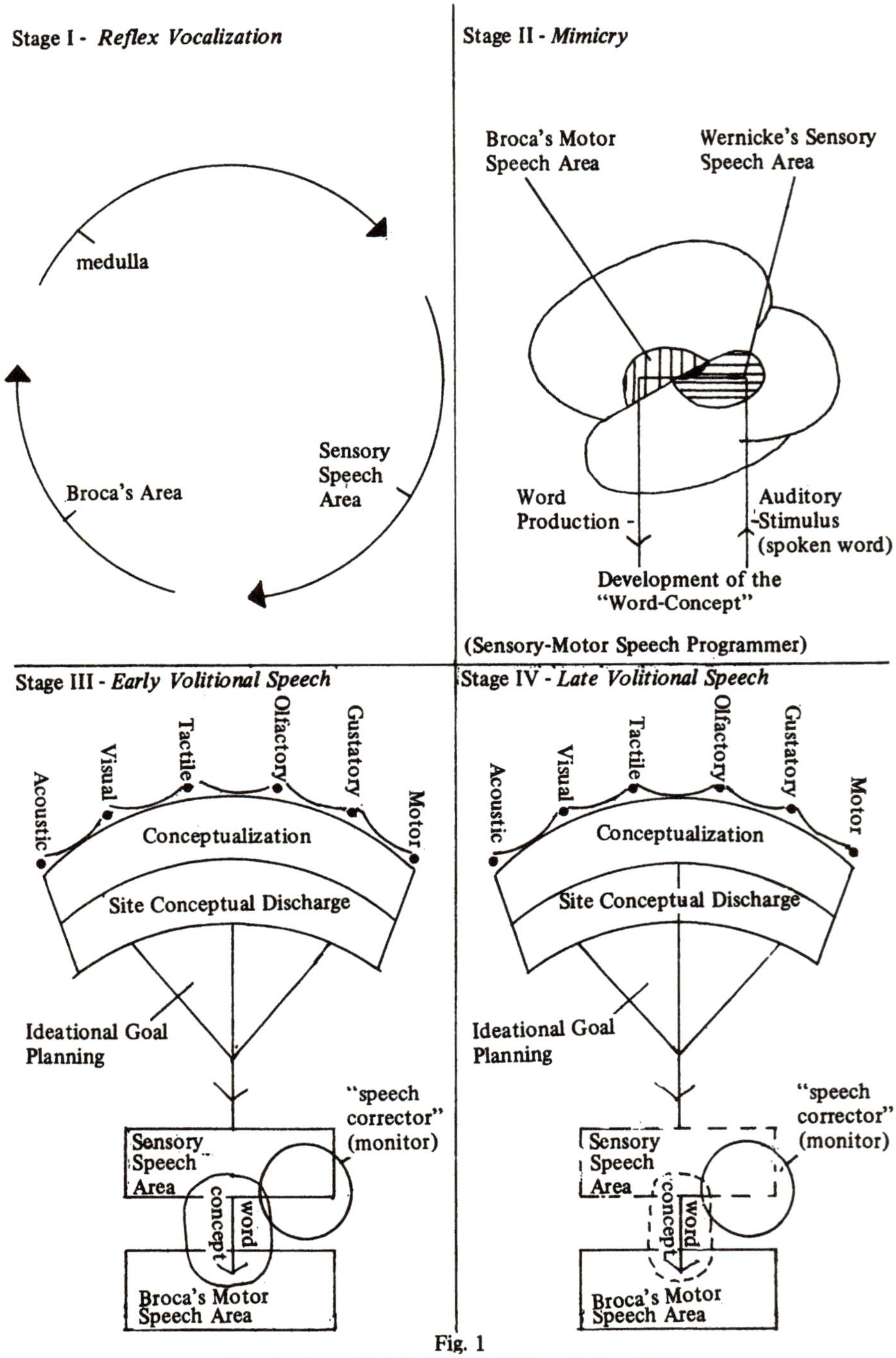

Fig. 1
The Wernicke Model: Stages of Speech Acquisition

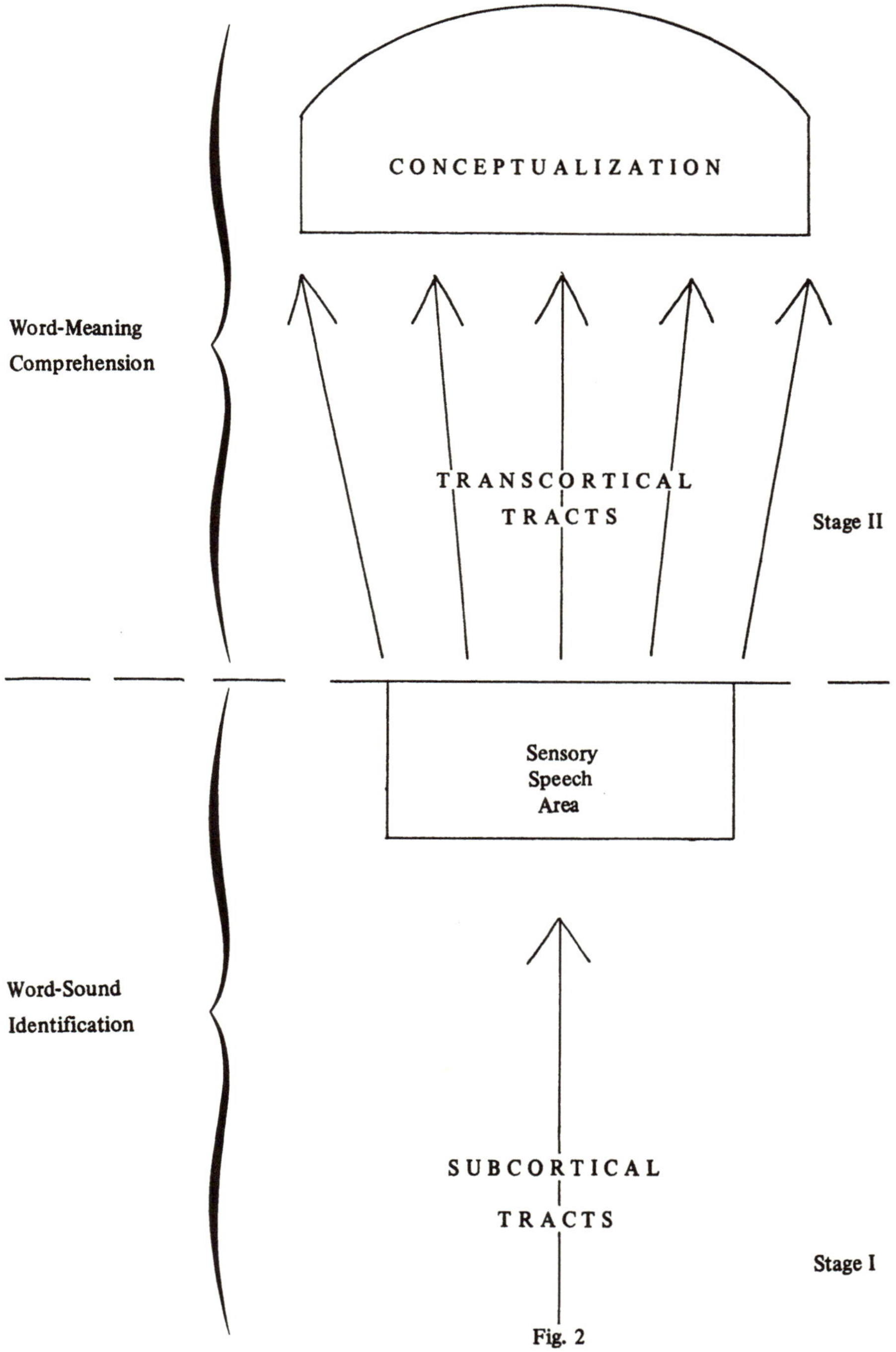

Fig. 2
The Wernicke Model: Auditory Comprehension

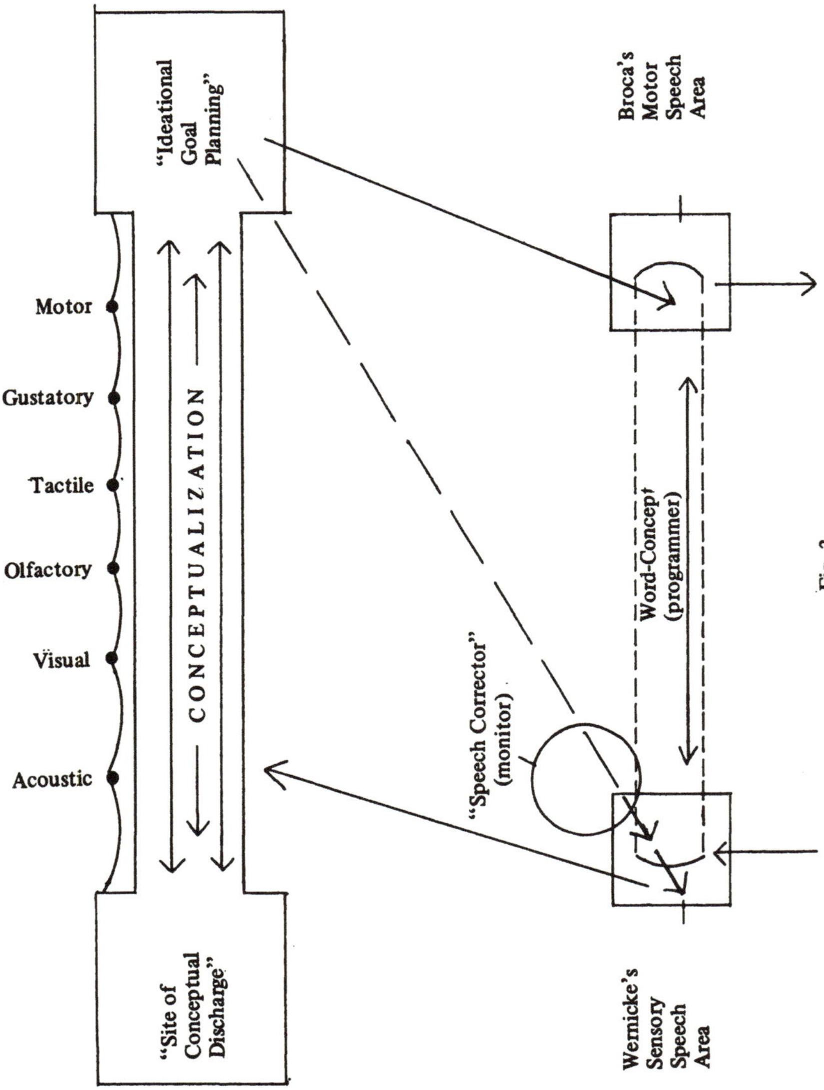

Fig. 3
Wernicke Language Model

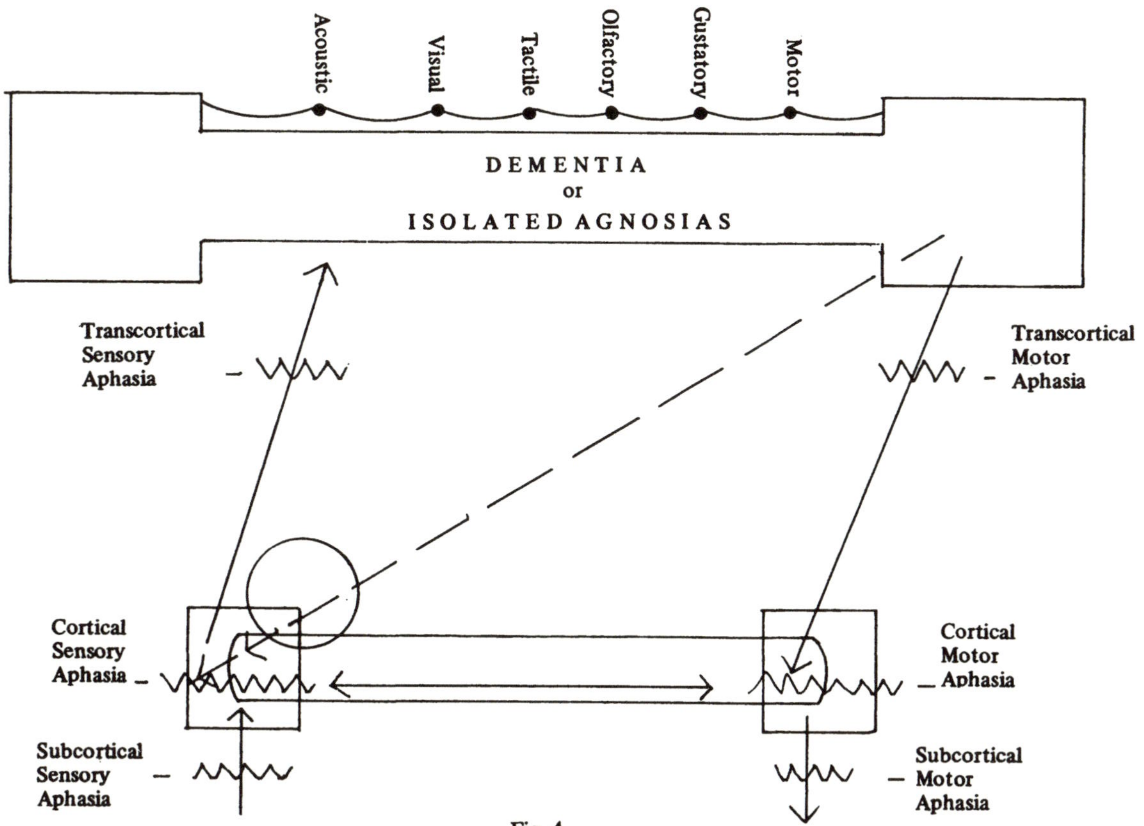

Fig. 4
Wernicke's Aphasia Model

Fig. 5 *The Wernicke Classification System*

THE APHASIAS

Subcortical *Sensory* Aphasia
CORTICAL *SENSORY* APHASIA
Transcortical Sensory Aphasia

Subcortical *Motor* Aphasia
CORTICAL *MOTOR* APHASIA
Transcortical Motor Aphasia

Conduction Aphasia

THE ALEXIAS

Subcortical Alexia
CORTICAL ALEXIA
Transcortical Alexia

THE AGRAPHIAS

Subcortical Agraphia
CORTICAL AGRAPHIA
Transcortical Agraphia
Conduction Agraphia

WERNICKE'S FINAL APHASIA PERIOD 1890-1905

Wernicke's Contemporaries and Connectionism

The preceding discussion has attempted to explore two new ideas, the word-concept and transcortical function, which were introduced during the Middle Period. These concepts formed significant elements of the Wernicke aphasia model.

However, the effects of the concepts advanced in "Recent Works" and those explored in Lichtheim's monograph did not really gain momentum until the last decade of the 1800's. This decade witnessed a marked increase in publication in the area of aphasia. Many of these studies were concerned with notions and issues raised in Wernicke's works.

By this time the aphasia scene was unmistakably centered in Germany and largely dominated by the Breslau Group. In addition to the Wernicke following, Arnold Pick from Prague, Lichtheim, Flechsig, und Freud numbered among the significant contributors to this subject. In the areas of anatomy and physiology,the localization approach was strongly supported by the works of Munk (1881) and Fritsch and Hitzig (1870), while Goltz (1888) held to a holistic view. Munk's ablation studies provided important findings in the area of psychic blindness and deafness. Fritsch and Hitzig's electrical stimulation experiments supplied a new mode of exploring the problem of cerebral localization. Flechsig's (1896) myelogenic approach led to his designation of primary projection and secondary association areas and to an interpretation of psychic function in the light of such findings.

In England, connectionism and "center-oriented" interpretations of aphasia had gained a firm foothold. Bastian (1898), a major figure in aphasia during this period, as well as his colleagues Broadbent (1879, 1905), Ross (1883), Bramwell (1897), and Hinshelwood (1900) espoused connectionistic concepts. Monographs by Wyllie (1894), Elder (1897), and Bateman (1890), published in this era, essentially followed the Wernicke schema and classification. The important works of Hughlings Jackson (1869, 1884), whose interpretations took an entirely different direction, did not gain strong support until several decades later.

Localization trends and connectionism also largely dominated the scene in France during these days, as is reflected in the works of Charcot (1883a), Pitres (1884), Ballet (1890) Mirallié (1896), and particularly, Dejerine (1892, 1897), who published the first clinico-pathological study of the syndrome of pure word-blindness in 1892. Ballet (1890), for example, has referred to Charcot as a "strong champion of the revolutionary doctrine" popularized by Wernicke and his followers in Germany. Charcot, in fact, contributed substantially to the adoption of such views in France and supported them with case studies.

In Italy, the problem of aphasia was explored by Mingazzini (1902) and

Sepilli (1884) during this time. Bonvicini, an Italian working in Vienna, contributed an important short monograph on subcortical sensory aphasia, examining in greater detail issues raised in Wernicke's description of that subform.

In America, Starr (1889; 1909), Mills (1898), and Meyer (1908) generally accepted and helped popularized the German classification system and schemas.

By the close of the nineteenth century, workers in Britain, France, Italy, and America largely followed the path broken by the Breslau-Halle school of aphasia.

Wernicke's 1906 "Aphasia Symptom Complex"

The third aphasia period was climaxed by Wernicke's final return to the subject of aphasia in his 1906 "Deutsche-Klinik" *Aphasia Symptom-Complex.* This monograph, reportedly written in 1903 and published posthumously 3 years later, and an essay on agraphia which appeared in 1903, represent a final summing up and recapitulation of the basic tenets of Wernicke's aphasia doctrine which had been previously detailed in his earlier works.

In this monograph, Wernicke reviewed his interpretation and description of the various aphasia forms. With the exception of a few modifications, he felt that his earlier classification had withstood the test of time. His previous description of the motor, sensory, and conduction aphasias and his threefold division into subcortical, cortical, and transcortical subforms was reaffirmed in this last work. Although transcortical aphasia lacked consistent pathological confirmation at that time, Wernicke continued to maintain its possible occurrence on a theoretic basis.

In the 1906 *Symptom-Complex* his earlier explanation of motor aphasia on the basis of disruption of the motor speech tract or lenticular nucleus was rejected. In this monograph he described the symptoms of motor aphasia in somewhat greater detail than in his earlier papers. These symptoms included the occurrence of emotional and automatic expressions, jargon responses, and recurrent utterances. The possible presence of verbal apraxia was also noted and defined as an inability to produce complex speech movements in the absence of paralysis of the muscles involved.

In the immediate post-Wernicke years the symptoms of motor aphasia were defined in greater detail. Such symptoms included perseveration, a telegram speech style, the predominant use of substantives, agrammatism and apraxia Pick (1894) drew attention to the blocking, laborious, stuttering-like pattern demonstrated in many motor aphasics, while Heilbronner (1907) and Kleist (1907b) noted the frequent difficulty in initiation of speech in this form. Later, Von Monakow (1914) attempted a further refinement of aphasia subgroups on the basis of pathological and clinical findings.

In the 1906 work, Wernicke presented a more definitive interpretation of sensory aphasia than had been described in his earlier writings. Bezold's (1897) studies on hearing had led Wernicke to interpret the impairment in auditory comprehension, which was characteristic of sensory aphasia, as a sequel to loss of phonemic perception. Bezold had established the speech range as a sixth tonal interval on the musical scale. Liepmann later expanded this interval to include an octave above and below this interval.

Wernicke localized the terminals of those branches of the auditory nerve which were involved in perception of the speech range to the posterior third of the first temporal gyrus. Impairment in auditory comprehension in aphasia was therefore based on loss of acoustic perception in the speech range. This interpretation was later found to be in error and rejected when studies confirmed Heschl's gyrus as the end-point of all fibers of the auditory tract.

The 1906 work also contained a review of the problems of alexia and agraphia, thus reflecting Wernicke's continuing interest in this area, which was first revealed in his original work on aphasia. In this review he continued to maintain his differentiation of verbal and literal alexia and agraphia and reaffirmed his classification of cortical, subcortical and transcortical forms of such disorders. Wernicke rejected the localization of a special writing center such as Exner had postulated in the foot of the second frontal gyrus as well as a special center for printed words in the posterior cerebral area. In his interpretation of the reading process, he called attention to the significance of "the fiber connections which mediate the visual written image associations with the unilaterally located speech center and that of the acoustic component involved". (1906)

In summary, Wernicke's final aphasia period witnessed a stabilization of connectionistic and localization concepts and was marked by further refinement and study of the clinical types, with greater emphasis on evaluation and interpretation of symptoms and more detailed pathological studies.

V.

A RETROSPECTIVE VIEW OF WERNICKE'S APHASIA

INTRODUCTION

This year marks the one-hundredth anniversary of Wernicke's discovery of sensory aphasia, and a short review of further developments in the area during the post-classical era may aid in tracing the course which has led to current interpretations and concepts.

Historically, the time was ripe for Wernicke's discovery. Localization of cerebral function was just gaining acceptance. As has been discussed in preceding chapters, Broca's discovery of a speech center in the anterior part of the brain, Fritsch and Hitzig's electrical cerebral stimulation studies, and Meynert's theory of memory imagery and his functional division of the brain into an anterior motor and a posterior sensory division had provided the necessary groundwork for promoting a cerebral localization approach of function. However, an important ingredient was missing for application of such a theory to language and aphasia. While damage to Broca's speech center might account for some of the symptoms present in aphasia, how could diametrically opposite symptoms be explained on the basis of damage to the same cerebral area?

Wernicke's discovery of a second speech area – a sensory speech center – offered a solution to this problem. It supplied the missing ingredient for an aphasia theory which could accommodate the symptom-picture of aphasia in its entirety. In his 1874 monograph Wernicke presents a broader and bolder purpose than the mere identification and description of a new aphasia form. A glance at the title reveals his underlying purpose. He did not call this work "Sensory Aphasia," "A New Aphasia Form" or something similar. But rather, his main title was "The Aphasia Symptom-Complex", focusing immediately on the diversity and complexity of symptoms housed under the term "aphasia".

In this study Wernicke tried to bring together the diverse and apparently conflicting symptoms of aphasia and attempted to organize them into some kind of coherent and orderly framework. The key to such an orderly organization could be found, he felt, in understanding the neuroanatomic basis of speech. This approach is reflected in the subtitle of his classic monograph –

"A Psychological Study on an Anatomic Basis". Such a neuroanatomic approach was founded on a sensory-motor dichotomy of language and was a necessary step in the evolution of aphasia theory.

Wernicke's discovery of a sensory form of aphasia stimulated a flurry of studies devoted to further investigation of this clinical entity. Some of these studies focused on the subdivisions of the syndrome designated in Wernicke's monograph. Many others were concerned with further exploration of specific aspects of the symptom-picture of sensory aphasia – auditory comprehension loss, literal and verbal paraphasia, paragrammatism, word-finding impairment, the alexias and agraphias. Such a significant segment of the work on aphasia in the post-Wernicke period was devoted to the investigation of various aspects of this new clinical entity that the history of aphasia of that era might, in fact, be viewed as the history of sensory aphasia. The following sections will attempt to briefly sketch the work carried out in exploring the primary symptoms – "the symptom-triad" – of sensory aphasia in the post-classical and noetic aphasia periods. This symptom-triad includes disorders in auditory comprehension loss, paraphasia, and word-finding impairment.

THE SYMPTOMATOLOGY OF WERNICKE'S APHASIA

Auditory Comprehension Impairment

A major impact of Wernicke's discovery of sensory aphasia was the highlighting of the problem of language comprehension impairment in aphasia and its localization to the left temporal area. This new interest in the auditory comprehension loss in aphasia, generated by the 1874 monograph, opened up a new area of study in aphasia research and stimulated further exploration of the localization of higher levels of auditory processing and the effects of cerebral damage on various aspects of language comprehension. Input to this area of investigation was provided by a variety of experimental approaches, such as the ablation studies of Munk, the myelogenic approach utilized by Flechsig, and the clinico-pathological studies of Von Monakow, Starr, Henschen, Nissl von Mayendorff and many others.

The post-Wernickean period witnessed not only further exploration of hearing and higher levels of auditory integration but attempted to specify more definitively the cerebral areas involved in such processing and integration. Moreover, Wernicke's classification system, which included such clinical subforms as the transcortical and subcortical sensory aphasia types, led to further detailing and exploration of the symptomatology and to the study of possible neuroanatomical correlations of such entities.

This era was indeed an active period in aphasia research, and this review can merely touch on some of the chief concepts regarding various aspects of auditory comprehension impairment in aphasia which emerged during that time.

Auditory processing, according to Wernicke's early interpretation, was divided into two stages. The first, "primary identification" of speech (word-sound comprehension) referred to the auditory perception of incoming stimuli without comprehension of meaning. In the second stage, "secondary identification" (word-meaning comprehension) such perceived sounds were associated with their respective concepts via the transcortical tracts, thus investing such input with meaning (Wernicke 1900; 1906). Wernicke referred to "primary identification" as a "fiction", indicating that such separation into stages of auditory perception and auditory comprehension was really an artificial division which would not occur in the normal brain. In certain kinds of damage to the temporal lobe, however, transcortical sensory aphasia could occur. The fact that such patients demonstrated intact auditory perception was indicated by the ability to accurately mimic what was heard. Such mimicry, however, would occur without comprehension.

In the post-classical aphasia period an elaboration of this division of auditory processing into stages can be found in the works of Liepmann, Kleist, Pick, and others. Liepmann (1898) hypothesized a three-stage model which included word-sound comprehension, word-meaning comprehension, and sentence-meaning comprehension. This was followed shortly after by Kleist's (1907-b) differentiation of three forms of auditory comprehension loss: (1) a word-sound deafness, reflecting a disorder in temporal sequencing of the components of the word; (2) a name-deafness, characterized by impairment in the comprehension of words as names (a disorder which involved a disturbance in the total naming process), and finally (3) a sentence-deafness with deficits in grasping grammatic and syntactic structures and relationships. Such impairment in the latter type of comprehension loss would be reflected in the expressive symptoms of agrammatism and paragrammatism. Of all models attempting to separate the stages of auditory processing into stages of increasing linguistic complexity, the best known is Pick's (1913) formulation of "the way from word to thought." This pathway, beginning with an initial stage of differentiation of speech sounds from the total acoustic experience, verbal and nonverbal, led through increasingly complex stages. These involved higher levels of auditory integration including phonetic perception, appreciation of the processing of prosodic elements and speech melody, the comprehension of speech sounds, and comprehension of grammatic and syntactic structures and relationships. This insightful formulation, which can be only briefly mentioned here, opened the door for later linguistic approaches to the aphasia problem.

During the post-Wernickean aphasia period, closer attention was given to observation and testing of the auditory comprehension deficits of aphasic patients. Heilbronner, (1910) an assistant of Wernicke at Breslau, made some interesting observations on this aspect of the problem. He stressed the importance of testing the hearing of aphasic patients and attempted to differentiate such losses in acuity from impairment in higher levels of auditory comprehension. Hearing testing at this time was limited to the use of pitch forks. However, in spite of the limitations of the test instruments available, some astute observations on certain aspects of auditory comprehension in aphasics were offered by this authority and others which continue to be valid today. For example, Heilbronner called attention to the difficulty and importance in differentiating auditory perceptual deficits from higher levels of auditory integration and comprehension. He felt that one valid indicator of intact perception was the ability of the patient to accurately mimic words spoken to him. Moreover, he reported that aphasics with integrity of higher levels of auditory comprehension could often compensate for damage to lower levels in auditory perception and grasp spoken language in spite of such perceptual impairment. Authorities of this period were well aware also of the greater difficulty experienced by some patients in comprehending language at abstract levels as well as the longer periods of time required for auditory processing of information. Heilbronner (1910) was perhaps first to point to the auditory neglect for speech sounds demonstrated by some patients who were, nevertheless, responsive to nonverbal auditory stimuli. Moreover, he also anticipated the observation made by current workers who have noted the aphasic's frequent ability to grasp the general meaning of statements while failing to retain or comprehend specific details.

This short sketch has attempted to indicate some of the early thinking and ideas of the complex problem of auditory comprehension loss in aphasia during the post-Wernickean period. Interest in this area continued in the years that followed, but the greater activity occurred after the second World War, and the past two decades have particularly witnessed many advances. Contributions from various spheres of interest, auditory physiology, speech perception, cerebral ablation studies, and dichotic listening research, to mention but a few, are providing significant and needed input to this important and complex problem. Certainly, our current methodologies are permitting more sophisticated treatment of this subject than could have been imagined by Wernicke and his followers. Such modes of approach will hopefully lead to promising advances in gaining new insights into an understanding of auditory processing and auditory comprehension loss. To Wernicke and his followers, however, we owe the debt of laying the groundwork and opening the door for further study and exploration of this intriguing but complex area.

Paraphasia

Paraphasia has been considered a primary feature of sensory aphasia since

Wernicke's first description of that syndrome in 1874. He recognized two types of the disturbance, "word-transpositions" and "word-confusions," later designated by Kussmaul as "literal" and "verbal paraphasia", respectively. The former term referred to a mutilation of the word itself by transposition, "verbal confusions," and the interchanging of sound elements within the word. In its extreme form, Wernicke felt that literal paraphasia might disintegrate into a pattern of jargon. The second type, verbal paraphasia, was used to designate the substitution of related or unrelated words or word groups for the intended word. Wernicke apparently included paragrammatism under the general sphere of verbal paraphasia. Paragrammatism was later discussed in greater detail by Kleist, who coined its name, and by others, such as Pick and Thiele.

Although the post-clinical and modern aphasia periods have witnessed the exploration of the problem of paraphasia by various investigators, the basic mechanisms underlying its occurrence still elude satisfactory interpretation. Wernicke explained paraphasia in sensory aphasia as a consequence of damage to the acoustic imagery located in the temporal lobe. He maintained that the acoustic imagery exerted a monitoring or regulatory effect on the expressive aspects of speech production, and damage to this monitoring system would be expected to result in paraphasic speech production. Such output would typically be copious, fluent, and in part correct because of the automaticity acquired early in life by the motor speech center. However, speech would still be marked by paraphasic errors because of the absence of the internal monitor.

Freud (1891) was among the first of Wernicke's contemporaries to oppose this interpretation for the obvious reason that such an internal rehearing or monitoring would occur too late to change speech output. No direct response to this criticism has been found in any of Wernicke's writings. If he did indeed regard this monitor as essentially a rehearing of the words, such criticism would certainly seem to be justified. However, two facts would seem to argue against this. First, Wernicke consistently describes this "corrector" as unconscious in nature and a rehearing would seem to involve considerable volitional participation on the part of the speaker. Secondly, it is felt that the key to understanding his interpretation of this monitor lies in an understanding of his notion of the "word-concept" or inner language. He emphasized that the presence of the word-concept in its entirety was necessary for production of spontaneous speech. This word-concept, which represented a precursor of current notions of a speech programmer, referred to the close association of acoustic and motor elements of the word, exclusive of its semantic aspects. Expression of the word was always accompanied by activation of the acoustic imagery during the period of early speech development in childhood. Wernicke maintained that the constant association of these two components led to a considerable degree of automaticity of motor production of speech in adulthood. Yet, in the event of damage to the acoustic components, as would occur in sensory aphasia, the lack of complete independence of the motor speech would typically be reflected in the occurrence of paraphasic errors. Wernicke states only that the acoustic imagery exerts this monitoring effect. The mechanisms by which this might occur are not described. This reluctance to speculate on mechanisms involved in memory imagery is found repeatedly in his writings. Such questions were usually dismissed with the observation that the issue was not yet ripe for scientific explanation.

Another and entirely different interpretation of paraphasia was suggested by Kussmaul (1877), an older contemporary of Wernicke's. He explained the disorder on the basis of diminished or disturbed attention. In addition to his terms literal and verbal paraphasia, he also coined the term "choreic paraphasia," which he specified as a condition in which the "flow of speech is smooth and continuous but the combination of words is meaningless, giving a confused picture." This impaired attention was felt to result in the arousal of associated words which resembled the intended word in meaning or sound.

Further exploration of the problem of paraphasia in the post-Wernickean period tended to take two directions. One school pursued Kussmaul's idea relating this disorder to impaired attention. Adherents of the second school expanded Wernicke's notion of a "word-concept" leading to development of the idea of a speech programmer.

Liepmann (1913) was first to pursue the latter course, applying his new model of apraxia to paraphasia. His model of the limb apraxias assumed the existence of a basic mnemonic or ideational plan fundamental to the production of normal limb movement and the synergy of isolated movements in formation of everyday actions. Relating this concept to speech, Liepmann postulated an "acoustic plan" as basic to normal speech expression. The ingredients of this word-plan consisted of the appropriate serial ordering of the acoustic components making up the word in close harmony with the specific motor elements of word-production. Liepmann regarded the acoustic elements of the word-plan to be of critical significance in the correct selection of the appropriate speech sounds and syllables in their proper sequential order. Damage to the acoustic components of the word-plan might therefore lead to "derailment" and disintergration of the word. Such deterioration would typically be reflected in an "ideokinetic paraphasia" characterized by the repetition or contamination of preceding sounds and syllables or the anticipation of sounds to be produced.

In his analogy of paraphasia to ideational and ideokinetic limb apraxia, Liepmann related ideokinetic paraphasia to the posterior cerebral areas. This form of paraphasia he states, is characterized by "syllable perseveration, premature production of syllables, word-slips with changes in sound and meaning, mixtures of appropriate word-segments and those mutilated in sound and meaning, word-perseverations and combinations of word-components evoked by chance sensory stimuli or associations" (1913).*

This concept was elaborated further by Kleist (1907b), Wernicke's young assistant at Halle, whose interest in paraphasia grew out of his studies of conduction aphasia. The latter syndrome shares with sensory aphasia this prominent symptom of paraphasia. Kleist identified two basic forms of paraphasia: 1) a literal form which was felt to reflect a disturbance in the finding and recall of the specific sound or sound elements making up the word and 2) a "word-finding" form which referred to the arousal of the word in its entirety. The first type was designated as "pure paraphasia". Together with Wernicke and Liepmann, Kleist's model anticipated contemporary concepts of speech programming. His "word-formula", which essentially represented an elaboration of Wernicke's "word-concept" and Liepmann's "word-plan", specified a synthesized organization or arrangement of speech sounds in a specific temporal rhythmic pattern. This word-formula contained acoustic as well as motor-kinesthetic components and was based on Kleist's concept of a special serializing or sequencing mechanism within the temporal lobe. He maintained that this mechanism governed the temporal ordering and patterning of "tonal images" and "acoustic engrams" of which the word was composed. Moreover, he regarded Broca's area as the substrate for a similar mechanism involved in the serial sequencing of the motor elements in discharge of the word. Normal speech production thus required an intimate association of these motor and acoustic patterning devices. Thus, Kleist viewed paraphasia as an impairment of the temporal acoustic serializing mechanism and its influence on that of the motor speech system.

As mentioned above, Kussmaul's hypothesis of a disturbed attention device mechanism, representing the other major school of thought on paraphasia, was most completely developed by Arnold Pick. Pick assumed the existence of an inhibitory mechanism in the left temporal lobe, postulating that damage to this mechanism, as characteristically occurred in sensory aphasia, would be followed by a relaxation of such a speech inhibitory control. This diminished inhibition would then be reflected in speech logorrhea, echolalia, and paraphasia. A decrease in specificity of word-recall would be caused by the lack of verbal inhibition and would typically result in the arousal and expression of words similar acoustically or semantically to the intended word. Such verbal paraphasic responses therefore revealed the inability to inhibit the awakening and production of such related but erroneous words. Literal paraphasia in Pick's schema was thus believed to be a consequence of impaired inhibition of the serial sequencing of sounds. Such disturbed control might typically result in the repetition, reversal, transposition or anticipation of sounds. Pick describes such modification of the word as anteception, metaception, and postception.

These early studies on paraphasia which in general reflected Kussmaul's or Wernicke's interpretations, were generally not restricted to investigation of this disorder in isolation but rather were viewed within the total context of expressive language symptomatology in aphasia. The close association of paraphasia with word-finding difficulty was observed by a number of early authorities and came into particular focus in Lotmar's work (1919-1935). His studies on word-finding also shed light on the problem of paraphasia. In the course of his examinations of aphasic patients on word-finding tasks, Lotmar noted the frequency of paraphasic responses. He labeled such responses "in between experiences", that is verbal mediators employed by the patient during attempts to evoke the intended word. Such findings were felt to support the purely verbal nature of word-finding difficulty, an issue which was a point of debate during the noetic aphasia period.

Goldstein's discussions of the problem of paraphasia bring us to the modern era. He differentiated two basic origins of the disorder. One form, designated as motor paraphasia, was attributed to motor difficulties. Describing this type Goldstein notes:

> ..... The patient has difficulty in pronouncing even sounds and letters correctly.... He hesitates, distorts letters, leaves one out because he is not able to pronounce it correctly, perseverates on others.... misplaces letters, etc. (1948, p. 83)

Impairment in inner speech was noted as another cause of paraphasic distortions. Discussing this form, Goldstein comments:

> In pathology the character of simultaneousness is lost, and the word is dissolved into different parts, into letters and syllables; or one part experienced before as background may gain the character of figure and gain abnormal importance. (1948, p. 99)

Goldstein accepted the common definition of verbal paraphasia as "the substitution of one word for another word". Both verbal and literal paraphasia were viewed from the perspective of his central concept of impairment in abstract attitude, the differentiation of figure and ground in psychological experience.

Unfortunately, the study of paraphasia was largely neglected in the postnoetic period. Recently, a refocus on this area seems to be occurring, particularly in the area of descriptive analysis of the disorder. The work of Lhermitte, Lecours and Bertrau (1965) has offered an innovative approach to the problem which appears promising. This study explores the "mechanisms of arousal, selection and seriation of linguistic units in normal and pathological speech." Burns and Canter (1974) have investigated another facet of the disorder, providing a description of phonemic errors in aphasic patients with presumed posterior lesions. This study focuses on particular error patterns demonstrated in Wernicke's and conduction aphasia in contrast to those found in presumed frontal lesions. The occurrence of literal and verbal paraphasia as components of the symptom-picture demonstrated by certain aphasics in verbal recall and production is another aspect of the problem currently under study with particular attention to recovery patterns (Eggert, G., Stewart, W., and Koenig, E., 1974). Much work leading to a clearer definition of the nature and mechanisms underlying paraphasia remains to be undertaken, and the next decades will likely see an increasing emphasis in study of this important facet of aphasia.

Word-Finding Difficulty

Although verbal amnesia or word-finding difficulty is found in most clinical aphasia forms, its particular significance as a primary symptom in the picture of sensory aphasia was first highlighted by Wernicke in his early description of that entity. In fact, it is regarded by some authorities as the chief characteristic in the final stages of sensory aphasia. Thus, the recovery profile of many severe sensory aphasics may follow a fairly predictable pattern through stages of initial jargon, followed by predominantly verbal and literal paraphasia, and may terminate in a fairly circumscribed syndrome of isolated word-finding deficit. This latter picture remains a residual disturbance which is particularly resistant to therapy and is regarded by some aphasiologists as a special aphasia subtype, that of amnesic aphasia. Such a clinical picture may persist long after significant or complete remission of the auditory comprehension aspects of the disorder have occurred.

Impairment in word retrieval, observed in various clinical types of aphasia, was reported as early as 1776. At that time Gessner (Kehrer, 1913) used the term "verbal amnesia" to refer to such disorders. Later, in 1853, Nasse attempted the task of classifying different sub-types of word-finding disturbance, calling particular attention to a special form of aphasia in which this was the primary and often the only feature. These observations anticipated the identification of a syndrome designated as amnesic or amnestic aphasia by Sanders in 1866. This entity did not, however, gain unanimous acceptance, and the attempt to isolate amnesic aphasia as a separate clinical form ushered in many years of controversy. Indeed, the emphasis of many investigations exploring this disorder during that period centered on attempts to resolve this particular issue, often to the neglect of consideration of other fundamental questions related to the problem of word-finding.

We shall not attempt to deal with the issue of amnesic aphasia as a special clinical form here but shall rather review various concepts relating to the problem of word-finding difficulty which emerged in the early post-classical and noetic aphasia periods.

Wernicke regarded word-finding difficulty as a mild motor transcortical aphasia. According to his schematic representation of this process, motor verbal production was stimulated directly by the complex processes of conceptualization. However, since motor and acoustic imagery were indivisible in inner language or the word-concept in Wernicke's schema, the participation of acoustic components in motor word-discharge could still be assumed. Thus, difficulty in word-finding was attributed to impairment in processes at the concept level which were necessary for activating the mechanisms involved in speech production.

Applying an approach which was not unlike Wernicke's in many respects, Kussmaul in 1877 attempted to explain verbal amnesia as "a disturbed arousal of the word image by the concept" and the constellations of subconcepts associated with the word to be evoked. The inadequacy of such word-excitation was felt to lead to the emergence of other words related in meaning or sound or to the awakening of fragments of such words. Kussmaul's approach was thus similar to Wernicke's with the exception that the former emphasized word-arousal indirectly via the acoustic speech center in contrast to Wernicke's more direct route from concept to motor speech discharge, as depicted in his schema.

Investigation of the problem of verbal amnesia in the early nineteen-hundreds led to various attempts to divide word-finding disturbances into different subtypes. One attempt by Kehrer (1913) classified such disorders into three forms: 1) word-sound amnesia, 2) word-motor amnesia, and 3) word-inhibition amnesia. Disruption of the inner acoustic experience of the word was noted to be the key feature of the first subtype, word-sound amnesia. Patients with such a disorder typically revealed difficulty in arousal and integration of the entire complex of sounds making up the word, although certain elements of the word, such as its length or the predominant vowel sound might be intact. The second form, word-motor amnesia, designated what might currently be considered a verbal apraxia. Characterized by integrity of the acoustic components of the word, speech breakdown in this type was assumed to occur in the translation of acoustic components to the corresponding motor elements of the word in verbal production. The third type, word-inhibition amnesia, referred to "complete derailment or inhibition" of word-arousal. Such errors apparently reflected either paraphasic verbal expression or a complete verbal block, resulting in no speech response.

During this period Freund (1899) called attention to a certain form of word-finding difficulty in which the patient characteristically demonstrated difficulty in naming objects presented visually. He labeled this problem "optic aphasia." Such patients, however, might be able to recall the appropriate names if objects were presented through some other channel such as the tactile, auditory, or olfactory modalities. These observations led to a more careful study and testing of the specific sensory modality which might be involved in certain kinds of word-finding difficulty and resulted in the isolation of a separate category of verbal amnesia, i.e., modality-specific word-finding impairment.

Two conflicting views of word-finding difficulty emerged in the early decades of the nineteen-hundreds. One school, headed by Binswanger (1925), included in its ranks Von-Woerkom, Bouman, Gelb, Goldstein, Head, and Wolpert. They regarded the problem of word-finding difficulty within the context of a basic thought disorder. The opposing camp, led by Lotmar, counted Isserlin, Kuehnberg, Kleist, and Pick among its members. The latter group stressed the verbal nature of word-finding difficulty. To refute Binswanger, Lotmar (1919, 1935) undertook a number of comprehensive studies of word-finding difficulty in aphasia. While they cannot be reviewed in any detail here, one must point with admiration to the detail and comprehensiveness of these studies. Lotmar, anticipating later linguistic approaches, recorded the responses of his aphasic subjects on various word-finding tasks in their entirety. Among the different aspects of word-recall studied were factors of latency, comparison of concrete and abstract word-retrieval, comparison of ease of recall of compound and simple words and the influence of the "depictability" of words on word-finding ability. Lotmar's studies in general supported his concept of the essentially verbal nature of word-finding impairment in aphasia.

Bridging the gap between the post-classical and modern periods in aphasia, Goldstein (1948) attempted to apply his concept of impairment in abstract attitude in brain damage to the area of word-finding difficulties. In describing this problem he states,

> Patients with this form of word-finding have not lost the words but are unable to use them in a categorial sense because they cannot assume the abstract attitude. When a patient truly names an object he has the experience of a word which means this object, considers the object as representing a category. (1948, p. 61)

Goldstein recognized two other forms of word-finding difficulty. One of these he related to "defects of speech instrumentalities". Paraphasic errors would be expected to result from such a disorder. A second infrequently occurring type was found in patients with acute brain injury or in individuals suffering from extreme fatique. Such patients might demonstrate difficulty in recalling proper names or words infrequent in use. Goldstein's work in the area of word-finding impairment spans the gap between the post-classical and modern periods.

As this short review has indicated, the problem of word-finding has occupied workers in the field for many decades. Early interpretations have relied on classical associationistic concepts, and the early studies were primarily descriptive in nature. The same observation might be made today. The focus of recent attention, as a brief scanning of current literature suggests, has been concerned with providing more comprehensive descriptions of the problem and its various facets. Contemporary workers, for example, are currently attempting to more specifically delineate the different varieties of naming disorders, (Geschwind, 1967) the effects of various stimulus-contexts on word-finding (Barton et al., 1969) and to explore possible correlations between word-retrieval and such factors as abstractness, word-frequency, and the "depictability" of words. Studies of word-recall in various clinical aphasia types and the exploration of modality specific word-finding disorders (Spreen et al., 1966; Goodglass et. al., 1968) have also been recent targets of investigation. In the area of diagnosis, construction of a test measuring verbal recall and production is currently underway. (Eggert, G., Stewart, W., and Koenig, E., 1974). Hopefully, such directions of research may provide clues to a clearer understanding of the basic processes impaired in this disorder, and perhaps eventually to the formulation of a theory of word-finding impairment in aphasia and related disorders.

SUMMARY

The preceding review has tried to sketch some of the developments which grew out of the studies of the symptom-picture of sensory aphasia in the post-classical period. As is well known, auditory comprehension loss, paraphasia and word-finding impairment may singly or in combination be found in various aphasia forms as well as in other disorders of higher mental processes. As a consequence, exploration of these symptoms had broader applications than merely contributing to the understanding of a single clinical entity. Viewed from this perspective, the study of Wernicke's aphasia in the post-classical and noetic periods contributed significantly to the history of aphasia and related disorders.

VI.

WERNICKE'S EARLY CRITICS

The fame which established Wernicke as one of the major figures in the history of the study of aphasia in the latter decades of the nineteenth century sustained a harsh blow as a result of Henry Head's publication in 1926. Although Wernickean concepts continued to permeate aphasia theory in the decades following his premature death in 1905, these ideas did not completely escape the critical eye of his contemporaries and later authorities. Kussmaul (1877), Freud (1891), and Flechsig (1896) in his own time raised questions on various issues. Somewhat later, Henschen (1918), the extreme localizationist, ironically became a caustic critic of Wernicke, one of the chief founders of the localizationist school. While the major point at issue was that of localization of language function, a number of questions of lesser importance also aroused attention at this time. The question of aphasia classification and the existence of the transcortical and conduction aphasia forms postulated by Wernicke, his application of Bezold's theory of hearing to auditory comprehension loss in aphasia, the problem of the extent of the cerebral speech area, as well as his interpretation of paraphasia and the related hypothesis of an internal language monitoring mechanism were among the issues of some debate. Such questions, however, were overshadowed by the major problem of localization of language function which absorbed much attention at that time.

Comprehensive analyses of the broader aspects of this controversy have been reviewed elsewhere and this discussion shall focus primarily on Head's attack of Wernicke's application of localization theory.

Pierre Marie's well-known assault on localization in 1906 caused considerable stir in French neurological circles but was apparently premature and did not effectively stem the tide of the localization movement in respect to aphasia. However, the soil was well-prepared for a new look at the entire problem by the time Head's work appeared in 1926. His two-volume publication was well received and became an important reference in aphasia in the years that followed. Its harsh review of localization of language function likely accelerated the decline of influence of the Breslau-Halle school of aphasia. This factor, of course, was not alone in bringing about such a decline. The political and economic conditions following in the wake of the first world war, the shift of scene in scientific research from the continent to America in the years that followed, the growing influence of Gestalt holistic concepts in the interpretation of higher mental processes, together with the general unavailability in English of the early German works in aphasia all contributed to the neglect and obscurity which befell Wernickean concepts and the work of his followers.

One must certainly acknowledge the merit and timeliness of Head's attempt to revive Hughling Jackson's contributions in his 1926 publication. Moreover, the time was ripe for a reassessment of the entire question of localization theory. Unfortunately, Head's biased and derogatory treatment of the problem weakened the potentially positive effects of such a reevaluation. In addition to this weapon of derogation, his arguments were based on isolated excerpts of the works of localization authorities, unfortunately interpreted out-of-context. This led to misrepresentation and in fact to frank inaccuracies in some cases. One may point to a number of instances where such errors occurred as a result of Head's out-of-context quoting of authorities such as Bastian and Wernicke.

Head's argument against localization focused on two areas, the primary and obvious one of association of language function to specific cerebral regions and secondly, the use of diagrams or schemas to illustrate the possible mechanisms involved in language and higher mental processes and the possible effects of damage to various cerebral areas.

However, a closer study of the works of eminent authorities such as Wernicke and Bastian reveals that neither took the simplistic view of mental processes attributed to them by Head. In respect to their views Head states:

> Moreover, all this school of observers believed that they could interpret the clinical manifestations directly in terms of anatomic tracts and centers. In reading these admirably written papers we are astonished at the serene dogmatism with which the writers assume a knowledge of the working of the mind and its dependence on hypothetical groups of cells and fibers. Most of the observers mentioned in this chapter failed to contribute anything of permanent value to the solution of the problem because they were dominated by a philosophical fallacy of their day... They imagined all vital processes could be explained by some simple formula. With the help of a few carefully selected assumptions they deduced the mechanisms of speech and embodied it in a schematic form... From diagrams based on *a priori* principles they deduced in turn the defects of function which must follow destruction of each center or internuncial path. They never doubted the validity of their postulates, based as they were on the rules of human reason (1926, pp. 57, 65).

A review of the works of authorities of the stature of Wernicke, whom Head later specifically includes in his diatribe, does not appear to support the latter's allegations. For example, in his 1874 ***Aphasia Symptom Complex,*** Wernicke cautioned against a strict application of localization of higher mental processes:

Primary functions alone can be referred to specific areas. Localization of visual perception to its central region and tactual sensation of the fingers to the central area of the ulnar nerve are examples of these primary functions..............
All processes which exceed these primary functions, such as the synthesis of various perceptions into concepts and the complex functions such as thought, and consciousness... are dependent upon the fiber bundles, that is, association. (1874) p. 92, this volume.

Reiterating this idea later in his second monograph, *Recent Works on Aphasia* Wernicke comments:

Any higher psychic processes exceeding these primary assumptions cannot be localized but rest on the mutual interaction of these fundamental psychic elements which mediate their manifold relations by means of the association fibers. Since that time I have become even more strongly convinced, particularly on the basis of clinical studies of aphasia, that we are not justified in going beyond this elementary premise. (1885-6) p. 177-8, this volume.

Moreover, the fact that Wernicke viewed language processes within the framework of function of the brain as a whole seems apparent in the following observation:

...Our interest in the speech mechanism, at least in the light of present knowledge, lies particularly in its role as an agent of consciousness. As was indicated in the conclusion of my discussion, the cerebral hemispheres as a whole, *in toto*, as an organ of consciousness function as the executor of the motor speech center in spontaneous speech production. The organ of consciousness *in toto* receives the message which is first translated to the sensory speech center... functioning as a receiving station for acoustic messages. (1885-6) p. 179, this volume.

Head frequently resorted to tactics such as sarcasm and ridicule in his attack on the localizationists. Even more damaging to their cause, however, was his tendency to cite selected quotations from their writings out-of-context to support his particular arguments. This led to frank distortions and misrepresentation of the ideas and concepts of localizationists who were victims of this practice.

A cogent example of such misrepresentations can be found in Head's reaction to Wernicke's 1903 essay on agraphia.

No better example could be chosen of the manner in which the writers of this period were compelled to lop and twist their cases to fit the procrustean bed of their hypothetical conceptions. Such a title (referring to Wernicke's article "A Case of Isolated Agraphia") can only mean that in this patient every other act of language could be perfectly performed except that of writing (Head then quotes symptoms from the case review which indicates presence of generalized aphasia in addition to agraphia but neglects to add that such symptoms essentially remitted at the time of Wernicke's first observation of the case). (Head, 1926, p. 63)

Head concluded:

Wernicke failed to recognize the wide-spread nature of the difficulty owing to the pre-

> conceptions with which it was approached; in the solemn discussion which follows that report we can only wonder at his clinical obtuseness and want of clinical insight. (1926, p. 63)

This paper reviewed the history of a patient who, following a cerebrovascular accident, presented a severe agraphia and some initial aphasic symptoms. Three years later, the aphasia, with the exception of "some difficulty in articulation" had largely resolved, leaving an agraphia as the predominant symptom. Relatively isolated agraphia had received scant attention at this time, and Wernicke used this case study as an example to introduce the general subject of agraphia.

In so doing he readily acknowledged the earlier symptoms of aphasia and the residual "difficulty in articulation". For the sake of discussion, however, Wernicke wished to focus on the problem of agraphia. Because the problem was relatively circumscribed, he apparently felt justified in titling this essay, "Isolated Agraphia." That he had no intention of ignoring the generalized earlier aphasic symptoms seems clear from the essay itself and his reference to it in his 1906 work:

> The second attack was followed by a transient disturbance in speech with moderate difficulty in articulation... Although we cannot ignore the moderate anarthia, for the purpose of this investigation it will be temporarily disregarded. (1906) p. 220, this volume.

Head's scathing critique of Wernicke's paper on agraphia completely misinterprets his clearly stated purpose in presenting this paper. Moreover, it ignores the fact that the aphasic symptoms had largely resolved at the time the essay was written. Furthermore, it unfairly charges Wernicke with covering up these symptoms and attempting to present an inaccurate picture of the patient's condition.

Head moreover, misinterpreted the postulation of a "concept center", included in the schemas of such authorities as Lichtheim and Wernicke. The latter, of course, did not thereby mean to imply a discrete anatomic localization of conceptual processes as Head erroneously assumed. This seems evident from Wernicke's statement:

> Now it is certainly understood that postulation of such a center is merely imaginary and only serves as a schematic simplification. In reality such processes involve areas which are located in various parts of the cortex. (1906) p. 237, this volume.

These excerpts from Wernicke's writings would then appear to refute Head's allegation that all representatives of the localization school "believed they could interpret the clinical manifestations directly in terms of anatomic tracts and centers." In fact, a search of the writings of localizationists such as Bastian or Wernicke would seem to fail to justify the charge that such authorities were ruled by "a serene dogmatism" which assumed". . . a knowledge of the mind and its dependence on hypothetical groups of cells and fibers." (Head, 1926) On the contrary, the excerpts from Wernicke's works quoted above would appear to point up his cautious approach to localization of speech function in which "the cerebral hemispheres as a whole *in toto*" were viewed as "an organ of consciousness functioning as the executor of the motor speech center in spontaneous speech production." P. 179, this volume.

The second focus of Head's attack on proponents of localization centered on the latter's use of diagrams or schemas to illustrate cerebral mechanisms. Thus, Head in his 1926 work comments:

> ...With the help of a few carefully selected assumptions they deduced the mechanisms of speech and embodied it in a schematic form... For every mental act there was a neural element... From diagrams based on *a priori* principles they deduced in turn the defects of function which must follow destruction of each 'center' or internuncial path. (1926, p. 65)

The diagrams and schemas designed by Wernicke, Bastian, and their nineteenth century contemporaries were intended to be used as teaching devices to clarify extremely complex processes. Caution was therefore necessary for their most effective use. The popularity of diagrams among Wernicke's contemporaries unfortunately led to indiscriminate application of such schemas and oversimplification in their interpretation by those who were eager for simple explanations to complex and obscure mental processes. However, the misuse of these schemas by those less gifted than a Bastian or a Wernicke does not diminish their intrinsic value. Wernicke clearly states the limitations of such diagrams or schemas in his comment:

> We must keep in mind that each schema, including our own, has value only as a mode of instruction and interpretation and loses its significance as soon as an easier or more accurate grouping of the data is found. (1900, 214-215)*

Thus a return to the original courses would seem to suggest that Head's assessment of the contributions of some of the major nineteenth century exponents of cerebral localization of language function such as Wernicke is flawed by inaccuracies and an apparent incomplete study of their works.

Although the question of localization was the primary target of Wernicke's critics, he was also challenged on a number of lesser issues. Among these, the existence and interpretation of the clinical entity of conduction aphasia advanced by Wernicke in the 1874 work was long the object of debate and in fact, continues to be so today.

Sigmund Freud, in his sole essay on aphasia was among Wernicke's contemporaries who questioned his interpretation of this syndrome. Conduction aphasia, characterized by intact auditory comprehension, fluent but paraphasic speech with impairment in mimicry, had been attributed by Wernicke to a disruption in the arcuate fiber tract somewhere along its course through the island region. Later, Von Monakow's studies indicated a more posterior localization of the lesion, deep within the parietal area.

Freud objected to Wernicke's interpretation of paraphasia on the basis of damage to the internal "corrector" or monitoring system. His discussion of this question suggests that he was unaware of Wernicke's notion of a word-concept. As indicated previously, an understanding of this notion is essential for an appreciation of Wernicke's interpretation of the internal "corrector."

Freud's 1891 monograph represented an early effort to temper the rising tide of the localization movement. Wernicke's theory, labeled by Freud as a "theory of centers and tracts," was viewed with suspicion. The latter interpreted Wernicke's emphasis in his later works on motor and sensory speech areas as evidence of his abandonment of the unified speech center he had advocated in earlier works. In an earlier essay, however, as well as in the 1874 monograph, Wernicke had stressed the unified nature of the speech region, an extensive area which included the entire "first primordial gyrus." Thus, sensory and motor areas as well as the supramarginal and angular gyri essentially formed a unitary region with the island as the pivot. That Wernicke did not later abandon this idea of a unified speech center seems apparent from this comment in his final work on aphasia:

> The entire first primordial gyrus, surrounding and embracing the Sylvian fossa region, may be counted as the speech area. (1906, p. 271, this volume)

Two other authorities who were quite vocal in their criticism of some of Wernicke's ideas may be briefly mentioned. In his 1896 monograph, *Gehirn und Seele,* Flechsig challenged Wernicke's lack of differentiation between the primary projection and secondary association areas. Flechsig's studies had led to his postulation of association areas surrounding the projection fields. He felt that Wernicke placed too much emphasis on the significance of the long fiber tracts in association processes, ignoring the multitude of short fibers connecting different association areas. History has proven the validity of both Flechsig's and Wernicke's concepts. The significance of the former's postulate of special association areas as well as the role of long fiber tracts in processes of association have won general acceptance.

Wernicke's interpretation of auditory comprehension impairment in sensory aphasia on the basis of loss of perception of sounds within a certain speech range was the target of sharp criticism from Henschen, writing some years after this notion had been advanced. This hypothesis was found to be in error as a consequence of studies which demonstrated that all auditory fibers terminated in Heschl's gyrus. Wernicke, it will be recalled, localized the area damaged in sensory aphasia to the posterior portion of the first temporal gyrus.

As this brief sketch of Wernicke's early critics reveals, his ideas did not escape challenge and even harsh attack from some quarters. On some issues, particularly those raised by Flechsig and Henschen, history has appeared to favor the position of his critics. However, on the question of localization of language function, a comprehensive study of his works *in toto* does not appear to justify or confirm the allegations of his strongest and most influential critic, Henry Head.

VII

WERNICKE'S CONTRIBUTION TO CURRENT CONCEPTS OF APHASIA AND RELATED DISORDERS

INTRODUCTION

The preceding chapters have attempted to trace the significance of the classic approach to the study of aphasia as reflected in the works of one of its chief exponents. In spite of the explosion of new information in recent years and rejection of some of the older material, these works continue to reveal a certain soundness and freshness. The current revival of such ideas is strong evidence of the relevance of such themes to contemporary thought on aphasia and higher mental processes.

The writings of Carl Wernicke take on an almost modern flavor when viewed in the light of current interest in connectionistic concepts. They represent a substantial contribution not only to the history of aphasia but also to current study and research.

Wernicke's works remind the contemporary researcher of the validity of a deductive, theory-oriented approach to the study of higher mental processes. They contain a wealth of clinical description and insight and offer an example of careful clinico-pathological methodology. Finally, the Breslau-Halle school has contributed model studies of the application of connectionism to the investigation of higher psychic processes. The following discussion shall attempt to briefly sketch the impact of the ideas developed in the works of Wernicke and his followers on contemporary thought.

Connectionism may be regarded as one of the major concepts originating in that period. It may be defined as an attempt to interpret the transmission and integration of auditory, visual, tactile, and motor data involved in higher mental processes by means of fiber tracts connecting specific cortical areas. This notion supplies the undergirding of the Wernicke aphasia schema and reflects his characteristic deductive approach to the resolution of scientific problems as well as his early absorption in the Meynert neuroanatomical doctrine.

The preceding chapters have attempted in part to outline the evolution of the concept of connectionism through various stages of its development in Wernicke's theory of aphasia. Conduction aphasia was the first disconnection syndrome to be described and likely furnished the model for development of the notions of subcortical and transcortical processes in language function and the effects of disruption of such tracts as demonstrated in the various aphasia pictures. Although connectionism was indeed a unique and important contribution of Wernicke and his contemporaries, it should be recalled that the disconnection syndromes formed only one segment of his aphasia model and classification system. There appears to be a current tendency among some contemporary workers towards emphasis on disorders which are related to the separation of intact centers, perhaps to the neglect of clinical syndromes caused by damage to cortical centers themselves. However, the Breslau-Halle school devoted considerable attention to the study of disturbances related to the involvement of such centers per se as manifested in the cortical motor and sensory aphasias. Indeed, the vitality and durability of the Wernicke model is felt to lie in its balanced emphasis on the interrelationships of subcortical, cortical, and transcortical processes, with appropriate value given to each component of the total model.

It is evident then that the current descriptions of disconnection and center syndromes had their origins in the classic period of aphasia and were most fully realized in the studies of Wernicke and his followers. These carefully detailed models, however, were essentially buried and neglected in the post-World War One period. The domination of holistic theories of psychology, the political-economic situation of the time in combination with the limited availability of these works in English, all contributed to the neglect of this important body of information. Moreover, Head's work, which stimulated a well-deserved revival of Jackson's ideas, unfortunately at the same time emphasized a negatively-biased and disparaging interpretation of localization concepts. This discouraged an impartial review and further exploration of the ideas generated in that period.

A REVIEW OF CONTEMPORARY CONCEPTS OF CONNECTIONISM

A dramatic return to connectionistic interpretations of brain mechanisms occurred in the early nineteen-fifties. Much of current research has focused on exploration of intra-and inter-hemispheric transmission and integration of information involved in higher mental processes. One area of emphasis has centered on the role of the corpus callosum in such information exchange and integration. In the interval between the classic period and the recent surge of interest in this area, ushered in by Myer's (1956) work, a brief flicker of attention to the possible significance of callosal connections in learning may be detected in work carried out in Pavlov's laboratory by Anrep and Bykov. Anrep's studies in 1923 on the dog had demonstrated "irradiation" of a conditioned response to tactile stimulation which was noted to be symmetrical in strength on both sides of the body. A repetition of these studies by Bykov

(1924) a year later on dogs with surgical transection of the callosum demonstrated an absence of such bilaterally equal response.

Myer's work on the cat in 1956 launched the current era of split-brain research. The initial experiments of this series focused on the mode of visual learning in the cat and the significance of the neocortical commissures in the transmission of such visual information. These studies attempted to explore the possibility of transfer of memory traces, apparently laid down in one hemisphere by means of input to one eye, to the opposite hemisphere. Further research investigated the possible effects of callosal sectioning on interocular transfer of such learning. These studies indicated that neither simple masking of one eye nor section of the optic chiasma prevented bilateral ocular learning. However, follow-up procedures, involving transection of callosal fibers together with the chiasma, demonstrated marked interference of such transfer and restriction of visual learning to one hemisphere. These early studies on interhemispheric exchange of visual information in the cat were later carried out on the monkey by Sperry (1958) and Downer (1958), with essentially similar results.

Such findings stimulated further exploration of the role of callosal fibers in transmission of learning through other sensory and motor modalities. In the somesthetic sphere Meyers (1960) found a high level of interhemispheric exchange in the learning of roughness and tactile form discrimination in the monkey with intact commissures. Transection of the callosal fibers, however, resulted in limitation of such tactile learning to one hand.

Split-brain research has also investigated the effects of olfactory perception in man following commissurotomy, revealing the significance of the commissures in the exchange of olfactory information. (Gordon and Sperry, 1969)

The probability of interaction between hemispheres in the auditory sphere has also been indicated by a number of studies. The complex bilateral subcortical representation of the auditory system complicates the assessment of the role of callosal connections in such interhemispheric transmission. Wegener (1964), summarizing some of the earlier studies, has reported the dependence on transmission at the cortical level in such tasks as tonal pattern discrimination, sound localization, and differentiation between auditory flutter and a steady auditory stimulus. Callosal fibers were felt to be implicated in the transmission of such auditory information.

The recent interest in dichotic studies has also pointed to the significance of the callosum in audition. In 1968, Milner, Taylor, and Sperry investigated the lateralized suppression of dichotically presented digits following commissurotomy in man. Shortly after, Sparks and Geschwind (1969) explored the possibility of interhemispheric transmission of auditory information in a patient who had undergone complete section of the commissures because of epilepsy. Their results appeared to demonstrate the particular importance of the callosal pathway in transmission of verbal material presented to the left ear in dichotic tasks.

A recent avenue of approach to the study of interhemispheric relations has involved analysis of patients who have undergone commissurotomy because of convulsive seizures. The earlier negative findings of the Akelaitis (1941, 1942, 1943, 1944) series, in which responses of epileptic patients who had undergone commissurotomy were explored, de-emphasized the significance of the callosum in the exchange of information between hemispheres. As Geschwind has pointed out (1965) the hazards of applying interpretations of possible relationships between cerebral mechanisms and language behavior based on studies of long-term epileptic patients is well known. In addition to the possibility of development of alternate neural connections in such subjects, limitations in test procedures or in the timing of administration of testing before spontaneous recovery of function has occurred are also factors which require consideration in interpretation of the Akelaitis studies.

During the past decade a number of studies have re-opened the question of the role of the callosum. The overall conclusions appear to have strongly confirmed the findings of the early classic studies which demonstrated the importance of such connections in interhemispheric transmission.

Research of Gazzaniga, Bogen, and Sperry (1965) on commissurotomized epileptic subjects has attempted to assess the nature and extent of interaction of the hemispheres in certain perceptual and mnemonic activities. The general conclusions of these studies suggest no disturbance in performance when visual input is limited to one hemisphere and the response requires the use of the contralateral hand. In such studies the manual performance is controlled by the same hemisphere to which the input has been relayed. When a visual stimulus is presented by tachistoscope to the left visual field (and therefore the right hemisphere), the right hand, (under control of the left hemisphere), fails in identification of the stimulus picture by choice selection. In contrast, no difficulty is demonstrated by the left hand in carrying out this task. Responses of a verbal nature, however, both oral and written can be accurately executed only if visual input is channeled to the left hemisphere. Some individual differences were noted in the quality of response of the two patients involved in this experiment. While later studies by the same group (Sperry and Gazziniga, 1967) have suggested greater participation by the minor hemisphere in verbal tasks than was previosuly anticipated, the basic conclusions supporting the important role of the callosum in interhemispheric exchange of information have been maintained.

Let us now briefly consider the significance of the concept of connectionism in relation to language production and breakdown. The processes of normal oral and written communication require integrity of the primary projection areas for input and discharge of language stimuli as well as intact function of the association areas necessary for processing, integration and formulation of such verbal information. Moreover, integrity of the fiber tracts participating in association and integration of such stimuli is requisite to normal language function. The summit of Wernicke's "primordial-gyrus," the supramarginal and angular gyri, may be regarded as the pivot in the union and integration of auditory, visual, and somesthetic stimuli. Workers in the classic era were well aware of the significance of this region in the mechanisms of higher mental processes and language.

The preceding section of this chapter has attempted a brief outline of recent research, in which the various clinical pictures related to disruption of intra- and interhemispheric integration are described and explored. The basic thrust of the Wernicke school aimed at a closer study of the cerebral areas and tracts involved in language function and higher mental processes and attempted to detail the various clinical pictures caused by damage to centers and their fiber connections. These classic studies of the agnosias, alexias, apraxias, agraphias, and various subforms of aphasia may therefore be regarded as early models of current research related to the involvement of intra- and interhemispheric integration.

The following section shall attempt to sketch representative classic studies of such syndromes which were carried out by the Wernicke school of aphasia and his nineteen century contemporaries.

CLASSIC MODELS OF DISCONNECTION SYNDROMES

Conduction Aphasia

Conduction aphasia, the first disconnection syndrome to be described, was initially discussed by Wernicke in his original work on aphasia. This syndrome was believed to be caused by disruption of fibers connecting the motor and sensory speech areas and was characterized by intact auditory comprehension and a paraphasic motor speech pattern with inability to mimic. Wernicke originally diagnosed, but later rejected, two cases described in his 1874 work as representative examples of conduction aphasia. At that time he localized the site of the lesion to the island area since he believed that the fibers uniting the motor and sensory speech areas were found in that region. However, he was unable to find the expected pathological confirmation of this symptom-picture in lesions of the island and later modified his position regarding this localization on the basis of Von Monakow's studies. These findings indicated that the arcuate fibers formed the chief link between the two speech regions. This tract coursed through the lower parietal lobe and, arching around the posterior end of the Sylvian fissure, ultimately terminated in the frontal lobe.

Pershing's case study reported in 1900 was among the early carefully documented clinico-pathological reports of conduction aphasia. His patient, a 45 year old man, suffered a stroke which resulted in a fluent jargon aphasia, and inability to mimic. Some impairment in auditory comprehension was observed during the first week, but this symptom completely remitted by the second week following the attack. Pathological findings revealed a single focal lesion "immediately above the Sylvian fissure, 6 cm. posterior to the junction of its vertical and horizontal branches." This lesion, according to Pershing's interpretation, completely disrupted fibers connecting the first temporal and third frontal gyri.

Other clinico-pathological studies of conduction aphasia were carried out in the early twentieth century by Heilbronner (1910), Kleist (1905), Liepmann and Pappenheim (1914) and others. Goldstein (1948) was also interested in this syndrome and renamed it "central aphasia." In the Wernicke era and in the years immediately following, conduction aphasia remained a controversial issue with varying interpretations of the clinical symptoms and cerebral localization. Lack of unanimity in regard to the localization, symptomatology and mechanisms involved diminishes the usefulness of this term. As is true today, many workers of that period regarded this syndrome as a stage in the recovery of sensory aphasia which was characterized by marked improvement in auditory comprehension. Clarification and further definitive study of this aphasia type would seem needed to enhance its usefulness in clinical classification systems.

Pure Word Deafness

Lichtheim (1884-85) was among the early workers to describe the syndrome of pure word-deafness. This syndrome is characterized by adequate hearing sensitivity in contrast to marked impairment in auditory comprehension, mild paraphasia, and difficulty in mimicry. The classic syndrome was assumed to be caused by lesions involving the left auditory radiation as well as callosal fibers from the opposite auditory center on the right, thus preventing sound stimuli from reaching the left sensory center necessary for comprehension of the spoken word.

Lichtheim's case, described in his monograph and earlier reported by Burckhardt (1882), involved a 55 year-old teacher and journalist who had suffered two cerebrovascular accidents. The initial attack was followed by fluent but paraphasic speech and paragraphia. There was gradual remission of these symptoms resulting in a picture of minimal impairment in speech, except for very occasional difficulty in word-finding. A second attack five years later resulted in a severe isolated loss of auditory comprehension but adequate hearing sensitivity, and essentially intact speech production. Writing was fluent and the patient was able to continue his work as a journalist. Lichtheim predicted a subcortical disruption of the auditory radiation on both sides. Wernicke regarded Lichtheim's description of this form as a major contribution and included it in his classification under the label of subcortical sensory aphasia.

Several years later Liepmann and Storch (1902) published the first pathological confirmation of a case of pure word-deafness which clearly verified Lichtheim's earlier predicted localization and which emphasized the significance of callosal lesions in production of this syndrome. Liepmann had earlier described this case in 1898. The Liepmann-Storch case, Gorstelle, a 67 year old carpenter, sustained a series of cerebrovascular accidents which ultimately resulted in the clinical picture of pure word-deafness. Wernicke himself carried out the autopsy findings of this case in which involvement of the auditory radiation on the left was demonstrated together with disruption of callosal fibers. This latter lesion prevented crossing of auditory stimuli from the right hemisphere to the auditory speech area in the left temporal lobe.

Pick (1892), Dejerine and Serieux (1898), Strohmayer (1902), Bonvicini (1905) and others explored various aspects of this syndrome and presented case-studies during the Wernicke era. However, many of these cases did not completely satisfy all the requisites of the clinical symptoms and the anticipated cerebral localization.

The infrequency of the occurrence of this syndrome is related to the peculiar type or combination of lesions needed to produce the classic clinical picture.

Motor Aphasia as A Disconnection Syndrome

The problem of a motor aphasia caused by disruption of subcortical tracts, essentially sparing Broca's area itself, was the object of much interest and controversy in the Wernicke era and the decades following. Henry Sachs (1893, p. 207) supported the hypothesis advanced by Lichtheim, Wernicke, and others of production of motor aphasia on the basis of the white substance beneath Broca's area. He particularly espoused Dejerine's notion of the role of callosal fiber disruption in producing such a motor aphasia. Wernicke's early hypothesis of a subcortical motor aphasia was attributed to destruction of a postulated motor speech path. However, later nineteenth century workers, including Wernicke who had modified his earlier views, explained such symptoms on the basis of a small lesion beneath the third frontal gyrus. Such a lesion would result in involvement of callosal fibers from Broca's area as well as fibers coursing to area 4 and the internal capsule. This type of lesion would cause isolation of an intact Broca's area from which speech impulses could reach the peripheral speech mechanism neither by its direct route nor circuitously, via callosal fibers.

Bonhoeffer (1914), one of Wernicke's assistants, provided a well-detailed study of such a case of a motor aphasia disconnection syndrome with alexia and agraphia produced by a subcortical lesion. The patient, a 51 year-old shoemaker, suffered a series of attacks in 1909 resulting in loss of speech, initial difficulty in mimicry, impairment in naming, essentially normal auditory comprehension, paralexia and paragraphia. A marked apraxia of the left hand and some lesser impairment in the right hand were also observed.

Pathological studies later revealed an old lesion of the anterior cerebral artery which resulted in destruction of the callosum up to the splenium. Bonhoeffer noted that there was absence of involvement of the third frontal gyrus, the foot of the central gyrus, the first temporal gyrus and its white matter, together with surrounding fibers of the corona radiata, the arcuate fasciculus, the island, and the lenticular nucleus, with the exception of a small area tangent to the capsular lesion.

Bonhoeffer interpreted the symptoms of motor aphasia on the basis of a subcortical lesion which had destroyed the anterior and superior portion of the internal capsule. This lesion, he believed, would result essentially in isolation of Broca's area, and in consequence, the clinical picture of motor aphasia. The callosal fiber destruction was also felt to be the basis of the apraxia involving the left hand and therefore supported Liepmann's careful studies carried out several years earlier.

Although the motor disconnection syndrome illustrated by Bonhoeffer's case included agraphia and alexia, the severity of which is not clear from his report, the subcortical motor aphasia of Wernicke represented a more isolated syndrome. This latter was differentiated from the cortical type by essentially intact writing and reading comprehension.

Contemporary workers have described subcortical motor aphasia as "apraxia of speech" (Darley, 1968) and "pure verbal apraxia" (Canter, 1969).

Visual Agnosia

Lissauer's classic work on visual agnosia was carried out in 1889 at the Breslau Clinic. This carefully documented study was preceded by Munk's (1881) animal experiments on psychic blindness as well as Wilbrandt's (1887) review of the problem. It reflects the characteristic Wernicke mark of thoroughness and detail, and the application of a theoretic approach to clinico-pathologic studies.

Lissauer's patient, an 80-year old businessman, sustained an essentially isolated impairment in the visual recognition of objects as well as loss of reading in association with essentially adequate visual acuity and absence of aphasia. In addition to the routine assessment of visual acuity and visual fields, the study included exploration of visual memory, the ability to judge distance and visual measurement, drawing from memory, copying of designs, reading, writing, visual-spatial orientation, and psychic reaction time to visual stimulation.

Lissauer differentiated two basic forms of visual agnosia.

1. Apperceptive visual agnosia was defined as an impairment in visual perception.
2. Associative or transcortical visual agnosia was characterized by disconnection between visual perception and the related psychic concepts such as tactile, acoustic, motor-kinesthetic, and verbal associations involved in comprehension of the object visualized. The patient thus was unable to attach meaning to his visual perceptions.

Lissauer hypothesized three anatomical levels of impairment corresponding to Wernicke's aphasia classification. These included 1) visual impairment of subcortical connections from the periphery to the visual cortical areas, 2) damage to the visual cortical areas, and 3) involvement of the transcortical tracts connecting the visual centers to the rest of the cortical surface and thus to all concepts related to the object visualized.

The case under study was interpreted as an example of the associative or transcortical type of visual agnosia. Lissauer predicted the presence of two focal lesions. The first implicated the visual radiation in combination with involvement of the transcortical fibers connecting the visual center to other cortical areas. In addition, he postulated the probability of a second lesion with involvement of callosal fibers because of the close anatomic relation between subcortical and transcortical fibers and the callosum.

Lissauer's premature death prevented his verification of the pathological findings of this patient. Hahn (1895), a fellow assistant at the Breslau Clinic, carried out the autopsy studies which revealed extensive involvement of the white matter and the association cortex of the parietal lobe, with simultaneous destruction of callosal fibers of the splenium and their termination in the occipital lobe. These findings therefore confirmed Lissauer's prediction of a transcortical or associative type of visual agnosia in this patient. Geschwind (1965) has suggested an interpretation of the Lissauer case as representing in effect a naming disorder, based on the disconnection of visual areas from speech areas with consequent inability to verbalize what has been seen. On the basis of Lissauer's protocol this interpretation may well be valid, although it is not clear if modes other than the verbal were employed in testing visual recognition in this particular patient.

Lissauer's case-study was among the first classic studies to be carried out by Wernicke's students. It is a model of thorough exhaustive observation and examination in combination with the characteristic Wernicke mode of interpretation of clinico-pathological findings within a theoretical framework.

Pure Word-Blindness

Pure word-blindness has been classically described as a syndrome characterized by a marked loss of reading in combination with essentially intact visual acuity, writing, language usage, and intelligence. The fluency and accuracy of writing stands in sharp contrast to the isolated severe loss of reading. Kussmaul first applied the label "pure word-blindness" to this disorder, while Wernicke preferred the term "subcortical alexia". Word-blindness, in contrast to pure word-blindness, referred to a combined loss of reading and writing with integrity of visual acuity, language, and intelligence.

Dejerine first localized the lesion responsible for pure word-blindness in 1892. His patient, a 68 year old man, presented fluent speech, normal auditory comprehension, and intact writing and language. However, he demonstrated complete loss of the ability to identify letters by name and the reading of words. Pathological study of this case by Dejerine revealed destruction of the medial and inferior aspects of the left occipital lobe and involvement of the splenium of the callosum. Dejerine interpreted the mechanism of word-blindness on the basis of isolation of the visual centers in the intact occipital lobe from the language areas in the left hemisphere. The destruction of the left occipital area prevented transfer of visual stimuli from that area to Wernicke's area on the left. The involvement of the callosum interfered with the transmission of such visual stimuli from the right occipital lobe via callosal fibers to the left language area. A right hemianopsia was a consistent finding in such cases which restricted vision to the left visual field (and right hemisphere) only. Dejerine's case represents the first disconnection syndrome in which the significance of involvement of the callosum was verified in pathological study.

Hinshelwood (1895, 1900), Edgren (1887), Bruns and Stölting (1894) and others during this period described cases which further detailed possible individual variation of symptoms presented. For example, certain patients retained isolated kinds of loss such as the preservation of reading of numbers or musical notes and demonstrated varied levels of reading performance in different languages.

Individual variation has also been reported in the ability to name objects. Dejerine's case, for example, apparently presented no specific loss in this area. Wernicke, however, had observed impairment in naming in certain patients with alexia. Because fluent speech is characteristic of this problem, this symptom may be easily overlooked unless specific testing is carried out. Some contemporary workers (Geschwind and Fusillo, 1964) have found instances of isolated impairment in color naming.

In addition to the symptoms commonly described in association with pure word-blindness, a case recently reported by Eggert and Canter (1968) also demonstrated involvement in the area of visual memory and a moderate impairment in naming. The first author has since observed other cases of pure word-blindness in which impairment in object and picture-naming was also present, although spontaneous speech was fluent with no evidence of word-finding difficulty. Involvement in visual memory as well as naming may not be noticed in such cases unless specific assessment of such areas is undertaken. These findings may underline the significance of internal verbalization in carrying out such tasks requiring visual-verbal associations such as spontaneous drawing, reproduction of designs from memory, and naming of objects from visual stimulation.

The syndrome of pure word-blindness received little attention following the early studies carried out in the classic era, and only recently has the revival of interest in connectionism again stimulated further study of this problem.

SUMMARY

This review has attempted to highlight early contributions to the study of cerebral disconnection syndromes. These careful clinicopathologic studies by late nineteenth and early twentieth century workers laid the foundation for our present understanding of many of the puzzling phenomena observed in aphasia, alexia, agnosia and apraxia.

Although contemporary research methodologies offer a much broader choice of approach to workers in this area, the detailed clinical and pathologic analysis of individual cases continues to be a valid and productive mode of exploring disorders of higher mental processes.

VIII.

CONCLUSION

This discussion of Wernicke's works together with the translations which follow represent an attempt to underscore the significance of the nineteenth century contributions to the study of aphasia as reflected in the writings of Wernicke and the Breslau-Halle school. A return to the primary sources is felt important to permit an objective and comprehensive assessment of the works of this earlier period and its relevance to current theory and research.

Let us briefly summarize the major contributions of Wernicke to the study of aphasia and related disorders.

His discovery of sensory aphasia and formulation of a theory of aphasia laid the basis for a scientific study of the subject which was to lead to further discoveries and a clearer understanding of the disorder. His descriptions of new aphasia subforms and his classification of the alexias and agraphias provided the impetus for further research by his students and contemporaries. Wernicke's works contain many small nuggets of information – brief insights. shrewd off-hand observations, which are included almost nonchalantly in the course of his presentations. One might point to his notion of a monitoring or feedback system in language production, his interpretation of paraphasia based on impairment of such a system, his description of motor speech imagery which in a sense foreshadowed current notions of motor speech programming, and his idea of a word-concept.

Together with Friedländer he published the first case of central deafness caused by bilateral temporal lesions and was first to localize tactile agnosia (Wernicke, 1895). The 1874 work on aphasia was among the first publications to emphasize the disorders of reading and writing and to place them within a total model of aphasia. Wernicke's observation of the poverty of spontaneous speech in transcortical motor aphasia led to a more complete study of this symptom by Kleist (1907) and others in the years which followed. Wernicke was first to apply a precursor of the currently popular linguistic method to evaluation of aphasia, as is evident in his mode of recording complete speech samples and conversations of his cases in the 1874 work. Traditional testing, until recently, has been commonly oriented to the eliciting of single-word responses and the use of pass and fail methods in the assessment of language performance. His careful, exhaustive approach to clinical examination and study has offered a model of the ideal combination of the clinician-researcher who could productively apply the art of hypothesis-testing to clinical work.

Moreover, Wernicke was the founder of a school of aphasia and his influence stimulated significant achievements in the works of his students. Although his followers carried the "Wernicke stamp." the Breslau-Halle school was not characterized by slavish imitation of its chief.

Perhaps Wernicke's most intangible and unique legacy may be found in the theme which provided the leitmotif to his life's work – the spirit of "Der Forscher," the researcher whose work betrays the effective blending of the daring theorist and the careful, persistent empiricist in his approach to science.

In marking this anniversary year of the discovery of sensory aphasia, one may well echo the closing tribute with which his colleague, Theodore Ziehen, commemorated Wernicke at the time of his death:

> In historical retrospect he will stand as one of the founders of our discipline, to whose works we may return again and again, to seek and find an endless store of learning and stimulation.*

BIBLIOGRAPHY

Akelaitis, A.

1941 Studies on the Corpus Callosum: II. *Arch. Neurol. Psychiat.* 45, 788-796.

1942 Studies on the Corpus Callosum: VI. *Arch. Neurol. Psychiat.* 48, 914-937.

1943 Studies on the Corpus Callosum. VII. Study of Language Functions unilateral following Section of the Corpus Callosum. *J. Neuropath. Exper. Neurol.*, 2, 226-262.

1944 A Study of Gnosis, Praxis, and Language following Section of the Corpus Callosum and Anterior Commissure. *J. of Neurosurg.*, 1, 94-102.

Anrep, G.

1964 *Proc. Roy. Soc. Bio.*, Cited in: *Ciba Foundation Symposium on the Function of the Corpus Callosum.* No. 20, Pp. 2-3.

Ballet, G.

1890 *Die Innerliche Sprache und die verschiedenen Formen der Aphasie.* (P. Bongers, Trans 7.), Leipzig: Deutsche. *Le langage intérieur,* Paris, Félix Alcan, 1886

Barton, Marusewki, M. and Urrea, D.

1969 Variation of Stimulus Context and its Effects on Word-finding Ability in Aphasics. *Cortex, 5,* No. 4, 351.

Bastian, C.

1869 On the Various Forms of Loss of Speech in Cerebral Disease. *Brit. and For. Med. Chir. Rev. April.*

1898 *A Treatise on Aphasia and other Speech Defects.* London: H. K. Lewis,

Batemann, F.

1890 *On Aphasia* (2nd. ed.) London: Churchill.

Bezold

1896 *Hörvermögen der Taubstummen.* Wiesbaden.

1896 Demonstration einer kontinuierlichen Tonreihe zum Nachweis von Gehördefekten. *Ztschr. f. Psycho. u. Phys. der Sinnesorgan,* 33.

Binswanger, L.

1926 Zum problem von Sprache und Denken. *Schweitz Arch Neur. 36,* No. 54.

Bonhoeffer, K.

1905 Die Stellung Wernicke's in der modernen Psychiatrie. *Berl. klin. Wchschr., 42,* 893-894; 927-930.

1914 Klinischer und anatomischer Befund zur Lehre von der Apraxie und der "motorischen Sprachbahn." *Mschr. Psychiat. Neurolog., 35,* 113-128.

Bonvicini, G.

1905 Über subcorticale sensorische Aphasie. *Jahrb. d. Psychiatrie u. Neurol. 26,* 126.

Bramwell, B.

1897 Illustrative Cases on Aphasia, *Lancet, 1,* 796, 868, 950, 1019, 1076, 1141, 1256, 1404.

Broadbent, W.

1879 A Case of Peculiar Affection of Speech with Commentary. *Brain, 1,* 484-503.

1872 On the Cerebral Mechanism of Speech and Thought. *Brit. Med. Journal, 55,* 145-194.

Bruns and Stölting,
Fall von Alexie. *Neurol. Zentralbl.*, 481, 1888.

Buesz, H.
1948 Carl Wernicke (1848-1905) ein Pioneer der Hirnpathologie. *Schw. Med. Wchschr., 24,* 604

Burns M., Canter G. and Trost, J.
1974 Phonemic Behavior in Fluent Aphasic Patients with Posterior Cerebral Lesions. Paper presented to the Annual Convention of American Speech and Hearing, Association. Las Vegas.

Bykov, K.
1924 Zbl. ges. Neurol. Psych., 39, 199, 1924. Cited in: *Ciba Foundation Symposium on Functions of the Corpus Callosum,* p. 2-3. 1964.

Canter. G.
1969 Paper presented to the Convention of the American Speech and Hearing Association, New York, N. Y.

Charcot, J.
1883 Des variétés de l'aphasie. Aphasie motrice. *Progrès med.*, Nos. 23, 24, 25, 27, 44. June.
1885 Cited in Wernicke, C. Einige neuere Arbeiten über Aphasie. *Fortschr. der Med.*, 824.

Darley, F.
1968 Paper presented to the Convention of the American Speech and Hearing Association, Denver, Colo.

Dejerine, J.
1892 Contribution à l'étude anatomo-pathologique et clinique des différentes variétés de cécité verbale. *Mém. Soc. Biol.*, 4, 61-90.

Dejerine J. and Sérieux P.
1898 Un cas de surdité verbale pure Revue de Psychologie. Cited in Goldstein, K., *Language and Language Disturbances.* New York: Grune and Stratton, 1948.
1914 Cited in Hinshelwood, *Congenital Word Blindness,* London: Lewis & Co.

Downer, J.
1958 Role of the Corpus Callosum in Transfer of Training in Macaca Mulatta. *Fed. Proc., 17,* 37.

Duchenne, G.
1883 *Physiologie der Bewegungen* (C. Wernicke, Trans.) Kassel: Fischer.

Edgren, Amusie.
1895 *Dtsch. Ztschr. f. Nervenheilk., 6,* 1.

Egger, V.
1904 *La parole intérieure,* Paris.

Eggert, G. and Canter, G.
1968 *A Case Study of Pure Word-Blindness.* Paper presented to the Convention of the American Speech and Hearing Association, Denver, Colo..

Eggert, G., Stewart, W., and Koenig, E.
1974 *The Symptom Profile Test of Word-Finding: A Preliminary Study.* Paper presented to the Convention of the Illinois Speech and Hearing Association Chicago, Ill.

Eggert, G.
1974 *The One-Hundredth Anniversary of Wernicke's Discovery of Sensory Aphasia: A Retrospective Look.* Paper presented to the Convention of the American Speech and Hearing Association, Las Vegas.
1976 *Liepmann's Works on Apraxia: A Review and Source-book.* in press. monograph.

Eisenberg, R.
1970 The Organization of Auditory Behavior. *J. of Speech and Hearing Res., 13,* 453-471, September.

Elder, W.
1897 *Aphasia and the Cerebral Speech Mechanism.* London: Lewis.
Flechsig, P.
1896 *Gehirn und Seele.* Leipzig: Veit.
Freud, S.
1891 *Zur Auffassung der Aphasien.* Leipzig.
1953 *On Aphasia.* (E. Stengel, Trans.) New York: International Universities Press.
Freund, C. S.
1899 Über optische Aphasie und Seelenblindheit. *Arch. f. Psych. 20, 276.*
1895 *Labyrinthtaubheit und Sprachtaubheit.* Wiesbaden.
Fritsch, G. and Hitzig, E.
1870 On the Electrical excitability of the Cerebrum. In: *The Cerebral Cortex* (G. Von Bonin, Trans.) Springfield: Thomas, 1960. 73-97 (Ueber die elektrische Erregbarkeit des Grosshirns) (*Arch. f. Anat., Physiolo. und wissenschäftl. Mediz.,* Leipzig, 300-332.)
Gazzaniga, M., Bogen, J. and Sperry, R.
1962 Some Functional Effects of Section of the cerebral Commissures in Man. *Proc. Nat. Acad. Sci. U. S. A., 48,* Part II, 1765-1969.
Gazzaniga M. and Sperry, R.
1967 Language after section cerebral Commissures, *Brain 90,* 131-148.
Geschwind, N. and Fusillo, M.
1964 Color-naming Defects in Association with Alexia. *Tr. Amer. Neurol. Ass., 89,* 172-176.
Geschwind, N.
1965 Disconnection syndromes in animals and man. *Brain, 88,* 237-294.
1966 Carl Wernicke and the Breslau School and the History of Aphasia. In: (E. Carterette, Ed.) *Brain Function Vol. III,* Proceedings of the Third Conference, November 1963, UCLA Forum in Medical Sciences No. 4. Berkeley: University of California Press, 1-16.
1967 The Varieties of Naming Disorders. *Cortex, 3,* 97-112.
1967 Wernicke's Contribution to the Study of Aphasia. *Cortex 3,* 449-463.
Goldscheider, A.
1892 Über centrale Sprache-Schreib und Lesestörungen. *Berl. Klin. Wchschr. , 64,* 100, 122, 144, 168,
Goldstein, K.
1948 *Language and Language Disturbances.* New York: Grune and Stratton.
Goltz, F.
1888 On the Functions of the Hemisphere. In: *The Cerebral Cortex* (G. Von Bonin, Trans.) Springfield: Thomas, 1960, 118-147. (Ueber die Verrichtungen des Grosshirns) *Pflüger's Archiv. f. die gesamte Physiologie, 42,* 419-467.
Goodglass, Barton, M. and Kaplan E.
1968 Sensory Modality and Object Naming in Aphasia. *J. Speech and Hearing Research, II,* 488-496.
Gordon, H. and Sperry, R.
1968 Lateralization of olfactory perception in the surgically separated hemispheres of man. *Neuropsychologia, 7,* 111-170
Gruhle, H.
1955 Wernicke's psychopathologische und klinische Lehren. *Der Nervenärzt. 26,* 505-507.
Head, H.
1926 *Aphasia and Kindred Disorders of Speech.* London: Cambridge University Press.
Heilbronner, K.
1905 Nekrologie Carl Wernicke, *Allg. Ztschr. Psychiat. 62,* 881-892.
1907 Zur Symptomatologie der Aphasie. *Arch. f. Psych. u. Nervenkr. 63,* No. 1, 234-298; No. 2, 698-758.
1910 Die aphasischen, apraktischen und agnostischen Störungen. In: *Handb. Neurol.* (M. Lewandowsky, Ed.), Berlin: Springer, *1,* 982-1093.

Henschen, S. E.
1917 Über die Hörsphäre. *J. F. Psychol. u. Neur. 22*, 319-474.
1920- *Klinische und anatomische Beitrage zur Pathologie des Gehirns.* 5-7- Stock-
1922 holm.
1927 Aphasiesysteme. *Monat. f. Psych. u. Neur., 65* 87-137.
Heubner.
1889 Über Aphasie. *Schmidt's Jahrbuch d. gesamt. Med. , 224.* , p. 220 Cited in Von Berg. M., Breitrag zur Kenntnis der Transcorticalen Aphasie. *Monatschr. f. Psychiat. u. Neurol., 12*, No. 5, 348-354.
Hildebrandt, K.
1924 Der philosophische Grundgedanke in Wernickes System. *Monatsch, f. Psychiat. u. Neurol., 54*, 210-215.
Hinshelwood
1895 Word-Blindness and Visual Memory. *Lancet, 73*, 1574-1580.
1900 Congenital Word-Blindness, *Lancet, 78*, 1506-1508.
1900 *Letter, Word and Mindblindness,* London: Lewis.
1917 *Congenital Word Blindness.* London: Lewis.
Isserlin, M.
1936 In: *Handbuch der Neurologie.* (O. Bumke and O. Foerster, Eds.), Berlin: Springer, 6, 626.
Jackson, Hughlings.
Selected Writings of John Hughlings Jackson. 2 vols. London: Hodder and Stoughton, 1931-32.
Jaspers, K.
1946 *Allgemeine Psychopathologie.* (4th ed.) Berlin: Springer.
1922 Cited in *Deutsche Irrenaertze,* Vol II (T. Kirchhoff, Ed.), Berlin: Springer, 238-250.
Kabelyanskaya L. and Viting, I.
1968 The Problem of So-Called "Transcortical" Sensory Aphasia. In: *Russian Translations on Speech and Hearing.* (R. West, Ed.) (S. Franklin, Trans.), *ASHA Reports,* No. 3, 407-422, March.
Kehrer, F.
1913 Beitrage zur Aphasielehre mit besonderer Berücksichtigung der amnestischen Aphasie. *Arch. f. Psychiat. u. Neur. 52*, 103.
Kleist, K.
1905 Carl Wernicke. *Münch. med. Wschr., 52*, 1402-1404.
1907a Corticale (innervatorische) Apraxie. *Jahrb. f. Psych. u. Neurol.*, 28, 47-112.
1907b Leitungsaphasie. *Monatschr. f. Psych. u. Neurol., 28.*
1959 Carl Wernicke. In: *Grosse Nervenaertze* Vol. II, (K. Kolle, Ed.), Stuttgart: Thieme, 106-128.
v. Koschütsky, R.
1959 Professor Wernicke, ein Charakterbild. *Deutsche Welt,* 1905, Cited in: *Grosse Nervenaertze,* Vol. II, (K. Kolle, Ed.). Stuttgart: Thieme.
Kussmaul, A.
1877 *Die Störungen der Sprache.* Leipzig: Vogel.
Lecours, A. R. and Lhermitte, F.
1969 Phonemic Paraphasias, Linguistic Structures and tentative Hypotheses *Cortex 5,* No. 3, 193.
v. Leyden, E.
1867 Beitrage zur Lehre von den centralen Sprachstörungen. *Berl. klin. Wchschrft.*, 4, 65, 67, 77, 89, February.
Lhermitte, F., Lecours, A. and Bertran.
1969 Aphasic Transformations of Linguistic Units. In: *Biocybernetics of the Central System.* (L. D. Proctor, Ed.) Boston, Little Brown and Co.
Lichtheim, L.
1885 Über Aphasie. *Deutsche Arch. f. klin. Med. , 36*, 204, 268.

1885 On Aphasia. *Brain,* 7, 433-484.

Liepmann, H.

1898 Ein Fall von reiner Sprachtaubheit. *Psychiat. Abhandlungen aus der psychiatr. Klinik in Breslau.*

1905 Carl Wernicke. *Cbl. Nervenh. Psychiat., 15,* 564-572.

1911 Ueber Wernickes Einflusz auf die klinische Psychiatrie. *Mschr. Psychiat. Neurolo., 30,* 1-37.

1922 Carl Wernicke, 1848-1905. In: *Deutsche Irrenärzte* Vol. II, (T. Kirchhoff, Ed.), Berlin: Springer, 238-250.

1969 Motorische Aphasie und Apraxie, *Monat. f. Psych. u. Neur. 34,* 485, 1913, Unpublished translation, G. H. Eggert.

Liepmann, H. and Pappenheim, M.

1914 Über einen Fall von sogenannten Leitungsaphasie. *Ztschr. f. die gesamt. Neurol. u. Psychol., 27,* 1-41.

Liepmann, H. and Storch, E.

1902 Die mikroskopische Gehirnbefund bei dem Fall Gorstelle. *Mschr. Psychiat. Neurol., 11,* 115-120.

Lissauer, H.

1889 Ein Fall von Seelenblindheit nebst einem Beitrag zur Theorie derselben. *Arch. f. Psychiat., 21,* 222-270.

Lotmar, F.

1920 Zur Kenntnis der erschwerten Wortfindung und ihr Bedeutung für das Denken des Aphasischen. *Schweiz. Arch. f. Neurol. u. Psychiatrie 5,* 206, 1919; *6,* 3.
Zur Pathophysiologie der erschwerter Wortfindung bei Aphasischen. *Schweiz. Arch. f. Neur. u. Psych.* 1933, *30,* 86-158; 322-329.

Meyer, A.

1908 The Relation of the Auditory Center to Aphasia. *J. Psycholog. u. Neurol., 13,* 203-213.

Meynert, T.

1884 *Psychiatry.* (B. Sachs, Trans.) New York: Putnam, 1885. (*Psychiatrie,* Vienna).

Mills, C.

1898 *The Nervous System and its Diseases.* Philadelphia: J. B. Lippincott.

Milner, B., Taylor, L., and Sperry, R.

1968 Lateralized Suppression of dichotically presented Digits after commissural Section in Man. *Science, 191,* 184-186.

Mingazzini, G.

1902 Klinische und anatomopathologische Beitrage ueber Aphasien. *Deutsch. Ztschrft. Nervenh.,* 386-394.

Mirallie, C.

1896 *De l'aphasie sensorielle.* Thèse de Paris, 1896. Cited in: Heilbronner, *K., Handbuch der Neurologie* Vol. *I,* p. 1069. 1910

Moeli, C.

1891 Über den gegenwärtigen Stand der Aphasiefrage. *Berl. klin. Wchschrft. 48,* 48, 1141, 1166.

v. Monakow, C.

1914 *Die Lokalisation im Grosshirn.* Wiesbaden: Bergmann.

Munk, H.

1888 On the Functions of the Cortex. In: *The Cerebral Cortex,* (G. Von Bonin, Trans.), Springfield: Thomas, 97-118. 1960. (Über die Verrichtungen des Grosshirns) (*Pflüger's Archiv. fur die gesamt. Physiologie, 42,* 419-467, 1888).

Myers, R.

1964 In: *Ciba Foundation Symposium on Functions of the Corpus Callosum.* (F. Ettlinger, Ed.), Boston: Little, Brown and Co., 1-17. (*Brain, 79,* 358, 1956).

1962 Transmission of Visual Information with and between the Hemispheres. In: *Interhemispheric Relations and Cerebral Dominance.* (V. Mountcastle, Ed.) Baltimore: Johns Hopkins Press, 51-73.

1960 Failure of Intermanual Transfer in Corpus Callosum-Sectioned Chimpanzees, *Anat. Rec., 136,* 358.

., and Hensen, C.

1960 Role of Corpus Callosum in Transfer of Tactuokinesthetic Learning in the Chimpanzee. *Arch. Neurol. Psychiat. 3,* 404-409.

Niessl von Mayendorf, E.

1926 Hugo Liepmann. *Psychologie u. Medizin, 1,* 257-277, August.

Pershing, H.

1900 Wernicke's Conduction Aphasia with Autopsy. *Proc. Amer. Neur. Assoc. Twenty-sixth Annual Meeting,* 53-58.

Pick, A.

1892 Beiträge zur Lehre von den Störungen der Sprache. *Arch. f. Psych. 23,* 896.

1894 Über das sogenannte aphatische Stottern als Symptom verscheiden örtlich localisierter cerebraler Herdaffectionen. *Archiv. f. Psych., 33,* 247-467.

1915 Zur Erklärung gewisser Hemmungerscheinungen. *Monatschr. f. Psychiat. u. Neurolo., 37,* No. 3, 143-150.

1913 *Die agrammatischen Sprachtörungen.* Berlin: Springer.

1931 Aphasie (Thiele, Ed.) In: *Handbuch d. norm. u. path. Physiol.* (Bethe, A. and Bergmann, Eds.), Berlin: Springer, *15,* 1416-1524.

Pitres, A.

1893 Considérations sur l'agraphie à propos d'une observation nouvelle d'agraphie motrice pure. *Revue de med., 4,* 855, 1884. Cited in: C. Wernicke, *Gesam' melte Aufsätze und kritische Referate zur Pathologie des Nervensystems.* Berlin: Fischer, 128-129.

Sachs, H.

1893 Bau und Tätigkeit des Grösshirns Breslau: Preuss und Jünger.

Sachs, H., Hahn, E., Schroder, P., and Foerster, O.

Atlas des Gehirns. (C. Wernicke, Ed.) 3 vols., Berlin: Karger, 1897-1903.

Saint-Paul, G.

1904 *Le Langage intérieur et les paraphasies,* Paris: Alcan, 1904 Cited in: *Handbuch norm. u. pathol. Physiol.* (Bethe, A. and Bergmann, G., Eds.), Berlin: Springer, *Vol. II,* 1439-1441. 1931

Schmidt,

1871 Gehör und Sprachstörung in Folge von Apoplexie. *Allg. Zschrft. f. Psych. 27,* 304.

Schroeder, P.

1939 Die Lehren Wernickes in ihrer Bedeutung für die heutige Psychiatrie. *Ztschr. ges. Neurol. Psychiat., 165,* 38-47.

Segarra, J. and Quadfasel, F.

1961 *Proceedings of the VII International Congress of Neurology. 11,* p. 377

Seppili,

1884 La sord. verbe l'afasia sens. *Riv. sper. di. Freniatria. 10,* 97, 1884. Cited in Henschen, Über die Hörsphäre. *J. f. Psychol. u. Neurolog. , 22,* No. 3, 404. 1918.

Siemerling, E.

1905 Carl Wernicke. *Arch. Psychiat. Nervenkr., 40,* 1016-1019.

Sparks, R. and Geschwind, N.

1969 Dichotic Listening after Section of Neocortical Commissures. *Cortex, 5,* 10-16.

Sperry, R.

1958 Corpus Callosum and Interhemispheric Transfer in the Monkey. *Anat. Rec.,* 131, 297.

Spreen, O., Benton, A., and Van Allen, M.

1966 Dissociation of visual and Tactile Naming in Amnesic Aphasia. *Cortex.*

Stamm, J. and Sperry, R.
1957 Function of the Corpus Callosum in Contralateral Transfer of Somesthetic. Discrimination in Cats. *J. Comp. Physiol. Psychol. 50,* 138-143.
Starr, M. A.
1889 The Pathology of Sensory Aphasia, with an analysis of Fifty Cases. *Brain,* 82-101.
1909 *The Diagnosis of Nervous Diseases.* 3rd. ed., New York: Lea and Febiger.
Storch, E.
1903 Der aphasische Symptomenkomplex. *Monatschr. f. Psychiat. Neurol., 13,* 321-341; 597-622.
Strohmayer, W.
1902 Zur Kritik der "subcorticalen sensorischen" Aphasie. *Deutsch. Ztschr. f. Nervenheilk., 21,* 371.
Thiele, R.
1928 Aphasie, Apraxie, Agnosie. In: *Handbuch der Geisteskrankheiten,* Vol.II (O Bumke, Ed.) Berlin: Hirschwaldsche.
1964 A Note on Auditory Discrimination Behavior of the Corpus Callosum. In: *Ciba Foundation Symposium on the Corpus Callosum.* (E. Ettlinger, Ed.), Boston, Little Brown and Co., 69-73.
Wernicke, C.
1874 *Der aphasische Symptomencomplex.* Beslau: Cohn und Weigert.
1875 Das Urwindungsystem des menschlichen Gehirns. *Arch. f. Psych. u. Neurol.,* 6, No. 1, 298-326.
1881-83 *Lehrbuch der Gehirnkrankheit.* 3 vols. Berlin: Fischer,
1879 Ueber das Bewusstsein. *Allg. Ztschr. f. Psych., 35,* 599
1882 Aphasie und Anarthie. *Deut. Med. Wchschrft.,* 163.
1884 Über die motorische Sprachbahn und das Verhältnis der Aphasie zur Anarthie. *Fortschr. der Med., 2,* 1, 405.
1886 Einige neuere Arbeiten uber Aphasie, Kritisches Referat. *Fortschr. der Med., 3,* 824, 1885; 4, 371, 463.
1887 Die Aufgaben der Klinischen Psychiatrie, *Breslauer ärtzl. Ztschr. 13.*
1890 Aphasie und Geisteskrankheit. *Verhandlungen des Congresses für innere Med. Wiesbaden,* 273.
1892 Grundzüge einer psychiatrischen Symptomenlehre. *Berliner Klin. Wchschrft.* , No. 23.
1893 *Gesammelte Aufsätze und Kritische Referate zur Pathologie des Nervensystems.* Berlin: Fischer.
1899/ *Krankenvorstellungen aus der psychiatrischen Klinik in Breslau.* 3 vols. Bres-
1900 *Grundzüge der Psychiatrie* in *Klinischen* Vorlesungen. Leipzig: G. Thieme.
1900 lau: Schletterische Buchhandlung.
1903 Ein Fall isolierte agraphie. *Monatschr. f. Psych. und Neurol., 13,* 241.
1906 Der Aphasische Symptomencomplex. In: *Deutsche Klinik am Eingange des 20. Jahrhunderts.* (V. Leyden u. Klemperer, Eds.), Berlin, 487-556.
1908 The Aphasia Symptom Complex. In: *Diseases of the Nervous System.* (Church, A., Ed.), New York: Appleton, 265-324.
Wernicke, C. and Friedländer, C.
1883 Ein Fall von Taubheit in Folge von doppelseitiger Läsion des Schläfelappens. *Fortschritte der Medizin. I.*
Wilbrand, H.
1887 *Seelenblindheit als Herderscheinung.* Wiesbaden: Bergmann.
Wyllie, J.
1894 *The Disorders of Speech.* Edinburgh: Oliver and Boyd.
Ziehen, T.
1905 Carl Wernicke. *Mschr. Psych. u. Neurol., 18,*

PART TWO

A TRANSLATION OF CARL WERNICKE'S MAJOR WORKS ON APHASIA

PREFACE TO THE TRANSLATIONS

The following translations include Carl Wernicke's major works on aphasia and related disorders. Each work has been preceded by a brief introduction by the translator to provide basic background information. While a strong effort has been made to offer a literal rendering of the original writings, occasional minor modifications have been necessary to provide greater readability and clarity of style.

I. WORKS OF WERNICKE'S EARLY APHASIA PERIOD

THE APHASIA SYMPTOM COMPLEX: A PSYCHOLOGICAL STUDY ON AN ANATOMIC BASIS

Original publication in: *Der Aphasische Symptomencomplex: Eine psychologische Studie auf anatomischer Basis, Breslau:* Cohn & Weigert, 1874.

Reprinted in: *Gesammelte Aufsätze und kritische Referate zur Pathologie des Nervensystems.* Berlin: Fischer, 1893, pp. 1-70

[This monograph, Wernicke's original work on aphasia, appeared in 1874 at the time when its youthful author was working as an assistant at the University of Breslau. The Wernicke aphasia doctrine was founded on the application of Meynert's theory of motor and sensory cortical areas connected by association fibers. The 1874 work confirmed the existence of a sensory speech area on the basis of Wernicke's pathological findings of destruction of the left superior temporal area in certain cases of aphasia.

The description of sensory aphasia in this work emphasized not only the impairment in auditory comprehension in association with intact hearing, typically found in such cases, but also the characteristic abnormalities in speech production. Speech expression in sensory aphasia was characterized by a copious, fluent, but confused speech output with transposition of sounds, syllables, words and phrases. In this work Wernicke drew specific attention to the expressive speech symptoms which differentiated the two entities of motor and sensory aphasia. He repeatedly stressed the fact that these two major features, loss of language comprehension and the confused, fluent speech pattern, were two aspects of the "unitary clinical picture" of sensory aphasia.

In the 1874 work Wernicke established his position between the extreme views of the Flourens holistic and the phrenologic localization schools. Although later historical references placed him among the strict localizers, Wernicke's appreciation of both holistic and localization aspects of psychic function was already clearly stated in his original work. "Only the primary functions, (perceptions) can be referred to specific cerebral areas. . . . All processes which exceed these functions such as thought, consciousness, etc., are dependent on fiber bundles connecting different areas of the cortex." (Wernicke, 1874)

In the 1874 work Wernicke reviewed a number of topics significant to the study of language. These include his neuroanatomic interpretation of speech acquisition and the development of reading and writing skills, his views of the significance of various types of imagery in language and concept formation, his notions regarding the effects of congenital and acquired deafness on speech development and production, and an introduction to the problems of alexia, agraphia, and asymbolia.

The 1874 work also contains a description of a new aphasia form, that of conduction aphasia. This form was assumed to be characterized by intact language comprehension and motor speech production but paraphasic expression. Lichtheim later added the symptom of inability to mimic. This hypothetical aphasia form was believed to be caused by an isolated disruption of the arcuate fibers, leaving both motor and sensory speech areas intact. Wernicke assumed that such fibers coursed through the island region, a hypothesis which he later rejected. He also rejected later his interpretation of two cases presented in the 1874 work as representative examples of this new clinical entity of conduction aphasia, although he continued to recognize the existence of the syndrome.

Of the ten clinico-pathological cases studies described by Wernicke, two cases (cases 2 and 8), which demonstrated the clinical symptoms of sensory aphasia, were found to have lesions of the temporal area. Another patient, who later recovered and did not come to autopsy (case 1) presented the characteristic picture of sensory aphasia with loss of comprehension in association with fluent but confused speech expression.

Although the pathological reviews presented in this work were tenuous and required further confirmation, Wernicke's study opened a new avenue for consideration of the aphasia problem, offered a theory for resolving the apparently conflicting clinical symptoms of the disorder and supplied a new direction for aphasia research. Produced just one hundred years ago, this classic work continues to hold a venerated place in the history of aphasia.]

I.

The genesis of a precise science of brain pathology may be found in Meynert's doctrine of cerebral fiber connections. His work sketches these early origins of the theory in broad, general outline form only. Yet this general outline is so unique, so basic, that even today it may be readily applied to the individual case.

The work here submitted is an attempt to provide just such a pratical application of Meynert's teachings of brain anatomy to the study of normal speech processes and the disorders generally recognized as aphasia. Such a study should certainly be grounded an anatomical principles, yet this fundamental pre-requisite has been largely neglected in the past.

Students of Meynert will readily differentiate a mere repetition of his theories from whatever is original in the work here submitted. The strict dependence on brain anantomy demanded by such a treatment of this subject has prevented acknowledgment to him throughout the study.

But at any event, whatever merit may be found in this work ultimately reverts to Meynert, for the conclusions here submitted issue naturally from a review of his writings and pathological studies.

The Flourens concept of the intellect as a single unity, claiming equivalence of all brain areas, has long proved untenable.[1] But not in the sense that the phrenologists held it to be untenable. On the basis of semantics they differentiate psychic functions – generosity, filial love, family-loyalty, etc., – and assigned them to localized cerebral areas. However, primary functions alone, can be referred to specific cortical areas. Localization of visual perception to its central region and tactual sensation of the fingers to the central area of the ulnar nerve are examples of these primary functions.

The cerebral surface is a mosaic of such primary elements whose properties are determined by their anatomical connections to the body-periphery. All processes which exceed these primary functions (such as the synthesis of various perceptions into single concepts and the more complex functions such as thought and consciousness) are dependent upon the fiber bundles connecting different areas of the cortex. Later, we shall see the implications of such processes in terms of our theory.

Sensory stimulation of the cortex is of greater *duration than excitation of the sensory organ itself. This stimulation permits an arousal of memory images, although of lesser intensity,* which is independent of the original stimulus. Therefore, neural excitation of the cortex itself must be differentiated from that occurring along other neural pathways and way-stations. In the latter case, all traces of the stimulus are erased at the time of excitation.

It is readily evident that memory is a unique, inherent feature of the central nervous system. This property has empirical support in the decreased resistance observed in frequently-used neural tracts. Reflex actions are most readily transmitted over such pathways and demonstrate consistent patterns of response. Moreover, the acquisition of frequently – practiced motor sequences. such as those involved in piano playing or the learning of certain auditory patterns while listening to a symphony, are based on this concept.

For example, if one should acquire epilepsy through a fall or blow to the head, a hypoxia of the pons could result in generalized convulsions.[2r] Thereafter, very minor stimuli might induce excitation of the neural pathway. Emotional excitement and its consequent circulatory changes may precipitate new convulsive attacks. The treatment of such a disorder becomes more difficult with increased repetition of attacks.

The phenomenon of after-images is based on the same principle. This is correctly emphasized in Meynert's teachings. Thus, the excitation of the sensory retinal cells continues after removal of the stimulus. The extinction of color sensation may likely lie in the inadequacy of the number of cells which continue to fire, and a new stimulus may be needed to extinguish the traces of the preceding stimulus.

Meynert estimates that the cortex contains some 600 million cells. This provided a wealth of storage areas for collection of countless sensory impressions. We need not regard the permanent molecular changes in the cortical cells, resulting from brief stimulation, as an uncommon property specific to them. This feature merely represents an analog of the characteristics found in peripheral nerves, although the unique anatomical conditions of the cortex allow such to be revealed in enhanced form.

We would like to label these residuals of stimulation with which the cortex is populated "memory images" and would emphasize the differentiation of such from the sensory stimulation itself. One must also hypothesize, on the basis of facts which shall be explained later, that the movements of the body, the muscular changes in response to stimuli, also cause the deposition of such memory images in the cortex. We would like to call such memory images of movement-sensation, "motor-images," an abbreviation of "movement-representation," (*Bewegungsvorstellungen*) or "movement-images," and consider them essentially equivalent to other memory images.

The entire cerebral cortex may be divided into two general areas which have important functional differences. The frontal area of the brain includes the entire region anterior to the Rolandic fissure of both hemispheres. The posterior area contains the temporal and occipital lobes. The first region is motor in function and is the site of motor imagery, while the latter is sensory, containing memory images of sensory impressions. The parietal area, lying between, represents a passageway for the transfer of processes which are still unclear.[3,4r]

This hypothesis, one of the fundamental tenets of the new brain physiology, is supported by the following facts. Meynert considers the frontal cortex to be the central terminal of that segment of the cerebral peduncle mediating conscious movement. Focal lesions of the frontal cortex produce convulsions and paralysis involving the opposite side of the body. General paresis, a specific motor psychosis, is one of the diseases of the cerebral cortex, which according to Meynert's assessment of brain weight is primarily related to atrophy of the frontal area of the brain.[5]

Experimental proof of localization of motor function to the frontal area of the brain was first produced by Fritsch and Hitzig, and later, by Nothnagel. They discovered that electrical stimulation of concentrated areas of the cortex located in the frontal regions of the brain produced paralytic-like symptoms of specific muscles groups. The remaining cerebral surface was not responsive to direct stimulation.[6]

The paralytic-like symptoms produced by ablation of these newly-found motor centers deserve our particular attention. Fritsch and Hitzig define such symptoms as disturbances in muscle-sensation, while Nothnagel frankly refers to them as ataxia. Both sides rejected an interpretation of these disorders as true paralysis. Empirically, however, destruction of such cortical areas in humans may produce paralysis, as one of Hitzig's cases has demonstrated. Moreover, this evidence is supported by the presence of a true paralysis in the syndrome of general paresis.

A critical study of Nothnagel's ideas, nevertheless, leads one to marvel at the ease and effectiveness of the production of bilateral movements by one hemisphere alone. This particularly applies to body parts which before have had common innervation. Voluntary stimulation from the left hemisphere alone is therefore adequate for production of bilaterally-equal speech movements.[7]

The novice piano player feels compelled to move the fingers of the left hand in synchrony with the right, and dissociation between the hands is accomplished only through many years of practice. Innervation of this action occurs only from the left hemisphere. However, the anterior spinal horn cells, which have previously been subjected to mutual stimulation and thereby have established strong associations, now operate together by means of these firmly-connected processes.

One may well call attention to the apparent paradox that presence of both hemispheres is not an absolute condition for simultaneous action of bilateral muscle groups, but rather of isolated movement of the same. In man, isolated movements of the upper extremeties may be practiced a thousand times, and yet innervation from one hemisphere alone is adequate to initiate movement of both extremities. How much more would this hold true for dogs and rabbits – animals in which conscious, isolated innervation of a single extremity rarely occurs?

Nevertheless, these incorrect interpretations of motor disorders in no way diminishes the significance of the experimental studies carried out by the renowned authorities mentioned above, an impressive contribution indeed. We refer to the evidence that *the very cortical area, stimulation of which produces motor response and so in the narrowest sense acts as a motor center, is at the same time the seat of muscle sensation and the area representing the degree and nature of muscle innervation.*

The generalized awkwardness of incoordination of gait observed in some paralytics provides examples of such kinesthetic disorders in man. These symptoms have formerly been interpreted as paralyses.

We have already recognized the existence of cortical motor areas connected with a centrifugal tract which function as centers of motor representation. However, if *a priori* we exclude the theory that ideas are innately present within the cortex, this puzzling question arises. How are motor images created within the cortex? Brücke and Lotze's physiological and philosophical deductions agree with Meynert's anatomically-derived conclusions in suggesting a solution to this problem. According to Brücke and Lotze, movements may be classified into primary and secondary types. The primary responses consist in reflex actions which long precede the establishment of conscious action in childhood. These are synthesized into motor images which in the second stage of their development may be aroused at will and in this way are converted into voluntary action.

A complex reflex mechanism, performed in the optic thalamus and quadrigeminal bodies, which functions independently following destruction of the hemispheres, has proven adequate for the production of all forms of reflex actions. The function of these ganglia is not dependent upon the presence of the hemispheres. Therefore, the chief significance of the fiber tracts coursing to the anterior portion of the brain, which make up a part of the anterior peduncle as well as a component of the internal capsule, lies in their function as a centripetal pathway. The sensations of innervation of reflexly-produced movements are discharged to the anterior portion of the brain by this route. Meynert has interpreted the function of these tracts in this way, and such an explanation thus provides a basis for our proposed theory.

The anatomic data definitely confirms the hypothesis that the temporo-occipital area is sensory in nature. All sensory nerves whose courses are known collectively terminate in the cortex of the temporo-occipital region. These include the olfactory nerve, the optic nerve, and that portion of the spinal cord which does not originate from the cerebellum.[81] The central pathway of the acoustic nerve has presently been traced only so far as the cerebellum; nevertheless, from a physiological standpoint, continuation of its course to the cerebrum cannot be questioned. Analogy with other cranial nerves would strongly suggest termination of the central acoustic nerve within the temporo-occipital cortex. This would also apply to the gustatory nerve whose central course is still completely unknown.

The hypothesis of the predominantly sensory nature of the temporo-occipital lobe is supported by the presence of a rich granular layer in a certain portion of this area. (This is particularly true of the region surrounding the hippocampal fissure.) Such a layer also predominates in other sensory areas – the olfactory lobes, the substantia gelatinosa of the trigeminal nerve, the retina, and the substantia gelatinosa of the tips of the posterior spinal horn cells.

Memory images of sensations as well as forms of motor response patterns function as elements provided by the outside world. Together they constitute the content of conscious thought. These generalizations lead to the formulation of a general interpretation of a primary conscious process such as voluntary action. Voluntary movement is also a characteristic of the lowest animals, and so as a model, satisfies the criterion of parsimony. Because it is the distinguishing mark of the animal organism, a detailed review of its unique significance is essential.

Two features differentiate voluntary movement from reflex action.

1. *Voluntary movement does not follow the stimulus immediately but owes its generation to memory images of earlier experiences,* coincidental with the external stimulus. Griesinger has emphasized this distinction as well as its analogy to reflex action in his essay, "Über psychische Reflexactionen" (A Consideration of Psychic Reflex Action). He attributes spontaneous movement, that is, "psychic reflex action", as well as reflex actions to stimuli transmitted to the cortex by the centripetal tracts. Residuals of sensory stimuli are clearly implicated in arousal of the same spontaneous actions which are attributed to the so-called instincts, such as mating and feeding, etc. The same is true of other spontaneous actions, although more numerous and complex perceptual processes may be implicated in their production.

2. Spontaneous movement may be differentiated from reflex action in its *specific, goal-directed features, i.e., the preformed motor-imagery–the representation of completed movements.* Such features, as discussed above, may be interpreted as sensory residuals of memory images.

We may now apply the schema of reflex action with its differentiating features to the process of spontaneous movement as demonstrated in the diagram in Figure 6. The stimulus (E) travels along the pathway (E-O) and releases a memory image at a point in the temporo-occipital area (O). The occurrence of a new external stimulus causes rearousal of the almost latent stimulus and transmission to a motor point in the frontal area of the brain (F) by way of a segment of the large fiber tract connecting the temporo-occipital area with the frontal region of the brain. Having reached this point, the stimulus traveling along the centrifugal pathway (F-B) produces movement.

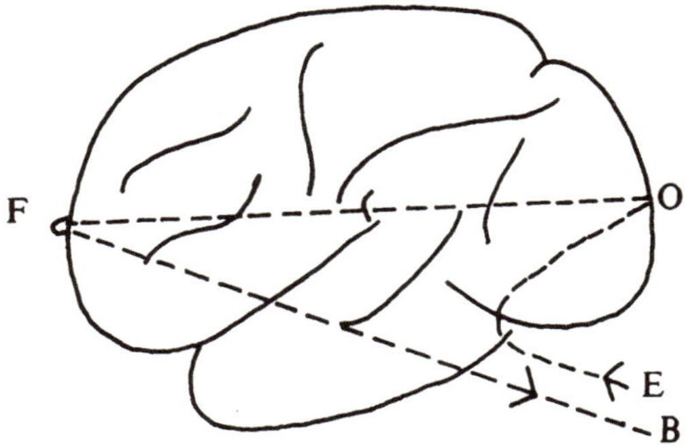

FIG. 6

Schema of Reflex Action
(E): Stimulus (O): Occipito-temporal area
(F): Frontal cerebral area
(B): Eye

This movement is invested with the second characteristic feature of the spontaneous motor process, a purposeful organization in which the points of motor discharge and motor image storage coincide in location. *Thus, pathway (E-O-F-B) adequately explains spontaneous movement in the mode of a reflex process.* Anatomic pathways which may mediate this type of reflex activity are present in profusion. The greater share of the white matter of the brain contains just such association tracts, at times simple and at times complex in course. Burdach (1825) has traced the routes of such tracts by means of fiber dissection with painstaking accuracy.

Transmission over these pathways, that is, the immediate stimulus discharge, is not a mere accident but rather demonstrates the consistent lawful association of the two brain areas which at one time cooperated in certain functions.

In Figure 7, (x) represents a cell of the quadrigeminal bodies which function as a reflex center producing internal gaze of the eyes designated by (B). Transmission occurs over the optic tract (E) involving stimulation of the motor cell (y). This process is not entirely unconscious but is mediated by tracts connecting the quadrigeminal bodies with the cerebral cortex. A sensory impression is deposited at (O) and a motor image at (F) in the cortex.

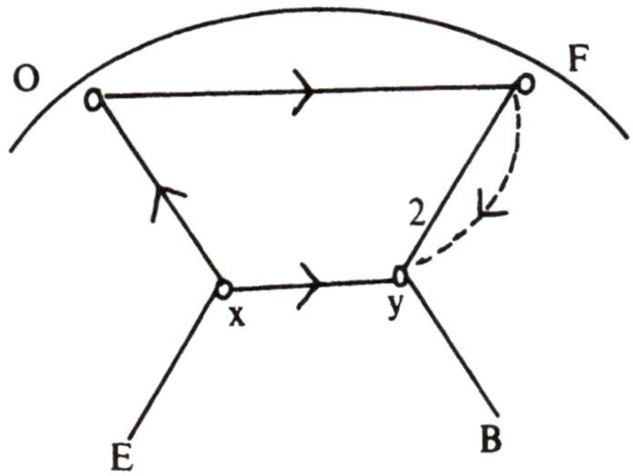

FIG. 7

Schema of Optic Reflex

(x): Cell of quadrigeminal bodies
(B): Eye
(E): Optic tract
(y): Motor cell
(O): Sensory memory image
(y-2-F): Motor path
(F): Motor memory image

A specific quantity of energy may be assumed necessary for neural excitation, and a share of such energy is claimed by the paths (x-O) and (y-2-F). These paths may be considered shunts in transmission of the stimulus.[9] The impulse must also pass between points (O) and (F), which are the terminals of the excitation process. If we compare excitation of a neural path such as one discharging from (E) with the initial oscillations of a fluid-filled conduit system, we might hypothesize this entire process to be electric in nature. However, this is not definitely established. Such an interpretation would help to explain the role of pathway (O-F) in the whole procedure. Because resistance of a neural conductor decreases during stimulation, the motor image (F) and the spontaneous movement itself could be readily activated by the sensory memory images (O) along the centrifugal path (F-y-B).

The generation of each spontaneous movement may be reduced to this simple schema. The number of memory images acting as the initial discharge points is clearly infinite. This schema may be applied to the most simple spontaneous motor response, i.e., innate instinctual movements.

The association of many memory images occurs simply by chance, because they are produced by a common external stimulus. In the same way, various images of motor patterns at the terminal of the reflex arc become associated with each other because they occur at the same time or in close succession. In this way different motor memory images may be called up into consciousness simultaneously. *The consciousness of a motor memory and the actual production of the action may represent different intensities of cell excitation. The actual movement can occur only if the stimulus is strong enough to overcome the resistance of the centrifugal path.* Motor images may be translated into action only if they have well-worn connections to many initial links of the reflex arc—provided that these links are of equal intensity—or if they have had a long association with *vivid* early memories. A low resistance of the conduction pathway is also a factor favoring ready translation of imagery into action. In the last two conditions the small number of stimuli may be compensated for by the intensity of the individual stimulus.

These features provide the possibility of selection of motor response. The number of choices available to the individual increases with the practice he has in memory association and the number of memory images at his disposal. The only true scientific definition of free will must be in harmony with this type of mechanistic interpretation of the genesis of spontaneous motor production.

2.

This initial review has attempted to illustrate certain general principles based on current anatomic and physiological evidence which may be applied to the lawful generation of spontaneous movement. All spontaneous motor action, including that of speech, is based on such principles. The fact that speech movement must be classified as conscious voluntary action needs no detailed explanation. The evidence clearly shows that speech production must be laboriously acquired during childhood. This is true of all spontaneous movement. Speech acquisition coincides so closely with the development of consciousness that it may be considered as a measuring gauge thereof. Motor speech production emerges only after the child has perfected many other conscious motor actions.

Before the development of consciousness, the primary speech movements, such as mimicry, are reflex in nature and are discharged to the same areas of the pons and medulla oblongata along the inner half of the cerebral peduncle tegmentum, which constitutes the origin of the acoustic nerve.[10] Numerous, large many-tailed cells may be found there, which apparently are processes of the facial, vagal, and hypoglossal nuclei. Meynert maintains that these cells are anatomically connected with the arcuate fibers associated with the origin of the acoustic nerve. Experimental evidence indicates that the respiratory center is located within this extensive area containing the origin of the acoustic nerve. The advantage of such a location can readily be seen in the new-born child, in that the medulla itself can produce the unarticulated cry, a unitary muscular response which in spite of its simplicity requires the combined action of expiration and adduction of the vocal folds.[11] Perhaps even the more complicated patterns of muscle action, those involved in formation of single words, may be first produced reflexly, although possibly in a more complex organ, the cerebellum. Because its functions are still incompletely known, we often try to use it as a convenient solution to fill all of the gaps in our knowledge. However, let us rather merely draw general conclusions from this notion and admit the difficulty of explaining the production of entire words by means of the reflex apparatus of the medulla oblongata. Whether the situation is such that complete words or merely word fragments are formed reflexly in the medulla, in any event, it appears that an acoustic image of the word or syllable is transmitted from the site of the reflex process to a sensory area of the brain, and the innervatory-sensation of the movement produced is transmitted as a motor speech image to the frontal area. The association of acoustic and motor images is then maintained by means of myelinated fibers (Figure 7). Production of the spontaneous movement, that is, the consciously formulated word would be brought about by rearousal of the motor image through the associated memory image of the sound. The stimulus is then transmitted along the tract within the foot of the cerebral peduncle, as is true of all other voluntary actions, until it reaches the speech musculature.

Before we try to suggest an anatomic basis for this interpretation of the speech process, let us pause and review some of the past attempts to localize a specific speech center within a definite anatomic cerebral region.

I shall pass over the host of older works regarding this problem, summaries of which may easily be found in detailed references and shall turn immediately to Broca. This author was first to reject broad, indefinite expanses of the cortex as sites of speech areas and instead ventured to designate a very circumscribed, anatomically-specific region as the seat of this function. As is well-known, he localized the faculty of speech to the posterior portion of the so-called third frontal gyrus, or the first,–according to Leuret's principle–in which counting proceeds from the Sylvian fossa. That is that portion of the most inferior and external part of the operculum, located in the frontal part of the central gyrus, just anterior to its juncture. In spite of the opposition to this view, which was very strong at the outset, such a large number of case studies of speech disturbance has been reported in its support, and the contradictory cases have furnished so little new positive evidence, that this theory continues to pave a constantly broader path and now boasts many followers.

In the meantime Meynert published a work which caused a great stir. In this study he demonstrated the connection of the acoustic nerve to the cortex of the Sylvian fossa by means of a fiber path which he called the acoustic tract (Acousticusstrang). This entire tract surrounding the origin of the acoustic nerve coincides to some extent with the region of the claustrum, which was designated by Meynert as an "acoustic field." He supported his hypothesis by a large number of post-mortem findings in aphasic patients demonstrating pathological changes either within the island-area itself or in the circumscribed portion of the Sylvian fossa.

Many well-known physicians, who were involved in the controversy, were inclined toward Meynert's view, particularly because it served to resolve the vaguely-felt need to relate the acoustic nerve to the speech process. Strangely enough, many continued to recognize the entire area of cortex surrounding the Sylvian fossa as a speech center, in spite of the fact that Meynert himself disclaimed such a function of the acoustic tract. He, indeed, expressed the view that the acoustic nerve was not directly connected to the cerebrum but first coursed through the cerebellum.[12]

Which areas then make up the immediate neighborhood of the Sylvian fossa? In answering this question we must call attention to that particular gyrus on the convexity of the cerebral surface which extends as an arc directed upward and backward, enclosing the Sylvian fissure, and which continues as the first frontal gyrus, according to Leuret's terminology, anterior to the central sulcus, terminating longitudinally in a clear line formed by the first temporal gyrus. Comparison with the animal brain, such as that of the dog family, suggests that this entire region might be regarded as a single gyrus. A review of comparative anatomy reveals that this feature is also common to the embryological brain structure in man. Thus an arc is traced by the gyri around the Sylvian fossa, with its summit facing the occipital pole and its two limbs extending to the frontal and temporal area in a more or less parallel course.

The summit of the first frontal gyrus in Leuret's terminology must be differentiated from its two side surfaces. Only the summit lies completely exposed on the convex cerebral surface. One of the two sides is turned medially, facing the sulcus of the second frontal cortex. The other side forms the direct continuation of the insular cortex and, projecting over the island, adheres flatly to it on all sides. Comparative anatomy thus reveals the entire first primordial-gyrus to be unitary in structure. Its internal structure reveals a characteristic which Meynert had earlier described. He observed that the island-facing surface of the claustrum extended from the island, projecting a considerable distance to the summit of the gyrus. The entire region of the first primordial-gyrus shares in the peculiar characteristic of the island-cortex in that the innermost cortical layer, that of the fusiform cells, is concentrated into a single gray mass.

Moreover, by fiber dissections, I have been able to demonstrate a typical feature of this area, namely the presence of white, densely-compact fiber tracts under the cortex on the surface of the first primordial-gyrus, facing the

Sylvian fossa. This same tract forms a continuous sheet of radiating fibers extending together with the medullary lamina of the first primordial-gyrus to the floor of the deep fissure which divides the first primordial-gyrus from the island (by means of the anterior superior and inferior sulci of Burdach). From this point it spans the fissure and ends in the island-cortex. The island resembles a large spider, whose fiber radiations from all parts of the first primordial-gyrus converge within its core, presenting the picture of a mighty control center, reserved for special functions.

The presence of the fibrae propriae, the arcuate lamina (Arnold), has also been demonstrated between the island-cortex and the gyral-system of the cerebral convexity. As far as I know, these fibers have not been previosuly described. Because they provide such significant evidence in support of the unitary nature of the entire first primordial-gyral arc in association with the island-cortex, they deserve a fairly detailed study.

The fibrae propriae are readily visible between the gyri of the cortical convexity and its medial surface. Therefore, one must question whether the Rolandic sulcus, which bisects the primordial-gyral system perpendicularly, is bridged by these fibers. The results of fiber dissection in this area are still very unclear. However, a different situation prevails in regard to the deep fissure which appears to tie off the island-region from the encircling first gyral-arc. Embryologically, the island is known to be an organizational midpoint of the entire convex surface of the hemisphere, its cortex forming a portion of the side of the ventricle of the hemisphere. Within, it merges with the basal ganglia, and its growth has been checked in such a way externally that a deep depression, the Sylvian fossa, has been formed on the convex surface of the ventricle.

Because of their location, a study of the fibers in this region is extremely difficult. Successful tracing of their course can be carried out only in alcohol-treated brains. But in such specimens, deflecting of the projecting portions of the hemisphere, which completely cover the island itself, is extremely difficult. If such dissection is not successful, one must work blindly and assume the most awkward and tiring postures to admit adequate light for visualization of the area. The region most easily dissected is that portion coursing perpendicularly, spanned by the fissure (Burdach's superior sulcus) first superiorly and then inferiorly, between the operculum and the island. This layer is also of considerable thickness, extending over one-half cm. in cross-section. Following this, the dissection can best be carried out in the anterior sulcus, between the frontal area of the brain and the island. The deep section which extends between this part of the frontal area and the operculum from front to back and above, is completely covered with the same type of fibers. The dissection of the temporal lobe presents the greatest difficulty of all, not only because of the deep position of the inferior sulcus which is spanned, but also because of the very narrow diameter of the arcuate lamina. This applies particularly to the deep sinus into which the rear terminations of the superior and inferior sulci converge.

In carrying out this dissection, it is recommended that the scalpel handle be first placed in the semi-elevation of the inner surface of the operculum. From that point, the cortex may be removed from above and towards the island. At the summit of the gyrus, the fibrae propriae branch out and can no longer be dissected. Moreover, the fibers cannot be traced within the island-cortex either, because they tend to interweave and lie deeply embedded within the claustrum.

In harmony with the preceding review, which considers speech development from the standpoint of conscious movement, *a priori* reasoning would view restriction of the speech center to a single area, namely, Broca's gyrus, as highly improbable. A consideration of the anatomic structure as described above, the support of numerous necropsy findings, and finally, the variability in the clinical picture of aphasia, all strongly lead us to the following interpretation of the data. The entire region of the first primordial convolution, the gyrus surrounding the Sylvian fossa in association with the island-cortex, serves as a speech center. The first frontal gyrus, (Leuret) which is motor in function, acts as a center of motor imagery; the first temporal gyrus, which is sensory in nature, may be regarded as the center of acoustic images; the fibrae propriae, converging into the island-cortex, from the mediating reflex arc. Therefore, the first temporal gyrus may be regarded as the central terminal of the acoustic nerve, and the first frontal gyrus (Leuret), including Broca's area, as the central terminal of the nerves controlling the speech musculature.

In the schema diagrammed in Figure 8, the letter (F) represents the frontal

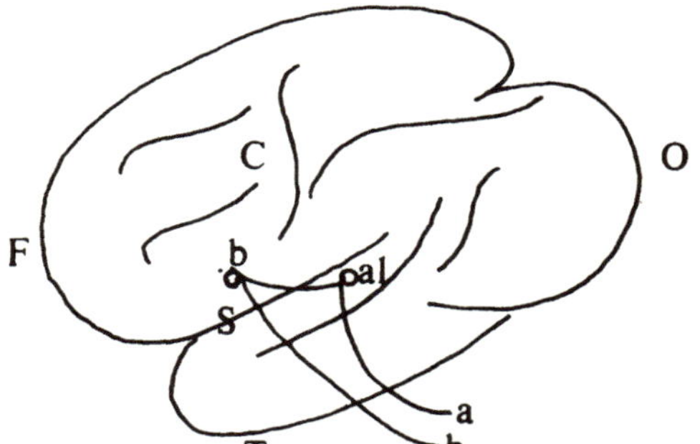

FIG. 8.

Schema of Spontaneous Speech Production

(O):	Occipital area	(C):	Central sulcus
(F):	Frontal area	(a1):	Central terminal of acoustic nerve
(T):	Temporal area	(a):	Acoustic nucleus in medulla
(S):	Sylvian sulcus	(b):	Motor imagery

area of the brain; the occipital terminal is designated by (O), the temporal terminal by (T), and the central sulcus by (C). The first primordial-gyrus extends around the Sylvian fossa, (S). Within the same is (a1), the central terminal of the acoustic nerve, (whose origin is in the medulla oblongata). The motor images, associated with speech-sound production in the frontal brain area are designated by (b). The association fibers (a1-b), coursing through the island-cortex, are connected with the motor images (b). The centrifugal pathway of the cranial motor nerves concerned with speech production extends from (b) to the medulla, where a large portion of the fibers terminate. (The accessory and phrenic nerves continue on down.)

Aphasia may be caused by any disruption of the pathway (a-a1) - (b-b1). The clinical picture, however, may vary considerably and is related to the specific segment of the pathway involved.

I. Let us assume that pathway (a-a1) is disrupted by some pathological process resulting in the destruction of the acoustic nerve at some site along its central course. Clinical experience shows that this would result in a primary deafness with no trace of aphasia. However, this would hold only for adults already in possession of an extensive store of earlier-acquired acoustic images which may be revived at will. Should this disrupting process occur during some period of childhood, before this store of acoustic images has been accumulated within the cortex, muteness would be an inevitable consequence. This is the common cause of deaf-muteness. The child has not yet developed the acoustic imagery from which the motor images may be activated.

The inevitable occurrence of muteness in congenital or early-acquired deafness throws an interesting sidelight on the significance of auditory sensation for normal speech development. There is a common, widely-spread error, championed especially by philosophers and speech investigators (such as Steinthal), that the formation of the concept, the sum total of sensory impressions of an object, is the most critical factor in speech development. The concept would then breed speech from an inner need, and its development would follow the same laws today as were originally operative in primitive man.

Speech then would not be regarded as mere mimicry but as an event which is self-activated, a process in which all sensory areas contribute essential elements necessary for development of the concept which is the fundamental prerequisite. An internal connection to a sensory area such as hearing would not then be considered relevant. If this were the case, muteness would occur more readily in the congenitally blind than in the congenitally deaf, since the eye, of all sensory structures, is unquestionably the most essential organ providing information regarding objects in the environment. All sensory areas associated with the tactual organs and those of vision and olfaction—in short, all areas essential to formation of the concept, would then need to be regarded as bound-up with the motor imagery activated during speech by means of a segment of the association system. (This shall be demonstrated later.)[13] However, the pathway (a-a1-b) alone is most critical of all for speech development because it provides the means by which the child learns speech.

The major task of the child in speech acquisition is mimicry of the spoken word. This is first learned in association with a specific meaning after the child has long been in possession of the word. The word is essentially a reproduction of the auditory image and not that of vision or the tactual sense; therefore, the learning of speech by the congenitally deaf is as little attainable as is drawing by the congenitally blind.

A typical example might be mentioned here. What is the effect of unilateral deafness on the child's development? Muteness may follow only if one assumes that the left speech center alone is capable of development, and that the right center atrophies perhaps because of constitutional causes or at least on the basis of functional disuse. Although we must concede that the child with right-sided deafness, who is therefore dependent on the right hemisphere for speech learning, may have more difficulty in speech development than the child with a left-sided deafness, yet one may definitely assume that the presence of the acoustic pathway coursing to the right temporal lobe will in itself be adequate to support speech development in childhood.

For purposes of comparison, a review of necropsy findings of this condition would be very important to provide an adequate explanation of the causative processes in many cases of aphasia with right-sided lesions. This question sharply points up the critical gaps in our knowledge regarding a definitive localization of the course of the acoustic nerve within the cerebrum. The termination of the left acoustic nerve within the right hemisphere is tentatively an arbitrary assumption.

The symptom-complex of deaf-muteness is so well-known that the coexistence of its two components is self-understood but has not yet been specifically studied in relation to the problem of aphasia. In contrast, the condition described by some as congenital aphasia, which may occur in children with intact hearing and good intelligence but who do not develop language, is a rare finding.

II. Let us now consider the condition caused by destruction of the area containing the acoustic imagery. This area is not identical with the broad central radiation of the acoustic nerve itself, since complete loss of acoustic imagery with intact bilateral hearing has been observed in aphasia. Perhaps the same situation applies to the central endings of the sensory cranial nerves as is true of the motor nerves, namely that their dispersion and termination in different areas of the cortex is consistent with their various functions. Thus, in spite of destruction of the central acoustic radiation, which carries the sounds of words, perception of noise and musical tone would still be intact.

Loss of area (a1), the cortex of the first temporal gyrus, would result in obliteration of the names [acoustic imagery] of all objects from memory. The concept itself however would remain fully clear, for in most cases, the acoustic image of a name is of secondary importance in relationship to the concept, while touch and tactual imagery, in contrast, are intrinsic components of the same. Disturbances of the visual and tactual imagery of the concept (Finkelnburg's asymbolia) are therefore not regarded as speech disorders, but as disturbances of the concept, that is, of the intellect. However, one must admit that such conceptual impairment may be divided into clearly differentiated subgroups.

It is obvious that integrity of the pathway (a1-b) in itself is of little value if the acoustic imagery is lost. In that event the word can no longer be activated by the acoustic image. Moreover, let us assume destruction of the path which connects the acoustic image with other sensory images of the object, i.e., the association fibers leading from the first temporal convolution to the other sensory regions of the temporo-occipital area. *In this event the patient would be able to neither repeat the spoken word, for that is the unique function of the pathway (a-a1-b-b1), nor would he be able to comprehend it.* The spoken word would be heard merely as meaningless noise. In cases presenting milder involvement, the word may be heard as a completely foreign language, with intact perception of individual sounds and gradual recovery of comprehension.

However, one possible means of activation of the motor speech images may still be available to the patient. Intellectual impairment is not a primary feature of this condition. The patient's ability to comprehend signs and gesture indicates intact recognition of sensory images of objects and of the concepts themselves. The associations of acoustic and motor imagery are so essential because they furnish the means by which speech is acquired. Shortly after the learning of oral production of the word, the desire to merely mimic and repeat sounds disappears and is replaced by the need to communicate a specific meaning. That is, the actual sensory image of an object is now able to activate the motor image directly. The capacity for speech production is maintained but with certain limitations. Observations of daily speech usage and the process of speech development indicates the presence of an unconscious, repeated activation and simultaneous mental reverberation of the acoustic image which exercises a continuous monitoring of the motor images. This monitoring device also functions in the deaf who demonstrate damage to the acoustic nerve alone.

The situation may be described schematically as follows. In Figure 9, which is similar to those previously presented, the tactual image (c) is associated with (a1) and with (d), the associated visual memory trace. The concept itself is represented by none other than the pathway (c-d). The child initially learns speech through utilization of pathway (a1-b), whose thousandfold use maintains a continuing significant control over the choice of the correct motor image. Later, the predominant use of this pathway is replaced by the shorter paths (c-b) and (d-b), and the mere presence of (a1-b), without its specific innervation, is adequate to assure choice of the correct motor image.

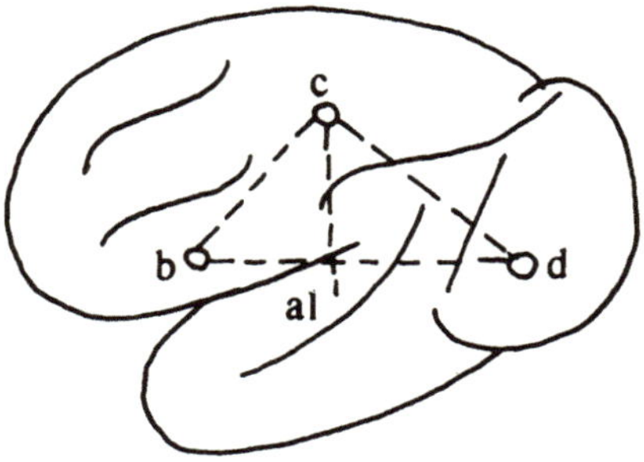

FIG. 9

Schema of Speech and Concept Association

(c): Tactual imagery
(d): Visual imagery
(b): Motor imagery
(c-d): Object concept
(a1): Acoustic speech imagery

Therefore, the sum total of (d+c+a1) always functions in harmony with the appropriate intensity necessary for correct selection of the word. However, if (a1) should be absent, the sum of (d + c) alone would be effective for such innervation with simultaneous suppression of the strong control of pathway (a1-b).

Apart from impairment in comprehension, the patient also presents aphasic symptoms in speech produced by absence of the unconscious monitoring of the imagery of the spoken sound. This lack is reflected in frequent word-confusion. The ability to name objects is retained, but this control tends to be very labile and is readily influenced by disposition and mood. There is no consistency of correct use of the word. The patient does not possess a vocabulary of specific words which are always used correctly. Furthermore, he seems unaware of the accuracy of his word-usage. Intense emotion may activate an explosion of words without the involvement of the associated memory image. Under such conditions, the monitoring device is missed least of all.

The severity of the symptoms will be dependent upon the degree and extent of the pathologic process involving the first temporal lobe. Diagnosis of the more severe forms, presenting loss of not only of the acoustic imagery of concrete objects and actions but also the connecting words necessary for sentence formulation, is dependent upon two factors, *the availability of words and the impairment in comprehension.* Such cases have not been observed up to the present, or at least have not been described in the literature. Apart from the infrequent occurrence of the condition, this lack stems from the erroneous interpretation of such symptoms as dementia by experienced and intelligent physicians, an error into which I myself have fallen in the past. The diagnosis, however, presents no difficulty at all to the psychiatrically-oriented, who are familiar with this specific form of confusion.

This diagnosis may be confirmed by the use of suggestion-questions in mild types of the disturbance, which present preservation of the form-elements necessary for sentence formulation, and in cases in which comprehension of questions succeeds merely by retained understanding of certain isolated words. For example, a glass may be presented to the patient with the question. "Is this a glass?" His response is usually not immediate. Frequently he may hesitate and reflect for a while and finally force a doubtful 'yes' or 'no'. Such behavior would place him in this category of aphasia.

The following points deserve attention.

1. In partial lesions of the sensory speech center a residual fund of consistently and correctly-produced and comprehended words will be retained. The extent of this word-store may be determined by the use of suggestion-questions. However, a tedious and lengthy period of observation is necessary to confirm the diagnosis in this partial form of sensory aphasia.[14r]

2. The primary feature of this particular form of aphasia is the retention of a sizeable fund of words. Cases whose word-store is restricted to a few simple words always belong to the category of motor aphasia discussed under section IV.

3. No evidence of hemiplegia.[15r]

4. Presence of agraphia. Writing is a conscious action, learned with close dependence on the sound and is always carried out under such acoustic control. Analysis by self-observation as well as clinical experience indicates an absence of direct connection between the written response and the concept itself, similar to that which must exist between the speech response and the concept. In cases of partial sensory aphasia a partial agraphia may also be anticipated.

5. Comprehension of written or printed letters of the alphabet presents an entirely different matter. This is related to the level of educational achievement and is independent of the presence of auditory imagery. The individual who has been exposed to minimal training in reading may comprehend the written word only after it has been heard. But the educated person, trained in this skill from early childhood, may be able to grasp the general meaning after a glance at the page without awareness of the individual words. The first case presents symptoms of an alexia apart from his aphasia. The second,

on the other hand, reveals intact comprehension of all written material in striking contrast to his lack of comprehension of the spoken word.[16r] Nevertheless, in oral reading the latter demonstrates as much aphasia as is evident in spontaneous speech.

Both conditions, agraphia as well as alexia, may also be caused by involvement of an entirely different area, that of the visual cortex, since the memory images of written signs are as indispensable to the writing process as to that of reading. However, one cannot deny the possibility that the images of written signs occupy a unique and specific cortical region through their intimate connections with the entire speech area. Therefore, the symptoms of a localized alexia with agraphia may occur on the basis of a very circumscribed cortical lesion. In such cases one would rather anticipate involvement of the entire visual sensory area. The symptom-complex would be complete if object recognition were also lost. However, this disorder is intrinsically not concerned with aphasia.

III. Now let us consider the condition characterized by involvement of the association fiber tracts i.e., pathway (a1-b), connecting the acoustic imagery to the associated motor imagery. In this condition the acoustic image (a1) and the motor image (b) itself are intact.

This patient presents a picture of *good comprehension in marked contrast to that which is typical of the form* of aphasia previously described. He speaks a great deal but shows a disturbance in his choice of words very much like the other type. The auditory image is intact. It is activated by the residual sensory imagery forming the concept. However, since pathway (a1-b) is disrupted, it cannot make its own unique contribution to the appropriate selection of the motor images, or it contributes but mimimally. While in the previous cases the total effect of (c + d) alone was active for motor innervation from (b), in this situation (c+d+a1) is operative. The latter, however, since it is designated as a part of the pathway (c-b), is normally of minimal significance. Word-confusion is also observed in these cases. While this symptom is not as marked as in the preceding form, it is still very much in evidence. Nevertheless, in this case another monitoring device may be operative which is little used in normal speech, namely, the gradual substitution of an unconscious process for one which is conscious. The acoustic nerve is intact and permits transfer of the sound of the spoken word to the undamaged area containing acoustic imagery. The spoken word can therefore be heard and its accuracy assessed. The patient has definite awareness of his error and therefore often becomes emotionally upset. If given a choice of words he usually chooses successfully, just as suggestion-questions are correctly answered. Such a patient is able to rehearse what he wishes to say by first quietly repeating the word to himself. If he is a strong-willed individual, capable of intense and keen vigilance, compensation may eventually develop by a conscious but laborious, and time-consuming monitoring mechanism.

In pure and complete forms the patient presents a picture which is very similar to that of sensory aphasia. He comprehends correctly, answers suggestion-questions accurately, and so appears more intelligent than he actually is. Hemiplegia of the opposite side is almost always present.

A moderate circulatory disorder may be the assumed cause of decreased neural transmission in milder cases. The symptoms of word-finding difficulty in these patients who show no signs of hemiplegia is more striking than the confusion of words. Their speech is very hesitant and is characterized by long pauses in which the patient gropes for expression. After a long period of search, he may give up and attempt a new sentence. The beginning of the sentence may be fluent, then follows the same hesitation, the same laborious effort. This experience also occurs in normal speech when a word suddenly cannot be found in the midst of conversation. One then tries to substitute another and must finally be satisfied with a word which may be only partly adequate. I have sometimes observed-even in intelligent individuals—the sudden occurrence of startling combinations of sounds in the midst of speech, as if they were speaking in an abbreviated manner during intense mental absorption. If Steinthal in his, *Abriss der Sprachwissenschaft,* ("Outline of Philology") found the process of thought to be highly complex in itself, how much more difficult would be simultaneous thought and speech. The functional hyperemia which causes facilitation in conduction between the continuously newly-aroused sensory imagery results in a corresponding anemia in the speech areas.[17]

The disturbance in reading and writing produced by aphasia of the island-region can only be understood by a detailed study of the means by which both are acquired. (Figure 10)

Reading is learned in the following way during childhood. The visual image located in area (c) (a portion of the entire visual sensory area) is brought into relationship with its acoustic image, thus forming a strong association. In this way the child learns to read aloud, since the sum of (c + a1) by means of the path (a1-b) activates the motor image (b). The union of the acoustic and visual imagery constitutes the entire concept of the letter. It is not endowed with other qualities.

In the event of disruption of pathway (a1-b), the same process does not apply to letters as applies to all other concrete object-representation, namely the activation of the motor speech image by the concept itself. Patients are therefore unable to read individual letters. To this extent alexia always accompanies the forms of aphasia just discussed. The patient's level of education determines whether such an alexia will also extend to entire words.[18r] If earlier reading achievement has been limited to the reading of individual letters, and words are formed letter-by-letter, the aphasia would cause complete loss of reading ability.[19r] If, on the other hand, this early reading achievement has been equal to that of educated classes, the concept can be revived by means of the written word. Under optimal conditions the word might then be comprehended and retrieved orally. Single letters, however, could not be read aloud by such a patient, because oral reading requires integrity of the pathway (a1-b). Nevertheless, if a choice of names of a number of letters are given to such a patient, he would be able to select the name of the letter he is attempting to read and reject all others offered. In this way he demonstrates complete comprehension of the meaning of the letter.[20r]

The educated individual with aphasia of the island-region therefore does not sustain impairment of comprehension of the written word. Unfortunately, this statement must be modified by the fact that in this form of aphasia, a right hemianopsia is a frequent complication.[21r]

Writing is learned in the following way. See Figure 10.

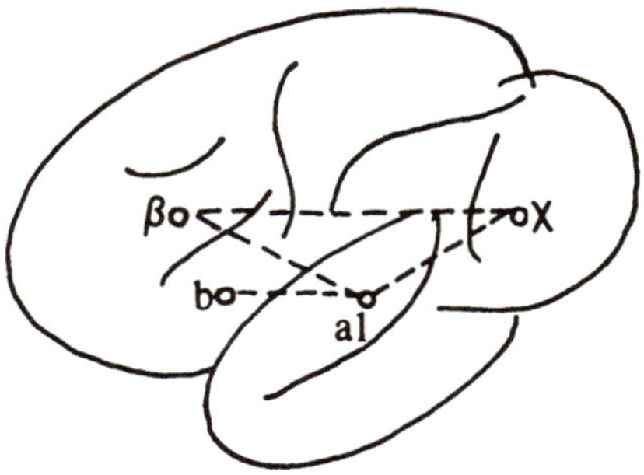

FIG. 10

Schema of the Acquisition of Reading and Writing

(χ): Visual letter imagery
(β): Graphic motor imagery
(b): Motor speech imagery
(a1): Acoustic speech imagery

The visual association image of the letter is copied by means of the path (χ - β). (β) is the center of graphic motor imagery. Only through intensive drill is association between the acoustic and motor imagery (a1-β) achieved, permitting us to write in the absence of a model. The original pathway (χ-β), by means of which we learned to write, maintains the same control of discharge of the written response as is exercised by the path (a1-b) in discharge of speech movements.

Because the motor center (β) is located in the frontal area of the brain, and the pathway (a1-β) is consequently a close neighbor to the path (a1-b), damage to this general area affects both simultaneously. This circuit provides the most direct route between the complex of sensory imagery constituting the concept and the motor writing center which activates graphic movements by means of the acoustic imagery. For this reason, aphasia of the island-region is frequently accompanied by agraphia. Nevertheless, the copying of letters and words may still be possible, since the pathway (χ-β) is yet intact.[22r]

IV. A completely different picture is presented in aphasia of the frontal lobe, caused by destruction of the motor speech images in area (b). *The patient presenting this condition comprehends all but is suddenly mute or has only a few simple words at his disposal.* These same words are used repetitively in reference to all objects, not because the patient lacks comprehension of their significance, but because they alone are available to him. This situation is similar to the dog's use of barking as a response to all commands. A single sound must serve to convey many meanings. The strong neural stimulation passing from (a1) and (c-d) to center (b) can find expression only is this single movement.

The absence of word-confusion in the pure motor form may be verified by means of suggestion-questions. These are always answered accurately by means of gesture. There is no difficulty in carrying out commands. The great majority of cases which have been reported up to this time belong to this category i.e., Broca's aphasia.

If the pathological process is extensive, the neighboring central area of motor imagery involved in written motor imagery, may also be involved, thus producing agraphia. One may well ask whether assumption of such a center is justified. The movements involved in writing are learned at a period after which the child has already developed significant and gross control of movement patterns. Therefore, the acquisition of new combinations of the motor images already present and refinement of muscular control alone is necessary. For that reason, one may not conclude that the graphic motor images are located only in the left hemisphere, since normal individuals are also able to write with the left hand, and not more awkwardly than is true of carrying out other actions with the left hand.

However, a process involving a large area of the frontal lobe would consequently also implicate the motor imagery of the opposite side, resulting in paralysis and a mechanically-produced agraphia. If a patient can place a pen with his intact left hand into his tightly-contracted, paralyzed right hand, and in this way guide the right hand, the writing would be really carried out by the left hand and not the right. This situation would in no way prove the presence of a left center for the movements involved in writing.

One who is accustomed to rehearse aloud what he is writing may be compared to the one who forcefully guides his pen with the intact hand. He would become agraphic because of the close association between the speech and graphic motor imagery, apart from the actual localization of the pathological process.

If the process disrupts those fiber tracts which emerge from the first temporal gyrus and connect the area of acoustic imagery with that of the graphic motor images, the patient would still be able to copy by means of the pathway (χ-β) but would fail in spontaneous writing. He would be partially agraphic.

Aphasia of the frontal lobe can never, except in the case described on page 108, abolish comprehension of script or printed letters.[23r]

V. Interruption of the pathway (b-b1) as presented in Figure 8, which primarily involves fibers from the first frontal gyrus converging into the great ganglion, would create an effect similar to the destruction of the specific cortical area itself.[24r] *Therefore, it would produce the same motor aphasia which has just been described.* One would hardly anticipate a process to destroy only this portion of the fibers radiating to the lenticular nucleus and corpus striatum alone, without damage to the remainder. In other words, this would produce a pure aphasia without any further paralysis. Such a situation would apply even more strongly to the fibers coursing throughout the lenticular nucleus and striatum.[25r] Destruction of but a very small area within the lenticular nucleus produces a dramatic change in the organization of the fibers. It is very probable that the various fibers concerned with different motor representations enter the lenticular nucleus from different cortical areas of the frontal area of the brain. Their arrangement there may be such that the area of one of the peripheral nerves is already represented in an adjoining circumscribed region by means of a specific quantity of gray ganglionic substance.

For example, it has definitely been established that the facial nerve in the lenticular nucleus is represented by two circumscribed but widely-separated nuclei. One of these contains fibers of the oral area which possibly originate from the first frontal gyrus and serve in production of speech movements. Or they might originate from some other region of the frontal area of the brain containing the motor images of mimicry. The other nucleus contains fibers concerned with the orbital region of the facial nerve regardless of the motor images to which they are related. In the same way, the tongue musculature has its own nucleus into which fibers from different cortical areas converge, concerned with production of speech movements as well as other consciously-executed movements involved in chewing and swallowing. Therefore, it follows that circumscribed lesions within the lenticular nucleus need not affect all speech movements simultaneously, but could produce a partial aphasia. Such an episode would present the appearance of a paralytic type of attack with involvement of innervation of the speech musculature, such as the branch of the facial nerve serving the oral region. Production of movements of the tongue and larynx used in the speech act would be intact and the word would continue to be intelligible.[26r]

It is very definite therefore that the difference between aphasia and alalia in regard to lenticular nuclear involvement is not one of kind but of degree. *Complete destruction of the left lenticular nucleus would therefore* cause aphasia as well as paralysis. This may be called "aphasia of the lenticular nucleus." This form deserves specific attention in contrast to the prevailing view, which I must emphasize is based on a very naive interpretation of the anatomic facts of this condition.

It should be clear from our discussion that disruption of the left cerebral peduncle must cause an aphasia.[27r] In fact, destruction of the inferior portion of the peduncle in itself can cause this condition, since the movements of speech are consciously learned, as has been discussed above.

It is self-evident that cases presenting two or three symptom-pictures in combination occur more frequently than the pure clinical forms caused by more or less isolated damage because the pathological process is generally very extensive. Undoubtedly, the typical pictures described, which adequately justify our formulation of a new clinical classification, actually do exist, (See the section describing clinical studies below.) I believe that the mere drawing of attention to such will result in the publication of many case histories supported by pathological findings. The mixed forms may readily be understood from the preceding discussion. If the psychic symptoms associated with aphasia of the temporal lobe are complicated by a right hemiplegia, one may predict involvement of both temporal lobe and the island-region. Combined lesions of the frontal area of the brain and the island-region are difficult to differentiate from those of the frontal area alone. Lesions of the entire first primordial-gyrus arc result in complete speech loss with impairment in comprehension, together with agraphia and alexia.

A correct diagnosis of aphasia requires a very detailed history of a specific period in the course of the illness. On the one hand, such diagnosis rests on remission of the generalized brain symptoms which accompany the onset of aphasia as well as other focal brain lesions. On the other hand, the duration of the condition must not have been of such length to allow substitution of function by the other hemisphere. Fortunately, both of these sources of error can be avoided, since substitution by the opposite hemisphere in aphasia of the frontal area generally occurs late. This form of aphasia produces the most severe generalized symptoms. Compensation in sensory aphasia however occurs early, and the generalized–symptoms are relatively mild. Unfortunately, only experienced examiners record the precise time of onset of the various symptoms, and then only if they have observed the case from onset of the condition. I need not stress the significance of this point in evaluating the pathological findings.

This newly-formulated theory of aphasia requires further elaboration lest one judge as inadequate the treatment of the precious material on which it is based.

I must now return to that hypothesis confirmed by clinical experience which offers a clear basis for a fruitful interpretation of the aphasia symptomatology. Speech is bred in mimicry of the spoken word. Speech is not identical with achievement of a specific level of mental development. Thought and speech are two independent processes which may be individually delayed. Daily observation supports this view. All children in the process of learning speech go through a stage in which they typically reveal the "Romberg-echolalia." They mimic questions put to them before answering. They play with words, experimenting with word-distortion in the process of achieving stable control of production of sounds. The meaning of the word at this stage is of secondary importance to them.

Casper Hauser, who grew up without human contact, did not develop speech although his brain development was normal. He showed much cunning and mental keenness in his struggles with animals. However, speech was learned rapidly when he eventually came into contact with other men.[28r]

Another pertinent example of this is supplied by the deaf-mute. Man normally learns speech by means of the acoustic nerve. Deprived of this pathway, he remains mute, regardless of his level of intellectual achievement. One must assume that the same factors are operative in pathological speech changes as exist in normal speech development.

Let us consider what occurs in deaf-mutes who may acquire articulate and clear speech by means of complex training methods. These cases merely confirm the existence of direct connections between the visual and tactual sensory areas and the region of motor speech-representation and prove that such connections are eventually adequate to support normal speech function. The fact that such cases can produce some speech and even learn entire sentences, in spite of loss of acoustic imagery, can be explained in no other way.

The speech learning process in other deaf-mutes who may achieve some limited speech by specific methods of training differs from that of the normal individual. In such cases visual and tactual association-images rather than the acoustic imagery may act as the initial links in the chain of the psychic reflex-arc. If such a deaf-mute achieves fairly adequate speech, even he may later become the victim of aphasia. Such an aphasia might be motor, sensory, or conduction in form, depending upon the location of the involvement.

But only in motor aphasia is the location of the lesion in the deaf-mute identical with that in normals, namely in the frontal area of the brain. This is well-supported by the available evidence. In sensory aphasia the tactual and visual imagery areas (c) and (d) as designated in Figure 11, may be lost. Their anatomic locations are not yet well-defined but are definitely not identical with the imagery of the first temporal lobe.

In conduction aphasia there must be disruption of the fiber tracts connecting the frontal lobe with the temporo-occipital area in the medullary tract of the hemisphere, particularly the superior longitudinal fasciculus of Burdach.

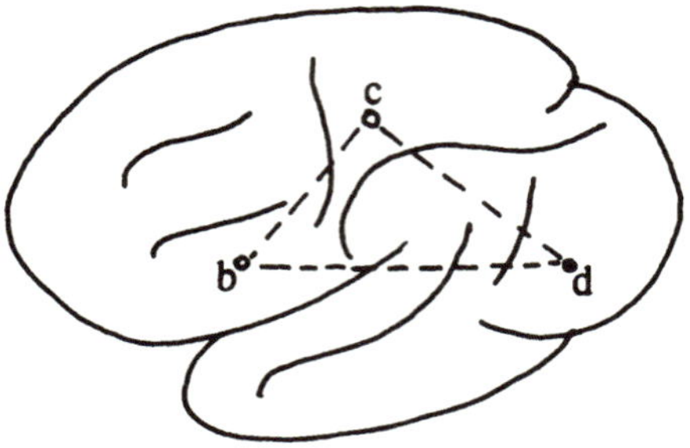

FIG. 11

Schema of the Association of the Concept and Motor Speech Imagery
(c): Tactual imagery
(d): Visual imagery
(b): Motor speech imagery

Further description of these three situations which may occur in deaf-muteness would be redundant. One might just point out that in deaf-muteness with sensory aphasia, an asymbolia (Finkelnburg) is inevitably present, and therefore the picture may become more complex and difficult to recognize. Pathological studies of such deaf-mutes as well as of those previously described would be of great value in formulating a model of aphasia.

Let us now consider the concept of asymbolia, not from the standpoint of our rather limited definition, but as Finkelnburg has described it. One of Finkelnburg's patients was no longer able to recognize familiar persons or places. The other presented impairment in comprehension of the spoken word. She confused various actions and no longer crossed herself during table-prayer. The third patient suffered tactual confusion and was no longer able to play the piano. The fourth, as frequently occurs in aphasia, no longer recognized different coins. In the fifth case, the symbols of worship, of state service, and forms of social convention were no longer familiar. Asymbolia, based on such case examples, might be defined as failure in recognition of the significance of objects and actions. Cases 4 and 5 are not particularly striking, since a large percentage of the mentally-ill demonstrate these same symptoms in their confused condition. Such symptoms may also accompany defects of intelligence.

The interpretation which is most damaging to the doctrine of aphasia is that which emphasizes the secondary intellectual deficits which often accompany aphasia as the primary feature of the symptom-picture. This type of error might be compared to the mistake of relating loss of consciousness occurring in an apoplectic attack to destruction of the lenticular nucleus. If our consideration of asymbolia is restricted to Finkelnburg's first example, we may formulate a suitable definition of this syndrome.[29] Asymbolia might then be described as a reduction or loss of the visual memory images of an object, or as the loss of a memory image essential for the conceptualization of the object. We cannot completely rule out the possibility of intellectual disturbance, but we have observed at least one form of circumscribed intellectual defect, the diagnosis of which–just as that of aphasia–was based on a focal brain lesion. In order to express myself even more clearly, I must take up a related topic which was mentioned earlier.

The spoken or written name of an object does not impart new qualities to the object. Therefore, it must be clearly differentiated from the unique sensory memory images of the object. The concept is fashioned only of the latter.

The concept of the word "bell," for example, is formed by the associated memory images of visual, tactual and auditory perceptions. These memory images represent the essential characteristic features of the object, bell. The spoken word "bell" is not the same as the auditory perception which calls up the picture of a bell, and there is even less similarity between the written characters and the picture of a bell. Only the most primitive writing systems, such as that of hieroglyphics, might provide an exception to this. The importance of preserving a distinction between the two is therefore clear. Impairment of the concept, of the elements involved in thought processes, are always disturbances of the intellect. Disturbances of speech, on the other hand, reflect only an interference in the use of the conventional tools used in communicating ideas.

We have relatively little anatomic evidence regarding location of the regions functioning as centers of visual and tactual imagery. It seems most plausible that the fiber arrangement observed in the brain stem may also be represented in the medullary tracts. This would imply that the visual radiation claims the most medial inner areas of the occipito-temporal lobe, with location of the sensory endings of the posterior column of the spinal cord lateral to these.[30r] In the outermost part of the first temporal gyrus which is a close neighbor, one may find the memory images which are not related to the speech process.

What significance do isolated lesions of this region have for speech? Let us consider the possibility of total destruction of these concept centers in both hemispheres. The lowest form of animal-like idiocy would result. Speech itself need not suffer, although its content would be complete nonsense. The telegraphic apparatus is in order, but the message has no meaning. In microcephaly, the mechanical production of speech is frequently intact. These patients may learn speech but lack comprehension. Their speech is essentially echolalia.

If the damage is limited to the visual sensory areas and involves both hemispheres, a very interesting form of alexia would be caused which differs essentially from the type already discussed.[31] The written signs would then be completely lost and could not be aroused by production of the sound. This would represent a complete alexia in contrast to the partial alexia which is only the by-product of aphasia. Moreover, agraphia would also follow. The written letters, however, have no priority over the other visual memory images. Therefore, recognition of the daily environment, including familiar objects, persons, and places would no longer be possible.

This disturbance in recognition which has presently been observed in partial form only, may be explained in the following way. In destruction of both occipital lobes, those memory images alone are lost which have representation on both sides, while in destruction of one hemisphere, the remaining images are still preserved. A case of this type has been reported in Gogol's excellent dissertation.[32] The patient bit into the soap and was incontinent. Thermometer, pitcher, compass, soap, and blotting-sand were all viewed as foreign objects. In an earlier carefully-observed phase of his illness, both the lack of intelligible expression as well as impairment in comprehension of the spoken word were established.

The pathological findings in this case (Ebstein) revealed the following.

> Up to 4cm. behind the Sylvian fossa, an ochre-yellow area is evident, with considerable softening of the brain substance, and difficulty in separation of the gyri is observed in the inferior layer of the third left frontal gyrus etc. As a result of the described softening process, the gyri (operculum) spanning the island of Reil are atrophied, leaving the island exposed. On the outer surface of the right occipital lobe, and even directly at the summit, an eight-penny-sized, ochre-yellow, scarred and retracted area is observed, with softening of the superficial layer of the cortical surface (Gogol, 1873).

3.

The clinical aphasia literature, rich as it may be, is of limited value for the support of any kind of anatomically-based theory. This is in part a reflection of the subjective nature of case interpretations supplied by most examiners. For example, in various case histories published by a single observer, the major emphasis is usually focused on one new, unique symptom, not previously reported in the literature. The complete psychic symptomatology, however, is neglected. Or, avoiding this error, we may find tedious, detailed, but objective reports with omission of the most important information. Such accounts are inadequate, since a comprehensive examination, especially of a psychic symptom-complex, dare not neglect assessment of the critical areas which furnish information needed to support the basic premises of the proposed theory.

A second problem is the inadequacy of the pathological studies. One cannot, of course, question the competence of the outstanding aphasia authorities such as Broca, Ogle, and Hughlings Jackson, whose exhaustive knowledge of cerebral anatomy permitted precise descriptions of localization of damage. However, the majority of examiners who furnished them with dissection material were very likely not able to provide adequately prepared brain sections. Therefore, it was necessary for each to work with questionable material, i.e., dissections permitting so many alternative explanations. The end-result was a mere gross interpretation of the pathological findings.

On these grounds I found it necessary to avoid an exhaustive use of clinical studies as a basis for my work. Fortunately, the few cases I myself have studied have provided adequate material to supply another kind of evidence. The great variability of the clinical picture of aphasia moves between the two extremes of pure motor aphasia and the pure sensory form. The demonstration of these two types must be regarded as conclusive proof of the existence of two anatomically separate language centers. Although pure motor aphasia has been so thoroughly reviewed in the literature that its relationship to involvement of the first frontal convolution is no longer questioned, the pure sensory form, on the contrary, to my knowledge has not been represented by a single typical case in the literature.[33r]

Two such cases have come to my attention, one of whom continues to be a patient on the mental ward of the Allerheiligen Hospital.

CASE 1

Suzanne Adam, nee Sommer, a laborer's widow, age 59 years, suddenly became ill from an unknown cause on March 1, 1874, with symptoms of vertigo and headache. However, there were no signs of loss of consciousness of the type which is often accompanied by confused speech. Correct speech usage was infrequent, and her answers to questions were completely confused. Although she was able to express her complaints regarding headache and dizziness quite accurately, the meaningless word "begraben" (buried) was interjected into whatever she said.

The patient had gone to bed following lunch as was her custom and on the next day was admitted to an inner ward of the Allerheiligen Hospital. There her condition was diagnosed as dementia, and since no physical illness was apparent, she was placed on a psychiatric ward.

On March 7, 1874, the following status was recorded. A frail, middle-aged woman, demonstrating a senile cataract on the right and a coloboma of the iris of the left. The patient's facial expression shows intelligence and cooperation. No disturbance is noted in gait. Handgrasp is bilaterally weak, with greater weakness demonstrated on the left. Some generalized decrease in sensation, tested by pinprick, is observed with minimal response demonstrated in fingers, toes, and face. Marked tortuosity of the veins, which are hard as ropes to palpation, including the superficial temporal arteries is evident. Heart and lungs are essentially normal. Hearing, tested by holding a watch to the ear, is well-preserved bilaterally. Glaucomatose excavation of the pap. optica is demonstrated on the left.

The patient could comprehend absolutely nothing which was said to her. However, caution was necessary to avoid giving clues by gesture. When called, she responded to unfamiliar names as well as her own by turning around and answering 'yes'. Superficially she gave the impression of dementia, not only because her answers to questions were inappropriate, but in that the sentences themselves were incorrectly produced, containing meaningless and garbled words. And yet, the overall meaning of a sentence, which could be grasped in a general way, was always reasonable. There was no trace of flight-of-ideas. Her behavior was calm and appropriate, while dementia, on the contrary, is generally accompanied by severe psychic deterioration.

Frequently, under the influence of strong emotion, complete sentences were correctly produced. The names of objects presented to her, such as a hat, pencil, clock, thaler, two-penny piece, handkerchief, etc. were often produced correctly. However, at other times she was completely unable to name them.

Examples of correct, appropriately-used sentences included the following.

"Today it tasted very good." "I hope that I will be well again." "The doctor has given me a two-penny piece." Many other sentences were correctly formulated. At one time she introduced her son who happened to be visiting the physician and said, "This is Richard, my fine son." "Is he not a fine boy?" Her morning and evening prayers, one of which was fourteen verses in length, were recited without error.

If one asked how she had spent the day, she usually recounted her activities correctly, and one may generally assume that she was in possession of an adequate vocabulary. Eventually, the patient could speak correctly but understood absolutely nothing. Care was necessary to avoid providing inadvertent clues such as a glance-of-the-eye, and the use of gestures was necessary to confirm this impression. When she was visited on daily rounds and asked to show her tongue, she responded correctly, but only because she guessed the meaning of the request and imitated the behavior of the other patients. For example, if one changed the request and asked her to close her eyes, she would respond by showing her tongue. If further commands were given without gesture, such as, "Take the glass from the chair," she would guess at the meaning, using trial and error by sticking out her tongue, closing her eyes, showing her teeth, etc., in short, actions which she has often observed other patients carrying out during ward rounds.

At this point of the examination she would say, "What am I supposed to show then? "What shall I smear (schmieren) now" etc. "of what use is it, since I cannot hear it?" Finally, she began to cry, "Will I ever be well again?" Gradually, she became calm when reassured by gesture.

She recognized the correct use of all objects and was able, for example, to put her eyeglasses on correctly, etc. When sitting at the table to write, she took the reversely-presented pencil, looked at it, and turning it around, grasped it correctly in an attempt to write. However, only scribbles and single strokes could be produced. The pen was also extended to her in a reversed position. After turning it about, she dipped it into the inkwell, and holding it correctly, attempted to write, but with no better success. After a few rows were written for her, the wet writing was extended to her and the sand-tray placed in her hand. She looked at the physician questioningly, "Shall I blot?" At his assent, she poured out some sand, sprinkled it on the paper as requested and poured the remainder into the sand-tray.

When she was successful in reporting something of importance to the physician, she would look at him and say, "Did you hear that?" and would look happy when he gestured an assent.

A complete alexia was present. Numbers could not be accurately comprehended, although they were correctly used in speech.

The patient's general condition improved rapidly. On March 15, 1874 she was presented to a number of colleagues. At that time fairly good comprehension was demonstrated if frequent repetition were given. She correctly responded to her name and ignored the calls of unfamiliar names. The total picture, however, continued to be consistently typical of this syndrome. Many words were spontaneously used correctly, but in contrast, only a few were comprehended well, and these only with great difficulty.

On March 18, 1874, the following conversation was recorded:

DR. WERNICKE – Good morning, how are things going?

MRS. ADAM – Thank you, things are fair.

DR. W. – How old are you?

MRS. A. – Things are going all right, thank you.

DR. W. – How old are you?

MRS. A. – Do you mean how I hei (neologism)... how I hear? (German: höre).

DR. W. – I would like to know how old you are.

MRS. A. – Yes, that I don't know at all. What my name ... (Wie ich so heiszen schwiere) (She has obvious difficulty and attempts to correct herself).... what I'm called- - -hear (German: höre).

DR. W. – Would you perhaps give me your hand?

MRS. A. – I don't know how I- - - (Presents no trace of comprehension.–

DR. W. – Where is Richard?

MRS. A. – (She thinks for a long time.) My sodom (neologism) - - - my Richard.

DR. W. – Do you need anything?

MRS. A. – Oh my, now who would anyone say something to me. - - - -(with friendly mien)- - - - - But I still do not know- - - to whom I should say someone.

DR. W. – Is this a pencil?

MRS. A. – I do not know now what it is called. I recognize it very well. I have already geschwollt mitte (paraphasia). I know very well how it really comes to be called. I cannot remember it.

A clock is presented to her.

MRS. A. – A watch (speaking quietly). . . a pocket. . . (speaking more loudly) . . . a pocket watch. . . a very fine one.

A pair of eyeglasses are given to her. She puts them on, looks at the clock and speaks.

MRS. A. – And yet, I cannot hear with it. A very fine clock. I like it very much (Shows pleasure.)

The watch is held to her ear, then held at a distance, and once again presented close to her ear.

MRS. A. – Yes, now I hear it. . . yes, now also, now I don't hear it. Now it appears a bit weak.

A button (German: Knopf) is presented to her.

MRS. A. – Yes, that I recognize. . . a Knurre. . . . a Knoppe (paraphasia).

One of her braids is touched.

MRS. A. – (Smiling) That is my. . . . .
DR. W. – Is that your hair (German: Haare)?
MRS. A. – Yes my clock (German: Uhr)- - - my Hore, my Haaruhre (paraphasia).

A three-penny piece (German: Dreier) is presented.

MRS. A. – Yes that is a Drekter- - - Droschen (paraphasia)- - -

She is given a two-penny piece.
That is two dokter (neologism) two Droschen (finally) "a two-penny piece."
The coin is given to her.

MRS. A. – That may I as many times as possible, what you have seen to me. I will thank you a many a dear time that you have told me this all, that you have been so good, so kind.

DR. W. – How is Richard?
MRS. A. – If he comes on Sunday and sees- - - -
DR. W. – How tall is Richard? (with gesture)
MRS. A. – Oh, he is very tall, taller than you. He is already 19 Tahr sohr (neologism). (After a while she cried:) Oh, dear Lord, if I only soon were well again.

By March 25, the improvement had continued. At first, she was unsuccessful in mimicking words. Eventually, however, accurate responses could be given, and she frequently corrected herself spontaneously. Her general condition was satisfactory.

April 20, 1874. Further progress was evident. The patient now comprehended almost everything said to her following several repetitions. However, only a few words could be produced in spontaneous speech, and she was unable to write to dictation. In contrast, she demonstrated fair success in copying from a model. Single letters were correctly produced. The agraphia is now her most striking speech disturbance.

This case strongly reminds me of one I have observed earlier. Unfortunately, however, my case-notes do not include many of the pertinent and specific details necessary for diagnosis, because at that time the true interpretation of aphasia still eluded me.

CASE 2

Susanne Rother, a 75 year old woman, the wife of a porter, was admitted to the Allerheiligen Hospital on October 7, 1873. She appeared to be in pain and presented all the signs of extreme senility with advanced atheromatous degeneration of all visible vessels. Persistent chills. No fever. Ambulation was possible only with support, apparently as a result of generalized weakness and dizziness. There was marked dragging of the left leg during ambulation. The patient lay in bed, huddled under the bed clothes, murmuring to herself much of the time and was incontinent.

Her mental condition at that time was regarded as dementia, complicated by aphasia. All questions were answered in complete confusion. She was unable to follow directions, or only in a very confused way, which at that time seemed to indicate an apraxia. (The attendant believed her to be deaf, because of her impairment in comprehension.) Moreover, she paid little attention to her surroundings, and in keeping with the severity of her illness, she showed little desire to converse. Consequently, her spontaneous fund of words seemed to be meager in comparison with the case just described, and yet the speech disturbance could definitely not be considered a motor aphasia.

The aphasia was characterized by mutilation and transposition of words. She often said correctly, "I thank you very much." At other times, "I thank you geblich (neologism) . . . . . I am quite ill." "Oh, I am so cold." "You are a very good man." These are examples of phrases frequently used. She often referred to the physician, whom she had called a good man, as "my little daughter," or "my little son," both with the same meaning.

November 5, 1873. Ophthalmoscopic examination revealed grey atrophy of the right papilla optica. Sensation appeared to be intact. Hand-grasp, equal bilaterally, was weak. Precise evaluation of sensation and motor function could not be carried out. Cardiac dullness was increased on the left. No abnormal murmur. There was no improvement in her mental and physical condition.

December 1, 1874. Death followed a lengthy intestinal flu which was associated with a two-day period of vomiting and complete prostration.

Pertinent history provided by relatives revealed a ten-year history of weakness of the left leg which gradually improved. Confusion of speech had occurred suddenly on November 2, 1873. Information regarding other aspects of physical or mental symptomatology is incomplete.

The pathological findings revealed edema of the pia and a mild internal hydrocephalus. The gyri and island-regions in both hemispheres were completely atrophied. Moreover, all cerebral arteries showed extensive atheromatous degeneration. The branch of the Sylvian fossa artery which extends below into the inferior sulcus of Burdach was occluded by a thrombus adherent to one of its arterial walls. The entire first temporal gyrus (adjacent to the Sylvian fossa), extending from its original union with the second gyrus, as well as the entire origin of the latter from the first gyrus (Bischof's inferior parietal lobe) and its outer longitudinal projection, had undergone changes, demonstrating a white-yellow pulp which was thick and firmly adherent to the pia.

The softened area disrupted a portion of temporal lobe fibers which radiate into the island area. The island lobe itself and the basal ganglia presented no changes. The boundaries of the softened area did not reveal any inflammatory type of induration, and its margins were of normal consistency. In the dorsal portion of the spinal cord, a segment of the left anterior lateral column demonstrated a grey degeneration and the same in the posterior columns of the lumbar area.

Permit me to make a few critical observations in regard to the two cases here reported. Both cases present the characteristic and primary symptoms of sensory aphasia. Each demonstrates a comparatively large fund of words in association with essentially complete loss of comprehension of the spoken word. They differ from each other, however, in respect to the progression of the disease.

The first case, one may assume, will experience essentially complete recovery, while the second, presented many generalized-brain symptoms eventually leading to death. Information regarding other diagnostic symptoms such as agraphia and alexia were absent in the second case.

Now it is my feeling, which essentially agrees with the findings of experienced brain pathologists, that a sharp differentiation between the concepts of focal and generalized brain damage cannot be adequately made. Among the many brain dissections of simple senile or alcoholic atrophy of the brain, which I carried out over a three-year period at the Allerheiligen Hospital, involvement of all gyri and specifically that of the island-area and first primordial arc was a consistent finding together with absence of specific focal symptoms during the course of the illness.

I observed this same finding in cases of extensive tubercular as well as traumatic meningitis. Marked shrinkage and atrophy (as described by Rokitansky) of all gyri secondary to pressure caused by the profuse exudate were evident in these cases, but, surprisingly, there were no significant focal symptoms during life. *The primary atrophy, which as part of the generalized atrophy had involved one of several gyral areas, did not, however, cause breakdown in the functions themselves. That is, it did not produce focal symptoms.* The consistent occurrence of these two findings may then be regarded as an established empirical law of brain pathology, and its explanation must be sought in the nature of the pathological process. Furthermore, neglect of this law has already caused much confusion both in pathological and clinical studies.

Therefore, we may state with some confidence that the only cerebral lesion in the case of Rother which might have produced the persisting focal symptoms of aphasia during the illness was the softening of the left temporal gyrus. The generalized gyral atrophy was due either to senility, or more likely, to a circumscribed focal involvement. Griesinger has quite appropriately stressed the destructive effect of focal brain disease on the nutrition of the entire brain. In this case, as is generally true, the anatomic basis can be found in the gyral atrophy.

The most striking focal symptom, i.e., the aphasia, in case 2, Rother, may be explained on the basis of softening of the left first temporal gyrus. We are likewise justified in assuming a focal lesion of the left first temporal gyrus in case 1, Adam.

A second point which should be made is the paresis of the left leg. This seems to suggest cerebral involvement on the right. The pathological findings, however, revealed a grey degeneration in the dorsal portion of the left lateral tract of the spinal cord. A review of the case history is important in evaluating the lack of relationship between these two symptoms, since the paresis of the left leg was of ten years duration.

Finally, we must call attention to the crossed-atrophy of the optic nerve.

This finding would support a hypothesis of complete crossing of fibers in the chiasm, if it were consistently observed in focal lesions of the temporal lobe.[34, 35r] The optic thalamus and quadrigeminal bodies demonstrated no changes in color or size.

CASE 3

The following case illustrates a typical example of conduction aphasia. I am indebted to Professor Foerster for referral of this patient.

Beckman, a 64 year old pharmacist, on the morning of March 15, 1874 noticed that he was no longer able to read properly and was even less able to write. Nevertheless, his vision was good, and he could see everything sharply and in clear outline. On the preceding evening after drinking a few glasses of beer, he had spent a restful night.

On March 18, he traveled to Breslau to consult an eye specialist. During that day the first symptoms of speech disturbance became apparent. There was not, however, the slightest evidence of generalized brain symptoms.

On March 20 I recorded the following observations in regard to the patient's condition.

A well-built man, in excellent health. Physically vigorous. No objective signs of advanced senile changes. Moderate rigidity of the radial artery. Pulse is strong and normal in rate, with interruption occurring every six to ten beats. No trace of paresis in the face or extremities. Area of cardiac dulness is increased on the left. Heart sounds are somewhat weak. No emphysema.

The patient comprehended adequately, and response to suggestion-questions was consistently accurate. His use and recognition of objects was appropriate. There was no trace of motor aphasia and no reduction in fund of words. Nevertheless, he had difficulty in finding the names of many objects. He would struggle to find the appropriate words, and in the process became irritated. If one provided the word for him, he was able to repeat it without hesitation. This same experience occurs functionally in many normals, and in the preceding discussion was described as conduction aphasia. He might speak fluently in conversation for some time, then suddenly come upon a word and hesitate, remain hanging for a time, struggle to find the word, but each attempt was inappropriate. He repeatedly corrected himself, but the harder he tried, the more frustrating the situation became. If one guessed the intended word and said it for him he would breathe a sigh of relief. "Yes, that is what I wanted to say." On the other hand, when he was relaxed, complete and essentially grammatically correct sentences would slip out with an entirely different meaning than he had intended. He would then become very angry and reject the sentence he had just spoken. He often asked in reference to what he had just said, "Was that correct?"

It is interesting to consider the relationship of aphasia to the disorders of alexia and agraphia. Both conditions can be observed in this patient, but in varying degree. If for example, a printed letter were presented to him for naming, he would likely be unable to recognize it, in spite of much effort. In his attempts to read it, he might look about the room for help, and if his glance should fall upon the title of a certain book printed in gold, he would immediately point to the title saying, "I can recognize this, the name is Goethe." Nearby stood another volume, that of Schiller. If he were asked to read that title, however, he would be unable to recognize the name in spite of persistent efforts, unless the two titles were compared.

While passing down the street he frequently read signs automatically, without conscious effort. However, if a specific word or letter of the alphabet were presented, he was unable to think of the name of it. A specific letter could be correctly although slowly selected from a group of letters and numbers. Moreover, he was usually aware if the specific letter sought was not among these. All isolated letters recited to him were accurately recognized. He proved this by indicating the correct letter and rejecting all others. To aid retrieval of the name of a specific number, he would fixate on it and count on his fingers until that number had been reached.

Impairment in vision as a cause of the problem in letter recognition was excluded by his ability to correctly recognize all other objects and photographs, etc. Moreover, he insisted that he could see all letters clearly. The letters of the alphabet were recognized as such. That is, they were not seen as foreign symbols such as Chinese or cuneiform letters, which must be the case in total loss of visual images. This was verified by the patient's ability to copy, although with difficulty, the letters and words he was unable to name.

Agraphia was also present. The patient was able to copy but could not write independently. Attempts to write letters spontaneously resulted in mere scribbles and lines. Greater success was observed in producing single-digit numbers. Two-digit numbers, however, were too difficult for him.

On March 25, 1874, Professor Foerster reported the following. A detailed examination of the visual fields revealed a specific hemianopsia on the right. No significant findings were evident on ophthalmoscopic examination. Further observation indicated a wide variation in the severity and consistency of the aphasia symptoms. At times it was essentially non-existent, and at other times it was severe. Moreover, only substantives, and among these particularly the names of places and people, were occasionally absent. Face-to-face with close relatives, the patient was much less aphasic than with strangers. The aphasia was always more marked during the medical examination, and it increased with his awareness of each new deficit.

The patient is still in treatment and his physical condition is excellent. There seems to be some improvement in the aphasia. At least it has not worsened. A second examination was carried out by Professor Foerster on April 9, 1874. Visual field testing, verified by perimetry, revealed further constriction of the visual fields in both eyes. The area lying to the right, between the mascula lutea and papilla, which had previously demonstrated clear vision, was now completely lost.[36r] In addition, the left border of the visual field on the right showed significant deterioration. This indicated that the process was progressive in nature.

An examination in May of the same year revealed significant clinical improvement. The patient continued to present the interesting symptom of intact ability in reading of entire words such as his name and those of his kin, but with loss of the ability to read isolated letters.[37r]

CASE 4

Kunschkel, a 50 year old goldsmith, suffered from urinary and fecal incontinence for a two-year period. For this reason he was admitted to the Allerheiligen hospital on January 27, 1874. His insolent and offensive behavior attracted the attention of nurses and doctors, and on January 29 he was transferred to the mental ward. The patient was surly and morose, demonstrating marked agitation and irritability without apparent cause, and complete bowel and bladder incontinence, which at times appeared to be deliberate. He seemed to be completely disoriented as to place. There were no symptoms of paraplegia or tabes. Skeletal changes as a result of rickets were also noted.

On March 26 he was involved in a quarrel which occurred in the men's hall, and before any one could intervene, he received a blow to the right ear. Following this, he spoke in a confused manner and walked with a staggering, unstable gait, dragging the right side of his body. On the next morning, a hematoma of the right ear, a marked aphasia, and paralysis of the right leg were found.

The patient staggered when ambulation was attempted and dragged the right leg. Hand-grasp was weak bilaterally, the left more so than the right. There was no evidence of facial paralysis. A moderate decrease in sensation was evident. The pulse was 90 and respirations rapid, about 22. Frequent cough without expectoration was noted. Rales were heard bilaterally over both lower lung areas. Hearing was intact.

The aphasia revealed itself in the following way. The patient spoke for long periods without hesitation, but frequently a wrong word, apparently added unconsciously, would slip out at the end of a sentence. If one questioned him about the word just spoken, he would attempt to correct it, and in the process produced meaningless combinations of words and syllables, a jargon which was difficult to record. In response to some interjected questions, however, he answered in complete and accurate sentences. His answers in so far as speech was possible were essentially correct and appropriate in meaning. Furthermore, his answers to suggestion-questions indicated a ready and intact comprehension.

Alexia was also observed. However, he responded successfully if given the task of designating a specific letter from a series. In the same way, single letters and numbers could be recognized if a series were presented orally. Agraphia was also present. He was able to write his first and last name correctly, but with an unsteady hand. The word, "goldsmith" could be written only as far as the letter 'd'. He then stopped and wrote a new word such as, 'well' where he had left off. At that point he was unable to continue, and further efforts led to meaningless scribbling.

The findings on visual field testing are questionable because of his inability to maintain attention. However, a right hemianopsia appeared to be present.

On March 30, I was able to record the following conversation.

DR. WERNICKE - What year is it?
MR. KUNSCHKEL - 44.
DR. W. - Is your father still living?
MR. K. - No, he died in 46.
DR. W. - And how long ago was that?
MR. K. - On the 29. . . zaten, daten. . . diten. (neologisms).
DR. W. - Do you have any money?
MR. K. - Yes, I have redeemed the lute and my things.
DR. W. - How much do you have then?
MR. K. - Close to one hundred thaler. If I would have 100 I would already (hesitates).
DR. W. - What would you have then?
MR. K. - Graetliche (neologism) hillock.
DR. W. - Is that to be used in a pub?
MR. K. - No, it is an emperor's palace.
DR. W. - What else?
MR. K. - Now there are emperor's kis katen (jargon) lebeln. There they have, for example, a kingly one from the Elizabethan coffer, that is from the common coffer.
DR. W. - Would you like to go home?
MR. K. - It has been four weeks since I have left this place.
DR. W. - What is this? (A handkerchief is presented).
MR. K. - That is a fine filil (neologism).
DR. W. - A filet?
MR. K. - No, it is not a netting, a netting is not as heavy.
DR. W. - What is it then?
MR. K. - It is called a handkerchief.
DR. W. - What else might one call it?
MR. K. - No, as one in noble. . . sections understand I move in nobility.

A pencil is presented (German. Bleistift).

MR. K. - I thought it might be a small kolinomitz (neologism) but it is not.
DR. W. - What is it then?
MR. K. - I have always had it under the Neuman. . . New. . . pencil.

Eyeglasses are presented. (German. Brille).

MR. K. - Those are called bridges, (Brücke). . . Brikke, one calls it.
DR. W. - What are they used for. . . amusement?
MR. K. - Oh no, in order to develop the mile the golden, to develop one's appearance.

The gait is clearly more stable. Ophthalmoscopic examination reveals normal papillary vessels.

On April 4, no tract of paralysis was apparent during ambulation. The aphasia was evident only in occasional uncertainty in the initiation of words and substitution of the wrong vowel in unaccented syllables of word endings, etc. The alexia had also disappeared. In difficult words such as 'Zugrundelegung' the final syllable alone was not clear. In contrast, unfamiliar or foreign words were repeated only in jargon, with correct production limited to certain syllables - the rest of which were supplemented erratically.

Complex numbers, such as 25, 394, were read correctly. Most striking was the impairment in writing, and a long period of thought was necessary before the patient began to write. He was able to write the beginning of a dictated sentence, but not the ending. When requested to write the word, "goldsmith," (Goldarbeiter) immediately after he had spoken of a pince nez, he began to write, "paen. . . " After awhile he became completely fatigued and could no longer muster the energy to attempt a new word.

The last two cases may be classified together. Both have intact comprehension of the spoken word and a large fund of words available. But the availability of this word-store is inconsistent and related to the situation and the patient's mood.

Beckman, case 3, is mentally completely intact, while Kunschkel, case 4, is mentally weak, verbose, and lacking in self-control and critical faculty.

During speech, Beckman frequently became blocked in the middle of a sentence and struggled for expression. Kunschkel, on the contrary, compensated for his errors by the use of meaningless words or new combinations or syllables. In this way he was able to complete the sentence. Moreover, he attempted to correct himself, although with limited success.

Each patient presented the same type of alexia, and in each, agraphia was more striking than the symptoms of aphasia or alexia. I think it very likely that a right hemianopsia was present in Kunschkel's case. If this were true, the similarity between the two cases, which must be based on the pathological findings, would be even less doubtful.

In our earlier discussion it was stated that conduction aphasia could not be considered the cause of alexia (with the exception of reading of letters of the alphabet)[38r] or at least not in the educated. Beckman appears to prove an exception. However, Beckman's situation, and perhaps also that of Kunsckel, is complicated by a right hemianopsia. Lacking this, Beckman might be expected to read without difficulty.[39r]

This was evident in his partial retention of this skill. He appeared to read automatically, as if only half-aware, without making a conscious attempt to fixate on the material. Apparently, the word fixated on was but half-existent to him, and therefore could not awaken the appropriate meaning within him. The ability to synthesize words from single letters was absent.

A striking example of his actual reading ability, apart from the Goethe incident recounted above, is the manner in which he glanced at a prescription. He barely threw a glance at it and remarked, "Here, this word says, aloe." Immediately underneath was the word (choloquinten). But in spite of much effort, this could not be deciphered. Perhaps, he momentarily read the word backwards or with a peripheral part of the retina, which still permitted a margin of vision on the right.

The rapid increase in constriction of the visual field with simultaneous improvement of the aphasia suggests that the progressive process had not implicated the island region itself, but had likely invaded the neighboring structures, perhaps the left optical tract, which represents the left halves of the retinas.[40] The encroachment into the external lateral portion of the right halves of the retinas can only be explained by assumption of an obstruction with invasion beyond the midline on the right.[41]

There is absence of paralysis and no disturbance in the patient's general status. All evidence suggests a focal lesion in the tuber cinerum, extending from the left to the initial portion of the Sylvian fossa (lamina perforata anterior), at which point the process has come to a standstill. The aphasia may be related only to the impaired circulation which involves the environs of the actual focal lesion.[42r]

Kunschkel's problem must be differentiated from that of Beckman, in that it was caused by trauma. The fact that the trauma occurred on the right, but the cerebral signs were on the left is consistent with the frequent observation that a blow to the side of the head produces a hemorrhage and softening in the opposite hemisphere.

Numerous cases of pure motor aphasia have been reported in the literature. At any event, the existence of the pure motor form has been well established and only requires confirmation by additional cases.

The following two case histories of aphasia are predominantly motor in nature.

CASE 5

Rosina Peter, a 78 year old coachman's widow, sustained a concussion two years prior to admission to the Allerheiligen Hospital, resulting in paralysis of the left extremities. This was followed by a rapid recovery, and after several days she was able to leave her bed. When ambulation was attempted, she dragged the left leg. There was rapid recovery of the left arm, which became completely functional. However, diminished sensation on the left persisted, and the extremities were usually cold to the touch. In addition, a general chorea followed the attack.

In October, 1873, her strong, uncontrolled choreic movements caused a fall from a chair and fracture of the neck of the left femur.

At the time of her admission to the mental ward on February 27, the following notations were made. A senile woman demonstrating random movements which primarily involve the right extremities and the face. The patient talks continually, producing a lalling, unintelligible mumble. The mouth and eyes are alternately open and closed. The tongue lolls in the mouth, while the hands agitate in the air, accompanied by meaningless jabbering and gestures. In short, she presents the picture of one possessed.

The patient presented dyspnea in the sitting position. A fresh fracture of the sternum directly under the angulus Ludovici was evident, apparently the result of excessive abnormal movement and crepitation. Hemorrhage was evident in the mediastinum. Irregular pericardial murmur. Cardiac arrhythmia. Inconstant fillings of the radialis. Veins extensively atheromatous. The left sternal area revealed signs of hemorrhagic suffusion.

The appearance is definitely maniacal. The patient dealt out blows and hurled containers extended to her. She was taken from bed and required to walk. Thereupon, she struggled violently, flinging the nurse from her with remarkable strength. Ambulation, possible only with support, was unsuccessful because she avoided bearing weight on the left foot.

The following day there was gradual quieting and a decrease in the dyspnea. She slept following a small dose of morphine administered subcutaneously. In the evening the temperature was high. (up to 39.5C.) Early in the day it was normal. Subjectively, she appeared to be in good health. She continued to become easily agitated, but in general was good-tempered and of an obliging disposition. The involuntary movements, which were constant when she was awake, disappeared during sleep and could be briefly suppressed by conscious effort.

Since March 19, there has been no evidence of fever. The general status is good. Some change in intensity of heart sounds in the mediastinal region was evident.

March 28, 1874. Vomiting occurred yesterday evening, but the patient passed the night quietly. Today there is recurrence of the vomiting. Nevertheless, she has no other complaints and has not lost consciousness. She is completely speechless and points to her mouth to indicate her inability to speak. The tongue can be protruded. She comprehends what has been said to her.

March 30. The patient spent a good night. Early in the morning, without warning or sound, she was suddenly unable to swallow. The mandible hung open, the tongue was protruded, and saliva flowed from the mouth. A right hemiplegia with facial paresis was present. The right leg was held in strong extension. Flexion could be achieved only with strong resistance. There was a marked paralysis of the right arm. Sensation, tested by pinprick, was generally diminished, particularly in the right hand. Ophthalmoscopic examination revealed greyish–red papillary vessels, without signs of congestion. She comprehended simple commands and attempted to carry them out with the left hand.

When entrance into the esophagus was attempted for mechanical feeding, she cried out, but extended her hand to the physician.

Death followed on April 10.

Pathological findings revealed pachymeningitic adhesions to the skull vertex, osteophytis of the inner cranial wall, and atrophy of the gyri bilaterally. On the left, a focal softening was noted extending to the union of the first and second temporal lines, chiefly involving the superior surface, to which the pia was adherent. From that point, the focal softening extended only slightly into the depths of the white matter posteriorly. From there it continued anteriorly in the white matter layer extending past Broca's area. This area was not itself involved, but rather, the entire outer part of the white matter into which it was depressed. The marrow of the central gyri was interrupted in the same way.

A small distance behind this focus there was similar softening of the white matter of the gyri forming a passageway to the occipital lobe (Gratiolet). On the right, an extensive area of the free surface of the convexity was involved. A large focal softening involved almost the entire breadth of the hemisphere behind the central sulcus. There was sclerosis of the area surrounding this focus and the grey substance of the gyrus there revealed intense red striations. Both gyri fornicati were intact, as was also the crura of the fornix. An old cyst, almost the size of a pea, containing serous fluid was found in the head of the right cuadate nucleus on the ventricle's surface.

CASE 6

Isidor Itzigsohn, a traveling businessman, 26 years of age, was admitted to the medical clinic on March 25, 1874. I would like to acknowledge referral of this case by Dr. Lebert.

The patient was taken ill on the morning of admission, and symptoms were limited to loss of speech. Several hours later, a paralysis of the right side was observed. Motor aphasia was the primary initial symptom. The patient appeared apathetic and mentally dull, symptoms which are not characteristic of this disorder. Total paralysis of the right arm was demonstrated, with dragging of the right leg upon attempts to walk. Ambulation, however, was still possible. Facial movement on the right side was sluggish. Sensation tested by pin-prick was intact. Reflexes of the paralyzed side were diminished. Vessels and heart were essentially nomral.

During the following days there was progression of the paralysis with eventual involvement of the leg. Mental status remained unchanged. Because the history revealed an earlier syphilitic infection, a smear treatment was ordered. The patient's condition improved rapidly, and by April 26, he was able to walk and had regained partial use of the right hand. Examination on this day revealed the following. In spite of full mobility of the tongue and lips, the patient was unable to speak a single word. Only syllables with the letter "a" and a mute appendage, usually "m" were articulated. Attempts to mimic a specific word resulted in verbalization which closely resembled the word in number of syllables and intonation.

The patient comprehended all simple commands and questions which did not require a high level of intelligence. Emotional lability and excitability, however, significantly impeded the examination. Impairment in comprehension of prepositions was evident. For example, the identical response was produced when the patient was requested at one time to place a book on top of the paper, and at another time, under it. He was unable to differentiate between the two directions. Commands in which the meaning was self-evident, such as "Climb on the stool" were carried out correctly. Comprehension of color-names was impaired, although matching of the color of a specific object to colors on a test chart could be accomplished. Some loss of acoustic imagery may be assumed.

Letters of the alphabet were accurately comprehended, and the patient was able to follow simple written directions. Furthermore, numbers of isolated letters of the alphabet could be recognized. Writing ability was limited to copying. The patient was unable to write his own name and most letters spontaneously or to direction. The alphabet could be written, but with frequent errors of transposition, and numbers were accurately produced in series. He did not show slavish dependence on the exact form of the model in these tasks. For example, a printed "r" was transcribed into its script counterpart.[43r] No hemianopsia was evident. Hearing and vision were intact. Ophthalmoscopic examination revealed normal findings.

Case 5, Peter, presents many interesting features. It should be noted first of all, that the chorea primarily involved the right extremities. This fact may be readily explained by the earlier occurrence of a left hemiplegia secondary to the first apoplectic attack. This supports Meynert's assumption of involvement of the foot of the cerebral peduncular tract in a choreic form of hyperkinesia. The hemiplegia was obviously caused, although indirectly, by the old focal softening in the right hemisphere which was accompanied by a collateral edema. The sudden deprivation of circulation involving such an extensive portion of the brain (as occurs, for example, in an apoplectic attack) results in the simultaneous occurrence of a collateral edema in the neighboring environs. One may, moreover, be fairly certain in assuming a collateral hyperemia in the opposite hemisphere.

The hemiplegia may be explained on the basis of the early pathological findings, while the more recent findings may account for the chorea. The chorea was then produced by a hyperemia of the tract of the foot of the cerebral peduncle, at some point along its course similar to the experienced hyperesthesia caused by cutting of the pia spinalis.[44r](Meynert)

The focal softening, of one year's duration, was joined by a second in the left hemisphere, resulting in an aphasia and a right hemiplegia, terminating shortly after in the patient's death.

The pendulous jaw, the complete immobility of the tongue, and the inability to swallow ought not to be interpreted as mere precursors of the approaching death, since the patient was fully conscious and well aware of her situation.

These symptoms, as well as the aphasia, may be considered secondary to destruction of the layer of white matter, since there was no involvement of the basal ganglia with the exception of a small cyst of the corpus striatum. Finally, one may point to the generalized gyral atrophy, which in this case was accompanied by focal brain involvement.

Itzigsohn's problem (case 6), a result of focal syphilitic brain involvement, cannot be regarded as a pure motor aphasia, since the latter would not typically include an agraphia.[45r] However, the agraphia in this case was incomplete, since impairment was restricted to spontaneous writing and writing to dictation. Preservation of copying indicates integrity of the pathway (α-β), and the agraphia is therefore explained on the basis of disruption of the pathway (al-β) which connects the acoustic imagery with the psychmotor center of writing movements.[46r] These findings suggest the probability of extension of the pathological process into the deep vascular sinus into which the anterior and superior sulci converge.

This would indicate a syphilitic encephalitis, since aphasia is but rarely caused by tumors, and even less often by adherent neoplasms. Moreover, the lesion extends over a considerable area of the sensory speech center.

The following case coincides well with the one just reported.

CASE 7

Karl Seidel, a day laborer, 60 years of age, became ill on May 7, 1874. The attack occurred as he was standing on a ladder. He managed to hold on until he could be helped down. The patient was giddy and speechless but still could walk home without being guided. There a right hemiplegia was observed.

He lay in a lethargic state for 24 hours and on the following day was admitted to the Medical Clinic where observation of him was graciously permitted me by Dr. Lebert.

On May 15, the following status was noted. A strongly built man, showing minimal senile changes, lying in bed, fully-conscious. Poor appearance. Yellow facial color. The arteries are tortuous but do not demonstrate generalized rigidity. Cardiac dullness is increased on the left. A systolic murmur is noted at the apex of the heart, and aryhthmia is present. The wrinkles on the right side of the face are absent at rest and the lips are open on the left. During speech the right side of the mouth reveals limited movement. Spontaneous use of the right arm is minimal. Such movements are slow and executed with marked resistance. Hand-grasp on the right is extremely weak. The right arm, is cooler to the touch than the left, with some evidence of cyanosis in the right hand. The right leg drags during ambulation but does not appear to be severely involved. However, when he attempts to get into bed, this leg must be moved with his hands. Sensation on the right, tested by pinprick, is unremarkable.

Mentally, the patient is somewhat apathetic and indifferent. His appetite is good. He produces essentially no spontaneous speech throughout the day, and responses to questions are limited to 'Yes' and 'No.' He is disoriented in his room, unable to find the lavatory and tends to confuse objects. A water glass is used as a urinal when the latter proves to be inadequate.

All simple communications and commands geared to his intellectual range can be comprehended and correctly carried out. However, his spontaneous speech is limited to 'Yes' and'No'. His responses to questions are for the most part unintelligible, although some well-articulated sounds can be perceived. He is able to mimic all words correctly but demonstrates some anarthria. The vowels and intonation of syllables etc., however, are clearly discernible. Closer observation reveals that only the consonants 'c', 'd', 't', 'z', and 'k' are difficult for him.

When asked to show his tongue, he merely opens his mouth. No better success is observed when this action is demonstrated to him. Lateral movements of the tongue can be performed, but only laboriously and inconsistently. Circular movements along the lip-border are not possible. Severe involvement of tongue mobility may therefore be assumed.

The following sample of conversation is typical of his specific speech disturbance.

DR. WERNICKE - Good evening.
MR. SEIDEL - Good evening.
DR. W. - How are things going with you?
MR. S. - Yes.
DR. W. - What is your name?

MR. S. - Yes
DR. W. - Is your name Thomas? Berthold? Schulze? Mueller?

The patient answers "No" to each name.

DR. W. - Is your name Seidel?
MR. S. - Yes
DR. W. - Say, Seidel?
MR. S..- Seidel, Seidel?
DR. W.- Say Berthold... Thomas... hospital... mental institution...bricklayer.

Each word is repeated correctly.

When asked if he could read or write, he answered, "No". And yet, he was able to write his own name and correctly wrote, Seidel. The name Karl was then written for him. He again wrote Seidel. On a new page the word, 'garden', (Garten) was written which he was asked to copy. His response was a mixture of "Seidel" and "Garten" in that he began with the 'S' and then produced a clear 'a' and 't'. In the meantime, the numbers 1874 were written on another page. In response, he wrote 1844. When asked to write the number 60, he wrote 1848. When attention was called to the error, he wrote 18 (that is, a two-digit number) and behaved as if this were now correct. When the number 60 was then presented to him for copying, he perseverated on the preceeding visual picture. The written image appeared to persist mentally for an abnormal length of time, and therefore disrupted production of a new response. He fatigued easily and then gave little further effort.

The patient was unable to read the date, 1874, which he had copied fairly adequately. During reading he fatigued easily and was extremely susceptible to perseveration. He was able to read the first few letters of a row, but not the remainder. The number 5 was read accurately, but not the 9 directly following. Five fingers were held up to him, and he was asked to name the number. After the question was repeated, he responded with the word "Fine". Two fingers were then held up, but he could not find the answer. When asked, "Are there five fingers? " he answered, "Yes". When the examiner questioned this saying, "You mean there are still five fingers?" he said, "Oh. yes."

A critical review of this case must take several factors into consideration. These symptoms can be certainly traced to embolism and resultant focal softening caused by the demonstrated mitral insufficiency. The focal softening apparently did not involve the area of the first primordial-gyrus and the island, since there is preservation of the entire psychic reflex arc (a-al) - (b-bl). On the other hand, one may assume disruption of the fiber tracts (c-b) and (d-b), since the concept is no longer able to activate the motor speech-imagery. Consequently, the white matter of the hemisphere was apparently involved in the focal softening, and the paralysis of the right side, particularly that of the tongue, indicates involvement of the lenticular nucleus.[47r] One must then assume a large focal softening with destruction of a part of the lenticular nucleus and extension into the white matter of the left hemisphere above the lateral ventricle.

The disturbance in reading and writing are of little diagnostic value because of the patient's limited education.

This case demonstrates a new form of aphasia, which in spite of its superficial similarity to the motor type, closely resembles aphasia of the island-region in symptomatology. This type is caused by disruption of the connecting pathways between motor and sensory centers, leaving the centers, per se, intact. No further proof is needed for diagnosis of Seidel's condition as aphasia, in spite of the accompanying symptoms of asymbolia. *The typical speech symptoms demonstrated can be explained only on the basis of disruption of pathways (c-b) and (d-b).* The additional symptom of asymbolia may be regarded merely as an incidental complication, caused by the extensiveness of the lesion and cannot account for the unique speech picture presented.

The following case, which is important because of its rare occurrence, provides a significant supplement to the case example of conduction aphasia, discussed under Section III.

CASE 8

Louise Funke, a 59 year old lady's companion, suffered an apoplectic attack on December 6, 1873 and was admitted on December 8 to the Allerheiligen Hospital. She demonstrated the characteristic picture of brain hemorrage. Hypertrophy of the left ventricle and some albuminuria verified this diagnosis. Paralysis of the right side and loss of speech were observed. Early in March 1874, the following status was noted. Complete right hemiplegia. The angle of the mouth on the right was lower than that on the left. The nasolabial fold was drawn to the left; the fold on the right was smooth. Movement was limited to the left side of the mouth. The tongue protruded very slowly, demonstrating some tremor. No deviation of the tongue was evident. Movement of the eyelids was bilaterally symmetrical, and closure on the right as well as the left was possible. The right extremities could be moved passively, but rapid movement was painful. Pulse was slow –48. Sensation of pain, in so far as could be assessed, was intact on the right or only slightly diminished.

The patient's vocabulary was limited to the word 'Yes' which was used in response to all questions. If she wished to utter anything spontaneously, the word 'Yes' was repeated indefinitely. She comprehended nothing which was spoken to her. The simplest questions and commands elicited only the repetitively-produced 'Yes'. One could communicate with her to some extent by gesture. For example, if a hand were extended, she would hold out her own; if one pointed to the mouth or demonstrated the action for her, she would respond by showing her tongue. All further examination foundered on her impairment in comprehension, which impeded definite elimination of the possibility of a unilateral or bilateral hearing loss. This case apparently indicates an extensive destruction of the lenticular nucleus and of the first primordial gyrus or its white matter.

CASE 9

Siegmund Zwettles, a 49 year old shopkeeper, three years prior to examination sustained a stroke resulting in paralysis of the right arm and loss of speech. (The leg was apparently not involved.) He was able to speak only his name and could write the same, although the capacity to read and write were otherwise completely lost. Since that time, complete recovery of the right arm as well as speech had occurred, with the exception that, upon occasion, words could be found only after much thought, and he could not immediately name objects presented to him.

His condition was complicated by a right hemianopsia. Because he was intellectually intact, it was possible for him to describe the effect of the hemianopsia on his reading ability. He indicated that he read letter by letter, combining the individual letters to form words. For this reason, reading was very slow and laborious. He found that as he walked down the street, he could read signs in an absent-minded fashion, and difficulty was present only when he consciously fixated on words.

He was successful in reading most letters individually. This was accomplished by mentally retaining the particular letter he sought. By recitation of the alphabet, he would then find the name of the specific letter he was attempting to read. These symptoms suggest the residuals of an earlier alexia. A four-digit number could be read only after much thought and experimentation. Special effort was required to differentiate between the unit and the tens place. These findings are in general similar to those of Beckman, case 3. An interpretation of that case was discussed above.[48r]

CASE 10

A shopworker, some 20 years of age, was admitted to the Allerheiligen Hospital on March 19, 1874. There he suffered an epileptic attack with a twelve-minute loss of consciousness. He complained of pain in the back and arms, which was particularly apparent at rest. An incidental suppurative parotitis developed on the left, with a persistent, long-lasting abscess formation. His state of nutrition had deteriorated. An impairment in speech developed ten to twelve days prior to death, but the precise time of onset of these symptoms was not adequately recorded.

On May 14, the following status was observed. A very anemic poorly-nourished individual with atrophied musculature, phlegmatic in facial expression, complaining of pain in the back and on the left side of the head. The pulse is 104, full and strong. Respiration is not rapid. Lungs are clear. The right side of the face is smooth, with erasure of the naso-labial fold; the angle of the mouth on the right is lower than that on the left. These symptoms are more apparent during laughter. The forehead shows symmetrical wrinkling. Lid-closure is intact. The right pupil is dilated, and reacts to light. No paralysis is observed in the extremities. Tapping on the left temporal area results in severe pain. There is a marked hyperesthesia, confined to the lower extremities. The gait is broadbased and laborious.

Ophthalmoscopic examination revealed a greyish color of both papillae with no obviously indistinct borders, without apparent congestion. However, a definite stage of choked disc could be discerned.

The patient comprehended most of what was said to him and had an unlimited vocabulary at his command. However, words were unconsciously confused when he spoke. Nevertheless, his speech was well-articulated and produced without mechanical obstruction. Object naming was inconsistent. For example, on one occasion he named a watch correctly, but then later a pocket-knife was called 'a watch'. When it was opened he referred to it as an 'open-watch.'

As is characteristic, the same speech symptoms present in spontaneous speech were also observed in oral reading. The lines were read fluently, but additional words were inserted unawares, which resulted in a meaningless mixture of correct and incorrectly read words.

His writing ability was not tested. On the basis of the symptom-complex just described, Dr. Friedländer, to whom I am indebted for use of this case-material, made a diagnosis of brain abscess of the left hemisphere. This was supported by the symptoms of mild irregular fluctuations in fever.

On May 18, a pneumonia of the left side was noted. The patient became comatose, and death occurred on May 21, 1874.

Pathological findings were as follows. The dura was unremarkable with no indication of skull injury. The pia was dry, pale in appearance, and mildly opaque. The sulci were infiltrated and poorly defined, with the gyri adherent to each other, particularly in the left hemisphere. Upon removal of the brain from the skull to observe changes involving the left temporal lobe, an area the size of a penny, greenish-yellow in color, was observed on the basal surface of the hippocampal gyrus. No specific involvement of the pia was noted. The left Sylvian fossa was exposed by careful removal of the pia and vessels.

The dissection revealed separation of the surface of the temporal lobe and operculum opposite each other in such a way that there was projection of the temporal lobe to the outside, and of the operculum inwardly, with sharp margins. The island-gyri were squeezed between the operculum and the temporal lobe, with a sharp shelf of the island projecting externally.

The entire brain stem on the left was squeezed together, compressed from above and beneath, and as a result, the cerebral peduncle was spread out on its undersurface in the shape of a saddle. The entire Sylvian fossa could be exposed without need of opening the abscess. The abscess itself involved the greater share of the temporal lobe, extending even to the outer and underside of the inferior horn of the ventricular wall, whose ependyma was intact. It contained foul green pus and was enclosed in an abscess membrane. The surrounding areas were macerated to such an extent that the boundaries of healthy tissue could no longer be determined. The marrow of the first temporal lobe manifested some softening in its deeper portions facing the layer of white matter; those areas located in the medullary ridge of the gyrus were still intact but edematous. The abscess extended within to the area where the temporal lobe merges with the island of Reil. At that site (at the point of union of the caudate and lenticular nuclei) a purulent infiltrate of the brain substance was observed with complete absence of a membrane. This disruption also involved the outer fibers of the cerebral peduncle. The left optical tract was partially softened and flattened.

Apart from the compression, all other portions of the brain, including the entire left frontal gyrus and the basal ganglia in particular, were normal. A circumscribed purulent meningitis was found in the posterior lumbar area of the spinal cord. The spinal cord itself was compressed by a thick purulent formation. The rest of the spinal cord revealed no abnormalities.

The case just reported presents so many riddles that a satisfactory interpretation of the results and the course of the disease hardly seems possible. In view of the absence of a right hemiplegia, the left basal ganglia, in spite of the compression, must be presumed to have been functional, or else the compression was very late in occurrence. If it were functional, the aphasia could definitely not be explained on the basis of compression of the third frontal gyrus. Therefore, this patient provides only negative findings which may be applied to a theory of aphasia. The basic question whether or not softening of the medullary substance was present during the patient's lifetime very likely cannot be resolved. It was certainly better preserved than the other temporal gyri. The clinical symptoms point to an aphasia of the island-region. However, they can hardly be used as an explanation if there was normal function of the basal ganglia, since the island-cortex and the basal ganglia suffered from the same compression.

On the other hand, symptoms of the onset of the aphasia were inadequately recorded. It is quite possible that there were earlier symptoms of sensory aphasia. In the meantime, the functions of the left temporal lobe might have been assumed by the other hemisphere, for this compensation occurs very rapidly in sensory aphasia. Moreover, a certain stage in the recovery process of sensory aphasia is characterized by fairly good comprehension, but continued symptoms of transposition and confusion of words.

This case yields evidence neither for nor against my proposed localization of speech centers. The pressure effect of abscesses, as is true of tumors, may cause changes in various areas of the brain, and operates according to laws completely unknown to us at this time . Therefore, this apsect of the case cannot be used to resolve this type of question. The finding of focal softening alone promises an explanation in regard to localized functions of the brain.[49r]

The paralysis of the right oro-facial musculature remains unresolved. Moreover, if the paralysis of the right oro-facial nerve is related to a partial destruction of the left motor ganglion, the area destroyed must contain the portions of the nucleus of the oro-facial nerve described in detail above.

The hyperesthesia of the lower extremities obscures the diagnosis. It may be readily explained on the basis of the cirumscribed spinal meningitis.

Here I would like to express my warmest gratitude to my colleagues at the hospital, Friedländer and Weigert, for their kind support and generous provision of material.

I am well aware that this presentation has not offered completely new insights into the nature of aphasia. Similar psychological and philosophic conclusions may be found in the writings of many aphasia authorities. Baginsky, for example, has expressed parallel views in his classification of centrifugal and contripetal aphasia. My conclusions differ from these earlier writings in the attempt to find a strong anatomical basis for the symptoms observed.

There is a significant difference between the invention of various theoretic centers (coordination center, concept center) – with complete neglect of their anatomic substrates, because the unknown functions of the brain up to the present have not completely warranted anatomically-based conclusions– and an attempt, based on an exhaustive study of brain anatomy and the commonly-recognized laws of experimental psychology, to translate such anatomic findings into psychological data, seeking in this way to formulate a theory by use of the same kind of material.

My interpretation of the speech process is merely the specific application of the process involved in spontaneous movement, the main features of which have already been well-established, to the movements necessary for speech. The sensory function of the temporo-occipital area and the motor function of the forebrain form the individual building blocks. Even, this fact, which still must be confirmed anatomically, the localization of sound images in the first temporal gyrus finds (apart from the autopsy evidence) indisputable anatomic support in the presence of the connecting fibers, which are evident in the claustrum as well as the fibrae propriae.

One might ask whether the use of still inconclusive anatomic and physiological studies is justified in the construction of a new theory. That answer must lie with the reader, for I have tried here to submit the material openly, without attempting to hide or embellish any of the evidence. If one recalls how daring and yet fruitful the still available but incomplete physiological material in some of the old handbooks, such as that by Romberg, proved to be in application to clinical practice, perhaps an attempt to finally risk the same thing in the area of brain physiology will not be too strongly condemned. However, the justification of our theory can be found in still other essential factors.

In dealing with this problem, I have never succumbed to the temptation to go beyond the basic elementary hypothesis which now can hardly be seriously challenged, that the central nerve endings are invested with the role of psychic elements. Thus many of the oddities in the province of aphasia must remain unresolved, such as the isolated loss of substantives or verbs, etc. *An interpretation of such unexplained symptoms on the basis of our primary anatomic elements was deliberately avoided, and it must be clearly stated here that whole areas of brain physiology and the odd symptoms observed therein, such as most of the emotional disturbances, at present are not accessible (in the medical sense) to scientific treatment.* A clear interpretation of this area, which we must forgo for the time being, is the most pressing challenge for the future progress of psychiatry.

The theory of aphasia, here proposed, permits a consolidation of the diversified picture of the disorder. The diverse variety of symptoms which formerly had presented new riddles to each investigators does not now seem so striking, but may be predicted according to the laws of symptom-combination.

However, one feature is common to all. The underlying basis of the disorder lies in a disruption of the psychic reflex-arc necessary for the normal speech process.
the concept of aphasia.

Just as the analysis of the normal speech process on the basis of different centers permits one to incorporate the manifold forms of aphasia within a broader framework, so it allows an explanation of most of the contradictions which up to now have seemed so striking. In the past these have been interpreted in part on the basis of differences in the observations of various examiners and in part on their differing theoretical orientations.

For example, one may cite the view of Griesinger and Sander who feel that aphasia represents a disconnection between visual and acoustic imagery in contrast to integrity of connection between acoustic and visual-imagery. This logical conflict is easily resolved by an analysis of Griesinger's acoustic-imagery in terms of a motor and sensory center. Moreover, the confusion of actions observed in aphasia patients may be explained to a great extent (in sensory aphasia) by the disturbance in comprehension of commands.

Aphasia falls under the broader concept of *focal psychic involvement.* An example may aid in understanding this idea. Meynert interprets maniacal movements on the basis of stimulation of motor areas by means of central pathways. If such maniacal movements are limited to a localized group of muscles and are constant over a period of time, one might be justified in assuming a circumscribed cortical lesion as the cause of the specific symptoms.[50]

Asymbolia represents one such focal disease which may be diagnosed only by means of psychic symptoms. Such forms of psychoses (commonly interpreted as insanity) which consist of auditory or visual hallucinations are probably caused, as is true of maniacal movements, by some type of stimulation of certain cerebral centers.

That the origin of sensation is referred to the sensory organ and so to the outside world, is as little strange as the referral of pain which the amputee transfers to the amputated toe. *Focal psychic diseases are therefore characterized by symptoms of the stimulation or loss of function of circumscribed groups of psychic elements.*

Focal psychic symptoms may be caused by disruption of the connecting fibers involved in the association of psychic elements, that is by disease of the cerebral white matter, as occurs in aphasia, which has been elaborated in such detail. Whenever lesions of the white matter remain undiagnosed, there is the possibility of falsely regarding such functions as insignificant. All higher psychic processes likely implicate the cerebral white matter.

Further investigation in the area of focal psychic disease must obviously be reserved for the psychiatrist. However, a true realization of pathological findings will only be possible if the anatomy of the cerebral white matter is adequately studied by means of prepared section specimens, since the fibers are otherwise poorly visualized.

The author is presently occupied in such an investigation, and since a study of material utilizing serial sections of dog and monkey brains is nearing completion, it is hoped that the results of these findings may be reported in the near future.[51r]

Breslau, May, 1874.

ADDENDUM

In the prologue to Hitzig's collected works, which appeared during the printing of the work here submitted, I found to my astonishment that the views there expressed concerning the significance of the cerebral cortex, and therefore in regard to aphasia, were identical to those I was just completing. It may perhaps not appear presumptuous then to mention my presentation of this theory of aphasia in November of the preceding year to a number of colleagues, with demonstration of the individual brain dissections for interpretation of the anatomical relationships.

This harmony of interpretation, moreover, fills me with even greater satisfaction, since it was achieved by entirely different methods. And this proves, furthermore, that anatomic and physiological experimentation, directed toward a deeper understanding of the brain, go hand in hand.

In the meantime, the death of Funke, (case 8), occurred. Pathological studies were carried out on June 23, 1874. Edema of the pia and general atrophy of the gyri were found. Apart from this, the right hemisphere was completely intact. A study of the convex surface on the left revealed an extended focus of yellow softening, which involved almost the entire primordial-gyral-arc and both margins of the Sylvian sulcus, above which the pia was adherent and opaque. The surfaces of the first primordial-gyrus facing each other were tightly adherent, and also adherent to the outer wall of the island. Exposure of the island and its resection could therefore be achieved only by careful dissection. There, thrombosis of the Sylvian artery could be observed, with conversion of the artery into a firm yellow, sinewy strand with anastamosis of smaller fibers. No trace of the lumen of the vessels could be seen.

The softening was limited anteriorly from the central to the first Leuret frontal gyrus, of which the anterior third alone was intact. A portion of the first primordial-gyrus into which the central sulcus terminates interiorly was also involved, as well as the inferior portions of both central gyri. The process extended broadly from behind these same gyri, occupying the entire lobe, which is formed by an anastamosis of the first and second temporal lines. The occipital pole and the more medial portions of the occipital lobe had maintained a normal consistency. The temporal lobe, on the contrary, was for the most part softened, the hippocampal gyrus alone revealing normal consistency. The island of Reil was reduced in all dimensions, presenting generalized, edematous softening.

A comparison of these findings with that of Rother (case 2) reveals in both cases a similarity in the involvement of the first temporal gyrus and its anastamosis with that of the second gyrus. Could this similarity be a matter of chance?

Finally, let us review the present status of various cases. The single persisting symptom in case 1, Adam, is agraphia. Beckman, case 3, on the contrary, is able to write fluently but continues to present a severe alexia. If improvement continues in both cases, as is anticipated, they will present respectively examples of isolated agraphia and alexia. Such symptoms appear to represent stages in the recovery of sensory and conduction aphasia.

APHASIA AND ANARTHRIA

Aphasie und Anarthrie

(Original publication in: Deutsche Med. Wchnschrft. 1882, p. 163)

[Wernicke's concept of a special speech pathway extending from Broca's area to the cranial nuclei and its implications regarding production of motor aphasia and anarthria were discussed at length in his 1884 essay "Motor Speech Pathway". Two years earlier he had presented this notion in a short paper "Aphasia and Anarthria". Wernicke later rejected the existence of such a tract specifically serving speech functions.]

Achieving an understanding of the relation of anarthria to motor aphasia caused by destruction of Broca's gyrus in the left hemisphere is beset with many difficulties. If this gyrus in reality represents a discharge point of the motor innervation necessary for the speech act, a fiber tract – which may be called the motor speech path – must exist connecting this point with the origins of the pertinent nerves in the medulla oblongata. The pertinent cranial nuclei on the floor of the fourth ventricle serves as the writing apparatus of a telegraph system with which the entire mechanism may be compared; if it is working, a third party may be able to read the telegram, i.e., in this instance, listen to it. More than this, it corresponds to the old-fashioned type of letter telegraph, and the disturbance in articulation (anarthria) relates to a loss of individual letters or certain sequences of letters of the ame. A motor aphasia would then result whenever that part of the motor speech path above these nuclei is disrupted; an anarthria, in contrast, always relates to a lesion of the nuclei itself.

Nevertheless, the axiom applies that only damage to the cerebrum itself causes aphasia, and that, in contrast, lesions in the pons or the cerebral peduncle etc. result not in aphasia, but anarthria, that is, an articulatory disturbance. This circumstance was earlier explained by hypothesizing the existence of an intermediate electrical switch in the lenticular nucleus. However, since that time, it has become evident that the anatomic structure of the lenticular nucleus opposes such an assumption. This, however, is completely incomprehensible and requires continued clinical confirmation. If one accepts this concept as conclusive, according to the principles which the author has presented in his text book of *Brain Diseases*, the following statements may be made:

1. Focal lesions are observed in the pons and cerebral peduncle in the presence of actual aphasia.
2. In a second series of cases, investigators expressly emphasize the disproportionately severe speech impairment – bordering on complete unintelligibility – in contrast to the minimal involvement of tongue and facial movement.
3. The motor speech path thus passes through the pons and cerebral peduncle, Superiority it follows an S-shaped course, its sagittally-directed mid-portion extending along the superior Burdach fissure; its anterior arm, the white matter of Broca's gyrus, and a posterior branch which courses obliquely down and inward, close to the sensory tract of the hemisphere, and continues on in the posterior branch of the internal capsule in its posterior half.

The motor speech path, including its source and terminal stations, forms an apparatus which functions, to a certain extent, independent of other neural input; thus, a motor aphasia is observed sometimes in isolation and sometimes in combination with a right-sided tongue and facial nerve paralysis. The latter paralysis also occurs alone, without aphasia, and is a common component-symptom of right-sided hemiplegia. But this independence does not extend further, and the integrity of the apparatus described does not.under all conditions insure normal speech production. If this were the case, a summation of bilateral focal symptoms, which is the basis of the so-called pseudobulbar paralysis, under certain conditions would leave speech intact, while for other movements, the tongue and lips would be paralyzed. Instead of this speech is always impaired to the same extent as other movements of the tongue, a circumstance which leads to confusion of the symptom-picture with an actual bulbar paralysis. As a consequence, under such exceptional conditions, the role which the right hemisphere obviously normally plays in the speech act is clear and, it supports the view, already expressed by Kussmaul, that a double stream of innervation courses from both hemispheres to the terminal bulbar apparatus, but that stream coming from the left hemisphere is by far the stronger. This moreover, explains the striking circumstance that aphasia not rarely occurs as an indirect localized symptom in acute focal disease of the right hemisphere. Of all functions of the left hemisphere those which normally require participation from the right hemisphere.

THE MOTOR SPEECH PATH AND THE RELATION OF APHASIA TO ANARTHRIA

Über die motorische Sprachbahn und das Verhältnis der Aphasie zur Anarthie

Original publication in: *Fortschr. der Medizin.* Vol. 2, 1884, p. 1.

Reprinted in: ***Gesammelte Aufsätze und Kritische Referate zur Pathologie des Nervensystems.*** Berlin: Fischer, 1893, pp. 71-91.

["The Motor Speech Path," a lengthy twenty-page essay, was published in 1884 in the last year of Wernicke's Berlin period. His interest in the problem of differentiation of aphasia and anarthia was first evident in a short paper published two years earlier on "Aphasie und Anarthie." Leyden's (1867) work on anarthia may well have stimulated Wernicke's further consideration of this problem.

In this work Wernicke hypothesized the presence of a motor speech path separate from the fiber tract serving other forms of voluntary action. The course of this tract was assumed to proceed from Broca's area posteriorly through the superior sulcus of the island close to the deepest fibers of the superior longitudinal fasciculus and the area of the inferior aspects of the parietal lobe in the posterior end of the Sylvian sulcus, from which point it coursed medially into the posterior part of the internal capsule and down to the cranial nuclei of the nerves serving the speech mechanism (H. Sachs, 1893).

Wernicke predicted the production of anarthia following partial destruction of the motor speech tract. The "transmission of concepts" in this event would still be possible. Total destruction of the tract above the cranial nuclei serving speech, however, would result in a motor aphasia. Moreover, Wernicke maintained that motor aphasia caused by lesions of the motor speech tract would inevitably be combined with symptoms of anarthia.

Several years later Wernicke rejected the existence of a special motor speech tract. His assistant, H. Sachs, reported in 1893 that in a personal communication Wernicke had modified his views on this subject and hypothesized that the speech fibers coursed together with other fiber bundles of the pyramidal tract involved in voluntary movement. This assumption was in part based on the absence of clinical evidence of intact production of speech in association with the absence of certain other voluntary non-speech movements of the speech mechanisms. This finding might be anticipated if the motor speech path did actually exist as a separate tract.

Apparently Wernicke was not aware at this time of a differentiation of the neural circuits of areas 44, 4, and 6. More significantly, the effects of small circumscribed lesions involving both fibers from Broca's area and the callosal fibers linking the frontal areas were evidently not known at this time. Such a lesion would result in the isolation of an intact Broca's area and the clinical picture of a subcortical motor aphasia. This clinical entity was confirmed several years later by Dejerine. Wernicke based his assumption of subcortical motor aphasia on the basis of disruption of the motor speech tract demonstrated in a number of case-studies. Among these was one reported by Andral in which a lesion of the tract was demonstrated, leaving Broca's area intact. (Wernicke, 1881, pp. 174-5). The location of this lesion or its combination with that of a second involving the right side suggests that isolation of Broca's area might have occurred, resulting in the picture of a motor aphasia.

The work also contains a brief review of other types of neurological disorders and concludes with a short discussion of left-sided dominance in language production.

Wernicke's hypothesis, therefore, regarding the neuroanatomical substrate of the clinical pictures of anarthia and aphasia, as discussed in this essay, is logically sound but inaccurate because of the limited knowledge of the neural circuits and their significance to speech production available at that time. Nevertheless, the paper is of historical significance because it represents one of the few discussions of this question which continues to tantalize workers interested in this area. Moreover, it clearly reflects Wernicke's characteristic creative and logical approach to scientific problems.]

1.

Older physicians will recall the great stir which was caused at the time when Broca's discovery became known in Germany, and was soon confirmed by numerous clinical observations. The question of the localization of cerebral functions had seemingly been resolved on the basis of negative findings. However, interest in the problem persistently revived, until it was finally quenched by the fresh perspective opened up by experiments conducted by Fritsch and Hitzig. I must now return to that time, which most of our colleagues will remember well, to get to the essential points of this subject.

Broca's primary thesis, it will be recalled, referred the loss of articulate speech which was often to be observed following apoplectic attack to a lesion of one particular area which has since been called Broca's gyrus. This claim was opposed by Trousseau who showed convincingly that a whole spectrum of speech disorders which he collectively designated as aphasia were caused by diversily located lesions. Elsewhere I have shown why the facts put forward by the two opponents could not be reconciled.

In spite of protect by Broca and Bouillaud, Trousseau's effective eloquence successfully invested the specific clinical picture described by Broca with an entirely different and much broader interpretation. As a result the two opponents were not contending on the same plane. What appeared to the public as a mere semantic dispute between the choice of two terms, Broca's aphemia and Trousseau's aphasia, proved on closer examination to be a conflict about things, not words since the two-terms referred to two different things. If Trousseau was conscious of his own behavior one might be permitted to say that it was a kind of feint whereby he appeared as victor in the argument. In any case we have him to thank for the unhappy fact that by the end of the decade Broca's opponents outnumbered his adherents and, moreover, that the question of localization was still open, as it had been at the beginning of the decade. It was soon obvious to anyone who studied the discussion that both opponents could readily be right. There was no true contradiction between Broca's claim that a sharply circumscribed localized lesion was the cause of a clearly defined clinical picture and Trousseau's that a broadly-conceived and compound clinical picture was attributable to manifold and variously located cerebral lesions. I have pointed out elsewhere that Trousseau's term aphasia embraces an entire complex of different clinical pictures of which Broca's aphemia represents only one.

An examination of the process by which one learns to speak leads to the conclusion that speech comprehension and the execution of the same, i.e. articulate speech, are in reality two independent processes. This independence can be demonstrated in pathological cases; either of these faculties may be lost without involvement of the other to any significant degree. Between the two processes only a bond of association exists, by which the child learns to mimic the speech sounds contained in words and by which adults also continue to be guided in the correct selection of those very speech movements which correspond to the intended acoustic effect. This analysis yielded three classes of speech disturbances: impairment of the passive aspect of speech (comprehension) the active aspect (the execution of speech) and finally only the loss of the capacity for association between these two aspects. One may then differentiate between sensory motor, and conduction aphasia; each of these impairments may be localized to different sites. Broca's aphemia is identical with one of these forms, motor aphasia.

In the foregoing I have given a brief outline of a paper published in 1874. Since then all of the essential features of this picture of aphasic disorders has been confirmed. It may be taken as an established fact that destruction of the so called Broca's gyrus always results in the motor form of aphasia while in the same way destruction of the left first temporal gyrus leads to the sensory form; on the other hand the location of damage finding expression in conduction aphasia can claim only relatively meager and inconclusive evidence. Even Kussmaul's textbook dealing with the disorders of speech in part reflects this interpretation viz in the sections of his work relating to clinical symptomatology. However, an exaggeratedly critical tendency which unconsciously permeates the entire work prevents him from assuming a decisive stand in regard to the localization of symptomatically discrete forms of aphasia.

One may be convinced of the accuracy of the facts presented as I am; however, it does not necessarily follow that only the designated sites need be the points of origin of the symptoms affecting them. Elsewhere I have censured the common error which holds that a specific focal symptom such as aphasia may be found only following destruction the relevant cerebral area itself. Quite the contrary, it occurs much more frequently in another way as an *indirect focal symptom*, as I have called it in that it is characteristic of most acute focal brain disease; in addition to the cerebral areas actually destroyed much of the neighboring environs are also damaged so that a temporary loss of function of these areas also may be observed.

The symptoms produced in this way characteristically show complete compensation after a time. Only in the event of certain breaks in connections do they become permanent. This brings me closer to my actual thesis. Broca's gyrus is commonly accepted to be merely the discharge point of the muscle movements by which articulated speech occurs. It thereby serves simultaneously as the source of a conduction pathway whose other known terminus is located in the motor nerve nuclei associated with the speech musculature. In speech, the facial hypoglossal, laryngeal and respiratory nerves are activated, and for this to happen the message dispatched from Broca's gyrus must first be transmitted to their source nuclei. Our problem, therefore, is to find the route, the telegraph line, by which the telegram is conveyed.

I have repeatedly stressed elsewhere that such a path must exist, and that its disruption must cause the same symptoms as the destruction of Broca's gyrus itself. I have pointed out that a series of observations which were in themselves indisputable and appeared to prove that not only Broca's area but others as well might be damaged in cases of chronic directly caused aphasia could only be interpreted, if one accepted the disruption of this path, as exceptions which proved the rule. For just as Broca's area functions as a speech center, it is equally certain that there must be a path leading from it to the nuclei named above. It is equally certain, again, that there must therefore be cases of motor aphasia caused by lesions in completely different locations from the normal. The actual existence of such cases, then, is more of a logical desideratum than something which could be brought forward against the localization of motor aphasia.

However, when we try to describe the exact nature and characteristics of this pathway, we come up against a strange obstacle. For this tract, which has been aptly named the motor speech path, can be regarded as a part of the collective motor tract of the left hemisphere, namely, it is a segment of that tract which transmits all voluntary impulses. For all other movements it is now thought that we have identified that pathway: it is none other than Charcot's pyramidal column and Flechsig's pyramidal tract; the characteristics which we know of this path will also, by analogy, have to be demanded of the motor speech path. Now, we know that the pyramidal tract is a direct pathway, and that it contains uninterrupted fibers which connect the motor areas of the cerebral cortex with the nuclei of the spinal motor nerves. If such a direct pathway also exists for speech movements, it follows that true motor aphasia does not arise simply from damage to the cerebrum, but from damage to any site above the bulbar nuclei associated with the speech musculature, as soon as it fulfils the condition that it completely severs the motor tract of the left hemisphere. Accordingly, true motor aphasia must also have been observed following destruction within the cerebral peduncle and the left half of the pons. Here, however, we seem to have run up against generally recognized clinical experience. That production of true aphasia can be caused only by focal cerebral involvement might be called a sort of article of faith, because it has been expressed so often and with such certainty by a large number of competent observers. This teaching holds that such cases occur less and less often the further the site of damage is from the cortex and especially, from Broca's gyrus. Moreover, it assumes that this form of aphasia does not occur at all in involvement of the cerebral peduncle or the pons. Any questioning of this dogma is regarded as a kind of heresy.

As is well known, it was Leyden's (1867) important findings that put the pertinent data relating to certain speech disorders caused by damage to the pons and cerebral peduncle in its proper place. He has demonstrated that the speech disorder so produced is not aphasic in character but rather amounts to a gross disturbance of the articulatory mechanism, which in true aphasia is usually left intact. For this type of speech disorder he has suggested the appropriate term *anarthia,* which has been commonly accepted.

If the motor speech path does in reality course directly to the bulbar nuclei, one might then ask why lesions of this tract are not aphasic in character in the lower section too? Why does the disturbance cease to be aphasia at a certain point and take on the appearance of anarthia? At which point and in what manner is this transition effected? Only a few years ago, before the direct course of the motor tract was definitely established, we were not faced with this dilemma. These facts first became commonly recognized through the work of Charcot and Flechsig. Earlier, Meynert's anatomical findings had seemed to resolve the problem, and it was held that the motor pathway which served voluntary function did not take the course previously described but functioned as a way-station in relationship to the great ganglia of the corpus striatum, the caudate and the lenticular nuclei. At that time, one could therefore logically hypothesize the occurrence of true aphasia only in the case of disruption of the motor pathway above these ganglia.

One might even still have held this hypothesis in regard to the motor speech path when the direct course of the pyramidal tract had been well-established. However, this assumption now seems untenable in view of my recent anatomic findings which demonstrate the lack of significant connections between the caudate and lenticular nuclei and the cortex, so that an anatomical basis for regarding these ganglia as a way-station also lacking.

Under these circumstances we must attempt to unravel the problem another way to test the accuracy of the evidence itself. This will require a comparison and differentiation of the characteristics of anarthia and aphasia.

The use of an analogy will help better than anything else to resolve the apparent contradiction which these facts present. Let us consider the passage of a telegram over two sections of telegraph apparatus. Broca's gyrus would then act as the dispatch-point, while reception and reading of the message would occur at the other area, the bulbar nerve nuclei. The dispatcher of the message is represented by the entire organ of consciousness, the cerebral cortex in toto. Destruction of Broca's area would prevent the dispatch, and an interruption in the connection would interfere with transfer of the message. Lesions of the nerve nuclei would result in garbling of the telegram. One might use the old fashioned letter telegraph as an example. If certain letters are missing in the apparatus, specific errors would be consistently repeated in the message. It is obvious that further interpretation would be necessary to complete the analogy, but this may suffice to indicate that total failure of the second apparatus has the same result as failure of the first, i.e. Broca's area. Therefore, we may conclude that sufficient *destruction of the related bulbar nuclei may cause true motor aphasia in addition to other symptoms.*

This statement requires some amplification. First of all, among such "other symptoms" we include the severe bilateral peripheral paralysis evident in the final stages of Duchenne's disease, progressive bulbar paralysis. A total inability to speak, or even, ultimately, to produce sounds at all, cannot in fact be differentiated in principle from true motor aphasia, with the exception of its consistent accompanying symptom of paralysis secondary to another cause, destruction of the nuclei. Whether residual expression, in the form of a few inarticulate sounds, is possible, and the degree of such expressive capacity, is dependent only on the extent of destruction. In certain cases in which the possibility of a motor aphasia in combination with bulbar paralysis may be entertained, diagnostic error can be avoided only by a careful review of the earlier stages of the illness. The difficulty involved in such diagnosis has long been recognized by writers who have studied the problems of aphasia in great detail. Intact writing ability in bulbar paralysis, in contrast to characteristic impairment of this skill in aphasia, is the main criterion which has been advanced for differential diagnosis of these two problems.

In my opinion, this statement is based on a fundamental error which assumes agraphia to be a consistent sequel to destruction of Broca's area, while this symptom does not necessarily follow disconnection of the motor speech path. The chief criteria in questionable cases, then, would be a typically gradual onset of the condition with transition of anarthia into aphasia.

The second condition for production of true aphasia on the basis of bulbar involvement lies in the acute, sudden onset of a specific disease process, and particularly, by processes causing softening of the areas implicated. (Hemorrhage does not come under consideration here because death rapidly follows.) In cases of the so-called apoplectic form of bulbar paralysis, traumatic destruction of the neural substance is so great that the entire nuclear area of the speech musculature is usually involved. As a consequence, complete loss of speech and inability to produce sound is observed during the early days and weeks of the illness in combination with other common bulbar symptoms. Again, in this event, differentiation between a more superior lesion interrupting the motor speech path, and a second lesion causing bulbar paralysis is not possible at this time on the basis of the actual pathology. This is particularly true if a marked right hemiplegia is present at the onset of the symptoms.

We have observed cases of aphasia which are equal in severity to a complete anarthia and which subsequently present a picture typical of a later stage of that problem. An essentially complete disconnection of the nerve nuclei is necessary for production of this condition. If impulses cannot reach these nuclei, the speech disorder retains the characteristics of anarthia. Such complete destruction of the nuclei, however, would be equivalent to total severance of the entire speech tract. It was this explanation which led us to interpret the severest level of anarthia as true aphasia.

This then leads to the question: How would partial destruction of the motor speech path just above the cranial nerve nuclei affect speech? Would such a speech disorder have the features of anarthia or of aphasia? Although one may try to invest the motor speech tract with various arbitrary yet unknown features, we must still admit that our knowledge regarding this tract is still very meager. However, it is definitely known that the motor-speech path is made up of various different kinds of fibers. One type of fiber, terminating uppermost, ends in the facial nucleus; the others can be traced to the nuclei of the vagal-accessory and hypoglossal nerves, and ultimately to those nuclei involved in respiration. All of these various fiber systems can then be found in this tract. Partial lesions of the tract, limited to this or that type of fiber, will result in the loss of specific nuclei only. This type of partial lesion would then produce anarthia.

We must emphasize, however, that we have as yet no picture of other partial lesions of the speech tract. In so far as it is possible to recognize partial motor aphasia it always consists in the ability to produce a limited number of words together with complete loss of the remainder of speech. However, one never observes a reduction of just one half of the patient's vocabulary. Preservation of one segment of the vocabulary with loss of another segment does not occur. Only in extremely isolated cases has the reverse of ordinary motor aphasia been observed, that is, consistent inability to produce specifically this or that word, while general expressive capacity is otherwise preserved.[52r] We may then essentially ignore the clinical existence of partial motor aphasia.

Therefore, it is not necessary to entertain the possibility of a partial lesion of the motor speech path, and we need only be concerned with the problem of differentiating between aphasia and anarthia. As has already been stated, anarthia must be caused by such lesions which involve fiber systems leading to their separate nuclei. If they are interrupted in toto, complete aphasia follows. It would be very interesting to trace the detailed course of these individual fiber bundles, and it would be particularly interesting to know at which level above the relevant nuclei the fibers leading to them diverge from the common speech tract. Only in this way can the various combinations of aphasia and anarthia which apparently so originate be determined. In any event the pertinent segment of the various fiber systems comprising the speech tract must be located in the area just superior to the nuclei, i.e., the pons, and we may assume that this tract is contained, in this split form, in a segment of indeterminate size in the superior section of the pons. It makes sense that focal disease of this area must preferentially produce anarthia, since only extensive lesions can completely disrupt a tract whose fibers are so diffuse, i.e. lesions which so significantly interfere with neural transmission to the nuclei on the opposite side that production of bulbar symptoms is inevitable. Therefore, the probability of aphasia without symptoms of anarthia is remote, while in contrast, a combination of aphasia with varying degrees of anarthia might occur quite readily.

This theory is so strongly supported by a number of case-studies that their observers are almost persuaded to label them as anarthia. However, in such studies the preservation of movement of the lips, tongue, etc. presents a marked contrast to the actual severity of the speech impairment. In these cases involvement of the left half of the pons was a consistent finding. The more superior the site of disruption along the motor speech tract, the more striking are the aphasic components of the disturbance and the less it is contaminated by symptoms of anarthia. After all, involvement of the cerebral peduncle, if severe enough to cause speech disturbance at all, customarily results only in aphasia. This is true only in involvement of the left cerebral peduncle. Lesions of the right peduncle do not generally produce speech impairment.

Sympathetic involvement of speech in the cases in question can occur only in a very specific way. Even if the possibility of a partial lesion of the speech tract is not entertained, one must still differentiate between various degrees of severity of impairment. A hemorrhage lying close to the path, but not disrupting it, may still interfere with transmission to such an extent that speech is impaired but not completely lost. The same may occur in focal softening. The type and mode of this condition has been discussed in my *Lehrbuch der Gehirnkrankheiten* [Text-book of Brain Diseases] in which all possible degrees of destruction from the mildest to the gravest have been presented. Just as indirectly produced hemiplegia may manifest itself in widely varying degrees of paralysis, so also with lesions of the motor speech tract. But since, as has been discussed above, the compactness of the speech tract would not permit the occurrence of partial lesions, one would expect in such cases to find complete loss of speech with equal impairment in all of its components. Thus, the resulting speech disturbance would present a consistent and specific clinical picture. For example, such patients would likely be able to utter but a few words in succession, and those only with great effort. Furthermore, one would predict difficulty in production of even minimal movements necessary for speech utterance. This is analogous to certain degrees of hemiplegia in which finger or arm movements can be executed only with great effort and are followed by marked fatigue. A special type of speech disorder, characterized by fading and decay of speech and voice, which has been discussed in my text-book, may, it seems to me, be included in this category. However, just as in a partial hemiplegia the impairment is limited preferentially to complex movements, so also decreased neural transmission along the motor speech path need not lead to complete or constant loss of speech. The more complex speech patterns will be more severely involved that the simple. This condition may result in another form of disturbance which I earlier described as lalling-speech, typical of childhood and characterized by the omission or substitution of those consonants which cause the greatest difficulty for a child learning to talk. The vowels, however, are generally completely unaffected.

A third form of speech disturbance which probably belongs to this general category is the slow, monotonous, but at the same time explosive type of speech pattern; however this may also be caused by a particular process, namely, that of sclerosis. One of its pecularities is that it produces symptoms of reduced transmission of the impulse, alternating with exaggerated motor effects.

This analysis permits us to formulate a more detailed concept of anarthria than was previously possible. Clearly the three types of speech disturbance just described do not belong to this syndrome. We shall instead have to look for the essence of anarthria in everything that points to a local disease process of the bulbar nerve nuclei or the branched-off fibers of the motor speech tract which represent them; and here the unequal extent to which the various nerve nuclei are involved in the speech disorder is just as crucial as the uniformity of the impairment of transmission in the motor speech tract is to that impairment of transmission.

2.

Let us now turn to the problem of tracing the course of the motor speech tract between the bulbar nuclei and Broca's gyrus. The detailed course of the speech path within the pons has not yet been definitely established for reasons which have been discussed above. There is a divergence of the tract in this area with significant transverse spread. It is not even known whether its course follows the anterior or posterior segment of the pons, and one can only roughly assume its position to be in the posterior portion of the lower half of the pons, but still in the anterior portion of the upper half, as is true of most of the other voluntary tracts. Cases of circumscribed focal disease of the cerebral peduncle are so rare that they likewise cannot be used to resolve this question.

However, one would not go seriously astray in suggesting that the following two statements are highly probable: 1) The motor speech path is contained within the foot of the cerebral peduncle. 2) At this point the motor speech path has already diverged from the remaining fibers of the motor pathway, the pyramidal tract. This assumption is based on evidence of the preservation of speech which has been observed in a number of patients with right hemiplegia caused by focal disease of the left cerebral peduncle. In contrast, another series of cases presented loss of speech in association with the hemiplegia.

The speech pathway can be found only in the posterior area of the internal capsule and lies fairly close to the sensory cerebral tract. This observation is based on the fact that only in focal disease of this area is chronic motor aphasia commonly produced in association with right hemiplegia and usually hemianesthesia. In many cases damage has been found in all other areas of the internal capsule including the anterior peduncle, the genu, and the anterior half of the posterior peduncle, viz. on the left side, without residual permanent motor aphasia. The observation that the right hemiplegia demonstrated by these cases is commonly accompanied by paralysis of the oro-facial nerve with deviation of the tongue to the right leads to the interesting fact that unilateral non-speech movements of the tongue, lips, and facial musculature are represented by cranial fibers other than those of the motor speech tract. It is believed that the cranial nerves may lie in the genu of the capsule in close proximity to the pyramidial tract. On this basis I had earlier assumed the likelihood of passage of the motor speech tract through this region.[53r] However, I am now forced to change this view since it has been disproved by the clinical facts, for while not a single example of motor aphasia produced directly by foci of the anterior areas of the internal capsule has ever been demonstrated, it is frequently found as soon as the posterior area becomes involved. Furthermore, it has been observed in a number of cases in which circumscribed foci in this posterior area have appeared among such mild generalized symptoms that one must assume the focal symptoms to have been directly caused. Moreover, indirectly caused motor aphasia appears to occur most easily in focal disease in this area and in the company of sensory disturbances. (Cf. my *Lehrbuch der Gehirnkrankheiten*, Vol. II, pp. 173, 176, 179.)

These statements may likewise be applied to the neighboring area of the foot of the corona radiata. To some extent this area parallels the posterior border of the lenticular nucleus, that area of the internal capsule which lies inward of it, and, higher above the foot of the corona radiata between the lenticular nucleus and the tail of the caudate nucleus. The sharp posterior projection of the island between the superior and inferior sulci of the Sylvian fissure corresponds to the same area on the outer wall of the hemisphere. From this point, the motor speech tract can only reach Broca's gyrus, its end-point by continuing along the superior Burdach sulcus, at the bottom of which it must turn to the front, possibly in the superior portion of the external capsule which lies alongside the upper border of the lenticular nucleus. However, in no event does it lie much higher than the superior border of the lenticular nucleus, since otherwise the many observed cases of disease in the medullary layer of the central gyri, which after all first turns upwards, would for the most part have been accompanied by aphasia, whereas in fact only unilateral paralysis of the lingual-facial area, or brachial monoplegias or combined monoplegias have been observed.

On the other hand, motor aphasia has been found in all cases in which the damage is not limited to the cortical substance but extends to an area beneath the level of the superior sulcus and to the uppermost part of the island gyri themselves even though Broca's gyrus itself is undamaged. The course of the motor speech tract along the upper border of the island gyrus can readily explain involvement of the island itself as the most consistent finding in aphasia apart from damage to Broca's area. In this connection, the reader may compare, for example, Kussmaul's (1877) discussion of speech disturbances in his *Störungen der Sprache,* pp. 141 and 144.

The extension of those same segments of the corona radiata containing the unilateral innervation of the face and tongue to the area of the genu of the internal capsule is consistent with the general radial arrangement of the corona radiata. The motor speech path follows a very different course. Here we must distinguish between a sagittal midsection extending longitudinally along the superior sulcus and two vertically directed limbs, of which the upper anterior, branch represents the medullary ridge of Broca's gyrus. The lower, posterior, limb courses downward and inward, along the posterior border of the lenticular nucleus to the internal capsule. The sensory tract follows this posterior elbow fairly closely. The sagittal midsection crosses, at the level of the central gyri, the unilateral facial and hypoglossal nerve fibers.

Let us now see if we can sketch all the consequences of this picture or whether we shall have to modify it, and if so how, in order to arrive at a complete and unambiguous account of the actual situation. If our information is accurate, the production of speech movement demands exclusively the apparatus described, including Broca's gyrus, the motor speech tract, and the bulbar nuclei,

We have then a tract which belongs exclusively to the left hemisphere, while the bilateral activity of the musculature used in speech is merely a consequence of the anatomic connections between the nuclei of both sides. Because of these connections, unilateral innervation from the left hemisphere is adequate to effect symmetrical muscular effects of both nuclei. According to this interpretation, these nuclei function as an independent mechanism, i.e. they are free of the right hemisphere as far as the production of speech is concerned. This then leads to the ultimate conclusion which I have consistently maintained in all of my writings dealing with the speech process, and which I must continue to hold, because it is in general an accurate reflection of the vast majority of data. The problem of the localization of the speech process in the left hemisphere must not be confused with the question of exclusive restriction of the organization of the speech apparatus to the left side. This frequent error has unfortunately hindered our achievement of a deeper understanding of the speech process.

Only by temporarily ignoring the exceptions relating to the localization of speech processes in the right hemisphere, and thus simplifying my task, could I hope to investigate successfully the principles applying to localization in the left hemisphere; the complexity of the question seems to me to require such a restriction of the field. However, it has never occurred to me to deny the existence of such cases, nor do I fail to recognize the great importance of this question. On the contrary, I have been well aware of the fact that even in partial brain atrophy, congenital or acquired, of the left Broca gyrus, speech is nevertheless generally acquired without difficulty. Furthermore, I myself have observed the fact that aphasia caused by destruction of Broca's area need not necessarily be permanent, but that the power of speech can be recovered. That therein I have been unable to see any obstacle, in principle, to the doctrine of speech localization follows from the view which I have steadily maintained in regard to the question of unilaterality of this localization. I have repeatedly referred to Hitzig's observation that the symmetrically working musculature of the tongue, face, jaws etc. can be made to contract bilaterally by electrical stimulation of only one hemisphere, and that in view of the existence of such pre-formed apparatus it would seem superfluous for the skills of speech to be learned by both hemispheres. On the contrary, one hemisphere would be sufficient, though I have again refrained from entering into the debate as to why it should normally be specifically the left hemisphere.

For the moment let us assume that the predominance of the left side is a matter of coincidence and consider more closely the mechanisms by which the relevant skill is achieved in the hemisphere. We already know that Broca's area contains a deposition of motor-representations necessary for speech which are finely perfected by means of training. Munk's findings have recently supplied more exact information in regard to the formation of such representations. The occurrence of speech movements is always simultaneously accompanied by simple and complex sensory impressions including such combinations as tactual, pressure, innervatory and kinesthetic sensations.

These specific combinations of persistently recurring sensations cause the gradual deposition of memory patterns in the cortex called motor-representations or motor images. The many varied types of movements which exist are reflected in just as many specific motor memory images. The child assimilates highly specific combinations of such motor representation during speech development. Once this has been achieved, production of speech is essentially independent of the sensations on which its learning originally rested. The pertinent motor speech images become then, once and for all, activating points of specific movement patterns. The trigeminal nerve thus plays a very significant role in this mode of speech formation, since it is without doubt that sensory nerve which transmits the fundamental motor, pressure, and kinesthetic sensations. That each hemisphere independently acquires its own movement patterns is a consequence of the fact that each half of the speech mechanism is supplied with its own trigeminal nerve whose central ending is located in the opposite hemisphere. It also follows that under certain conditions, the right hemisphere may also be predisposed to act as the discharge center of such movement. There is no fundamental reason which might refute the view that first one, then the other, then both hemispheres produce motor speech action; the complete symmetry of these movements makes it plausible that the left hemisphere alone is adequate for carrying out this activity.

Let us now return to our original assumption that it is coincidence which determines which of these conditions shall prevail. We have stated that the left hemisphere is the choice in the majority of cases. Indeed, it seems definite than in most people (i.e., those who are right-handed – the reverse is true of the left-handed) integrity of the left hemisphere is completely adequate to activate the speech mechanism. Right hemisphere lesions of almost any location or extent do not generally impair speech, or only temporarily. The latter, for example, may occur in a left hemiplegia sustained secondary to apoplectic attack. Although motor aphasia may often be observed in such instances, it is of very brief duration. As I have discussed in my textbook, this phenomenon provides the only indirectly-caused focal symptom of involvement of the left hemisphere. Complete recovery of speech is observed in such cases within several days at the latest, and even articulation remains only mildly impaired, even if there are marked symptoms of a left paralysis of the left facial and hypoglossal nerves. These facts appear to be in complete accordance with our earlier picture. Nevertheless, they only prove that in certain circumstances the participation of the right hemisphere in speech can be dispensed with, or that such loss on the right side may be substituted for by greater use and compensation by the left. This commonly occurs very rapidly.

Cases with acute bilateral focal involvement indicate that in other circumstances the contribution of the right hemisphere may become completely indispensable. Such cases often present exactly the same clinical picture of speech disturbances as is found in advanced stages of progressive bulbar paralysis. If the facts actually are as we have described above, and if the bulbar nuclei do indeed possess the supposed independence and capacity to be innervated by the left motor speech path alone, one would inevitably expect to find a case demonstrating intact speech but with the other side effects of bulbar paralysis, such as paralysis of the tongue, lips, pharynx, and larynx. If Broca's gyrus and the motor speech tract should be undamaged, the site of the lesion might be such that a combination of symptoms is presented. Such a picture might show paralysis of the *right* facial, hypoglossal etc. nerves, caused by a lesion on the *left,* and paralysis of the *left* facial, hypoglossal etc. nerves caused by a lesion on the *right,* though the speech act itself may remain completely unaffected. Instead of this, in all cases of pseudobulbar palsy we find the same degree of impairment in speech movement as is demonstrated in all other types of movement governed by the bulbar nuclei, and we never see even the faintest sign of the condition hypothesized under our first assumption mentioned above. Moreover, had such a case ever occurred, it would certainly have been recorded in the literature. The absence of such reported evidence would therefore lead one to assume that such a situation does not occur. In addition to this, there is the curious combination and the sequence according to which speech impairment becomes evident in such cases of bilateral focal damage. We know of cases which first demonstrated a right hemiplegia with involvement of the facial and hypoglossal nerves and aphasia. This was followed by compensation of the right-sided symptoms and gradual recovery of the aphasia, although autopsy revealed that the latter was produced by direct destruction within the Broca area. A new attack then followed with symptoms of left hemiplegia and a complete and permanent loss of speech. Necropsy studies revealed a second lesion in the right hemisphere, so situated that it produced disruption of the right facial hypoglossal tract. In this case the aphasia following the first episode was apparently caused by involvement of the left hemisphere, while the second was caused by involvement of the right. Wherein other cases, there was paralysis restricted exclusively to the facial and hypoglossal nerves, that is, facio-lingual monoplegia; the loss of articulation was concurrent with the other paralytic symptoms.

Even if we must therefore in any event attribute to the right hemisphere a certain measure of participation in the speech act, so that there is a bilateral downward flow of innervation from the hemispheres, there appears nevertheless to be a wide variation in the effectiveness of participation by the right side in this function. This has been demonstrated by studies of the persistence of aphasia in destruction of the left Broca gyrus. Complete destruction most frequently result in permanent aphasia, and the difficult art of speech cannot be relearned. In other cases, the combination of a gifted intellect and persistent effort over a period of years may be effective in developing a considerably primitive and clumsy mode of expression. A third group may present relatively rapid and more or less complete return of speech within a period of a few months, though agraphia usually persists over a longer period of time. In left-handed individuals the major innervation arises from the right hemisphere. All of these variations may be explained by the fact that the degree of participation by the right hemisphere is related to individual differences and is apparently dependent on circumstances still largely unknown. As the anatomic substrate for acquisition of motor speech representation is present in both hemispheres, but dominance of only one hemisphere is required for the actualization of speech, this kind of changing relationship can easily arise.

Now it is easy to explain why such severity of speech impairment is observed in most cases of focal disease of the pons. A well-defined aphasia would require restriction of the focal effects to the motor speech tract in the left half of the pons alone, without crossing over to the right half or disrupting the connections to the individual nuclei. Instead, on the one hand a lesion in the left half of the pons damages both the motor speech tract and the connections to the nuclei, and on the other hand, the connections on the other side do not escape the trauma, so that there is now a summation of bilateral effects, very similar to that of pseudo-bulbar paralysis. All such cases present a speech disturbance demonstrating the bulbar characteristics of anarthria, and the only variable is the extent to which transmission of the motor speech tract is still possible. If this tract continues to function well, pure anarthria is the result. However, should it too be involved, a mixture of aphasia and anarthria occurs, in which under certain conditions even the aphasic component of the speech impairment can be dominant.

Another circumstance which is now easily explained is the observed fact that in the case of apoplectic foci in the right hemisphere it is precisely the power of speech which is so relatively often affected sympathetically, so that it is not uncommon, in the period immediately following the attack, to find the combination of left-sided hemiplegia and aphasia. After a number of hours, days, or perhaps a somewhat longer period, there is usually complete remission of the aphasia with residual left hemiplegia, thus showing that the aphasia is only an indirectly produced symptom emanating from the left hemisphere. I have consistently interpreted such a finding in this way and have defended this hypothesis in my textbook. It still has to be explained, however, why of all the functions of the left hemisphere it is precisely that of speech which suffers when the right hemisphere suffers apoplectic damage, and why further symptoms of right-sided hemiplegia do not also occur, as a sign that the whole left hemisphere has been subjected to a particular trauma.

As has been discussed above, under normal conditions, the hemispheres work together in speech production, although in unequal proportion, with the greater share of innervation falling to the left hemisphere. If we now assume this to be, on average, 3/4 or 4/5 of the entire innervation necessary for speech, then 1/4 or 1/5 of the total would be supplied by the right hemisphere. If an apoplectic episode should start from the right hemisphere, this latter fraction of the total innervation would in any case be substracted from the whole. Moreover if there is any sort of involvement of the left hemisphere as a secondary effect of the trauma naturally that function would be involved which had already in part been impaired as a result of damage to the right hemipshere. However, movements which are under the exclusive control of the left hemipshere, such as function of the right arm, are least affected. To some extent an analogy may be made between this peculiar condition and that which prevails in other movements. For example, lateral eye movements are not exclusively under control of one hemisphere. Although lateralization to the right is primarily controlled by the left hemisphere, nevertheless, participation by the right is not completely lacking in this function. For example, in the event of a right-sided apoplectic focus, a conjugate ocular deviation to the right will follow as a consequence of involvement of the right hemisphere in many cases and as a consequence of the excessive participation of the left hemisphere, whose control is decisive for lateralization of the eyes to the right. The possibility of turning the eyes to the left, however, by means of strong effort, is not completely lost, since the left hemisphere is also invested with the capacity, albeit to a lesser extent. Nevertheless, in exceptional cases there may be an actual inability to lateralize to the left, particularly initially, or during the first few days following a severe attack. The same movement, then, is lost whose production normally depends 3/4 on the right hemisphere and 1/4 on the left. The traumatic effect on the left hemisphere, therefore, must now be evidenced in disturbance of this function, while the other functions of the left hemisphere may still be intact.*

* The work referred to forms the subject of a paper presented by the author at a session of the Association of Internal Medicine and reported in *Deutsch. med. Wochenschrift*. No. 13, 1882.

A CASE OF DEAFNESS AS A RESULT OF BILATERAL LESIONS OF THE TEMPORAL LOBE

by Carl Wernicke and Carl Friedländer

Ein Fall von Taubheit in Folge von doppelseitiger Läsion des Schläfelappens

Original publication in: *"Fortschritte der Medizin."* Vol. 1, No. 6, 1883
Reprinted in: *Gesammelte Aufsätze und kritische Referate zur Pathologie des Nervensystems.* Berlin: Fischer, 1893.

[This clinico-pathological study was carried out by Wernicke and his colleague Friedländer and first published in 1883. It is significant in that it represents the first detailed report of a pathologically-confirmed case of central deafness caused by bilateral temporal lesions.

Wernicke used this case study as an opportunity to reiterate his 1874 findings regarding temporal lobe function. The clinical picture of sensory aphasia is reviewed with the symptoms of specific abnormality in speech expression typically associated with this syndrome. The case under study presented such a picture before involvement of the right temporal lobe which was followed by deafness. Wernicke also used this opportunity to refer to the probability of crossed-deafness carried out by Munk and others. It should be remembered that auditory testing was still relatively gross at this time.

The controversy between Kussmaul and Wernicke regarding the appropriate designation of sensory aphasia is also alluded to in this paper. Kussmaul had renamed this clinical entity "word-deafness" in a monograph which he published three years following the 1874 "Symptom-Complex." Wernicke strongly objected to the use of this term because he felt it neglected the disturbance in oral expression characteristic of the syndrome. The impairment in auditory comprehension, as he repeatedly stressed, formed only "one part of that which we regard as an indivisible, unitary picture." The use of the term "word-deafness", moreover, tended to be confused with "pure word-deafness," a completely different and separate entity, clinically and pathologically.

This review is among the few case-studies published by Wernicke, who as Liepmann has commented, limited his publications to cases which presented new findings or which clearly illustrated particular problems which he felt required attention.]

This case review concerns a 43 year old woman who first suffered convulsions at the age of eighteen. This condition lasted for a period of one year and was accompanied by falling and loss of consciousness. Good health apparently then prevailed until September, 1879, at which time she complained of headaches involving the frontal and parietal areas, nausea, vomiting, and the reappearance of convulsions. The latter were epileptic in nature, occurred several times per week, and lasted up to fifteen minutes in length. Gradual development of awkwardness and a tremor of the left hand when it was used was then observed. For example, the patient often dropped a cup, though she could still grasp objects firmly.

In the first part of April 1880, the attacks assumed a specific form. Prior to an attack, the patient noted depression of mood followed by tremor and shaking of the left hand, after flexion of the elbow and extension of the wrist; the jerking then progressed to the shoulder area. The patient could manage to say "The thing has again come upon me", after which loss of consciousness would follow with generalized convulsions. During the same period the patient began to consume unusually large quantities of water, indeed by the pailful. She complained of constant thirst and passed conspicuously large volumes of urine. During this time those around her noticed that she became motionless, presented the appearance of stupidity, and was hard of hearing. She did not always understand even when shouted to and answered inappropriately, without doing what was asked of her. She excused this behavior by saying that she was unaware of it. No impairment in vision or hearing had been observed prior to this. She was still able to busy herself with handwork.

One June 22 the patient appeared to suffer an apoplectic attack. Aphasia and a right hemiplegia were demonstrated and she was admitted to the city hospital. Initially speech was limited to the production of inarticulate sounds, although there had been a complete return of consciousness. During the next weeks improvement of all symptoms was observed. By the time of her discharge on August 4, it was observed that, although speech was possible, the patient could not make herself understood. A moderate right hemiparesis involving the arm was still fairly marked. The patient's landlady observed that she spoke in a confused manner and initially thought her to be insane or drunk. It was impossible to understand the patient, nor did she understand what was said to her. Communication was completely impossible.

On September 10 the patient was readmitted to the hospital with a mild paresis of the left arm which particularly involved finger movements. Nothing more was observed of the paralysis of the right side. The patient appeared to be confused and was completely deaf, so that it was impossible to communicate with her. Moreover, her speech was apparently impeded by excessive saliva secretion in the mouth, and was unclear. During October symptoms of a severe leukemia were noted, followed by repeated vomiting of blood in large quantities. Death followed on October 21.

Section was carried out on October 22, by C. Friedländer.

Anatomic Diagnosis

Syphilis. Viscious softening of both temporal lobes. Proctitis ulcerosis with perforation into the vagina. Gummata of the liver. Significant enlargement of the spleen. Leukemia, moderate in degree. Hemorrhage noted in the stomach and intestine.

A well-nourished individual. Extensive panniculas. Mild edema of the lower extremities.

The bone marrow of the femur was greyish-red in color containing many nucleated hemoglobin-colored cells. The ratio of white to red blood corpuscules was 1:7.

Little blood was found in the heart. The lungs were likewise pale although clear, as was the pharynx. There were enlargements of the spleen which was more than four times greater than normal. (Length: 210; Width: 130; Depth: 40) Trabecula: pale red. Follicle: unclear. Spleen: tenacious in consistency.

One-half liter of bloody content was observed in the stomach with occasional coagulated blood. The gastric mucosa was bloody and firmly adherent. No defects. Blackish content of the lower part of the ileum. Both kidneys were very pale, otherwise clean.

Some atrophy of the liver was noted with marked scarring on the surface. On cross-section, more pea-sized, cheese-like deposits, streaked with scar tissue, were evident.

The rectum demonstrated ulcerous scarring on the surface, moderate constriction, and a perforation in the fossa navicularis of a size which readily admitted the scope. Normal mucuous membrane could be seen in the lower end of the scope with sharp margins on the ulcerated surfaces.

The dura mater was under only moderate tension and was firmly adherent to the pia and brain substance of both temporal lobes and the projection portions of the inferior aspects of the right parietal lobe, extending on both sides almost to the size of a one-mark coin. Softening of the brain substance, which was partly white and partly brown in color, was noted in the area of the adherent coverings, and its environs.

No abnormalities were found in the brain.

On microscopic examination after the brain had been hardened the inner aspects of the dura revealed large-celled granulation tissue with homogeneous, minimally-fibrillar, intercellular substance. There was a complete lack of normal cortical substance, particularly of the ganglia cells in the area of the involved parts.

The brain was then preserved in Mueller's solution, and the following pathological study was carried out by C. Wernicke.

On cross-section of the left temporal lobe, somewhat behind the mid-point of its longitudinal extension, a neoplasm was found which involved the entire mass of the first and second gyri and a neighboring portion of the fusiform gyrus. The corona radiata of the temporal lobe in its entire expanse was likewise involved.

Narrowing somewhat, the neoplasm extended anteriorly, confining itself to the substance of the first and second gyri up to the boundary of the anterior and middle third portion of these gyri. Here the dura mater merged completely with the pia mater and the brain surface. Macroscopically, the cortex and medullary lamina revealed changes characterized by partially scarred and partially gelatinous looking tissue. In regard to its posterior border, the process

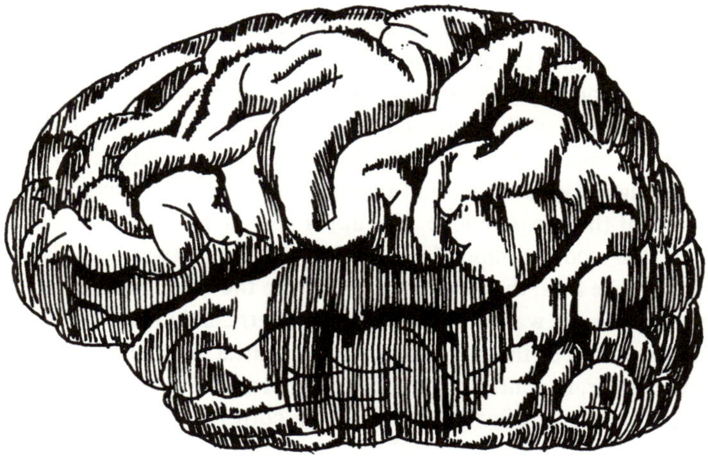

FIG. 12

Left Hemisphere
Bilateral Cortical Deafness

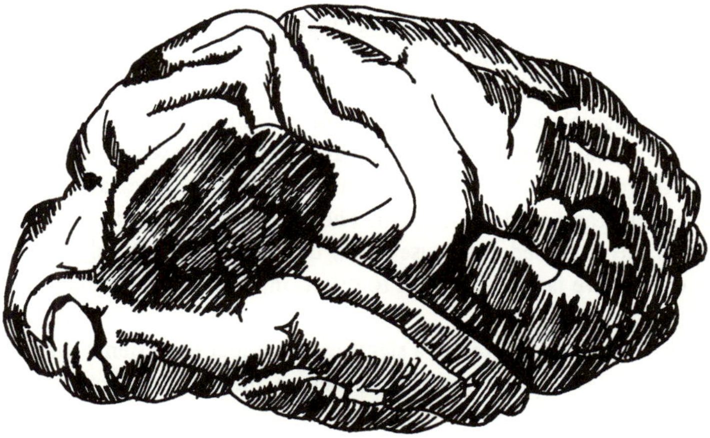

FIG. 13

Right Hemisphere
Bilateral Cortical Deafness

extended longitudinally somewhat posteriorly into the substance of the second gyrus to a point approximately one-half inch from the inferior occipital sulcus, the rear boundary of the temporal lobe.

In the right hemisphere there was involvement of only the most superior and posterior areas of the temporal lobe, bordering on the parietal lobe. The chief changes implicated the inferior parietal lobe, extending from that point along the angular gyrus to a point superior to the anterior occipital sulcus in the origins of the occipital lobe. The upper parietal lobe and the inferior branch of the second temporal gyrus remained completely uninvolved.

In this entire area, the dura was adherent to the brain surface. On cross-section, the process was found to be more superficial in the posterior portion with no extension of the neoplasm into the sagittal layer of white matter. Farther anterior, in contrast, the process penetrated deeply, extending into the area of that layer of white matter which corresponds to the merging of the corona radiata of the temporal lobe and that of the parietal lobe. Even in the preserved, hardened brain the softened, half-viscious consistency of the corona radiata of the inferior parietal lobe could be recognized. At the level of the central gyri everything was essentially back to normal, and the rest of the brain demonstrated no changes.

1. The outstanding interest of this case lies in the bilateral lesion of the temporal lobe and the resultant total deafness. The causative relationship between the two symptoms is not in question. It is most clearly seen in the fact that the hearing difficulty developed only at the onset of the brain disease and worsened during the course of the illness. The fact that the patient's hearing had previously been good was well-established. Apart from brain disease such a rapidly-increasing deafness could be explained only by new and rather marked changes of the middle and inner ears on both sides. Because such a chance complication might not be beyond the realm of possibility, although obvious changes were not evident on fresh section of the petrous temporal bone, further examination, which we would like to acknowledge with gratitude, was willingly carried out by Dr. Luca and proved negative, except for a mild dry catarrh. Therefore, involvement of the auditory apparatus was excluded as a cause of the deafness. This left only one other possible causative factor still open to question, that of intracranial involvement.

It has been demonstrated in a significant number of patients that bilateral deafness may develop as a symptom of severe, increased skull compression. Some cases of this type involve tumors of the posterior skull cavity. In the others, there is always a marked internal hydrocephalus which extends into the fourth ventricle. The pathological findings in our case indicated that increase of skull compression of any note was definitely not responsible for the problem, since viscous infiltrate of the brain often occurs without any evidence of pressure-effects. Therefore, one might rather be inclined to attribute it to the softening rather than to a tumor. The deafness could then be explained only on the basis of the two lesions of the temporal lobe, presenting essentially a central deafness in its narrow sense.

The anatomic basis of this symptom must still be interpreted. We have repeatedly referred above to both temporal lobes, although the right temporal lobe appeared superficially to be only mildly involved, while in contrast, the chief damage implicated the inferior parietal lobe. In reality, however, the findings in the right hemisphere amounted to significant destruction of the temporal lobe. Detailed examination revealed evidence of major extension of the lesion in its inner deep aspect at the boundary between the inferior parietal and the temporal lobes including the corona radiata.

Interruption of the corona radiata of the temporal lobe results in loss of sensory communication with the outer world and if the acoustic tract has its central area of spread there, this amounts to the same as severance of the acoustic tract. It will be recalled that there was disruption of the corona radiata in the left temporal lobe. However, in this case, a not insignificant destruction was simultaneously found in the cortex of the temporal lobe.

Our knowledge of temporal lobe function is still new.* I first reported in 1874 the first case studies demonstrating that destruction of certain areas of the left temporal lobe in man was followed by a characteristic disturbance in hearing, in which the spoken word was heard but not comprehended. On the basis of these findings it was concluded that the memory images of auditory sensations were deposited in the temporal lobe, and from that it was further concluded that the auditory nerve must reach the temporal lobe. This work was the starting point of a splendid series of experiments by which Munk obtained more detailed information on the central projection areas of the optic and acoustic nerves and, specifically in regard to hearing, confirmed my views by showing that destruction of one temporal lobe in the dog results in a crossed-deafness.

Strangely enough, although many years have passed since that time, clinical support of this finding has been lacking. So far we have one case, reported by Hutin in 1877, in which a significant loss of hearing in the opposite ear consequent to softening of the temporal lobe, and a second case reported by Schiess-Gemuseeus (1870), in which there was likewise a tumor of the left temporal lobe and complete contralateral deafness. However, in both of these cases there was inadequate proofof the normal functioning of the auditory organs themselves, and in the case of Schiess-Gemuseeus, the deafness was expressly described as having been of long standing. Only very recently (1882) has Vetter reported a case of contralateral deafness following a lesion of the internal capsule. However, in this patient also, the examination of the hearing organ itself was inadequate.

* From this point onwards the article is the work of Wernicke alone.

Therefore, complete crossing of the acoustic tract in the hemispheres in man cannot yet even be considered to have been definitely established. Our case can prove nothing in regard to this either. However, as the result of an uncommonly happy coincidence of circumstances, this patient does present evidence that the acoustic nerves do reach the temporal lobes, since bilateral lesions of the fiber bundles of this lobe, as observed in this case, produced complete deafness. Therefore, the temporal lobe in man may be definitely designated as the central abodes of auditory sensation.

2. However, in addition to this, the particular type of speech disturbance presented by the patient demands our attention. I do not refer to the speech disturbance which occurred in connection with the right hemiplegia secondary to the apoplectic attack, for this, as is also true of the paralysis, must be considered as an indirect focal symptom, independent of the site of the tumor. The fact that speech was lost and the patient unable to speak, or able to utter only a few simple words, is consistent with the notion of the transience and indirect production of the right hemiplegia. Evidence of *motor aphasia*, as it may most appropriately be called, was again only transiently present in our patient. Very different indeed was the chronic impairment of expressive language which the patient maintained until her death. This is in keeping with the findings of a series of cases presenting destruction of the first left temporal gyrus. We have already alluded to this point above, but it must now be pursued in even greater detail.

Ever since publication of my first work (1874) there has been repeated confirmation of the fact referred to above, that loss of memory images of auditory sensation simultaneously affects speech expression. Patients who do not comprehend the spoken word produce a seemingly confused type of speech with the result that they are often, as in this case, regarded as mentally ill. However, the rest of their behavior completely contradicts such a diagnosis, and a careful analysis of the nature of their speech enables us to establish the basis for this appearance of confusion.

Such a patient typically has many words at his command but often substitutes incorrect words for the appropriate expression. Repeated misspeaking, a characteristic of these patients, may prevail to such an extent that entire sentences are inserted in the wrong place, and slips of speech occur in the heat of the moment, resulting in complete distortion of meaning. This problem may be inconsistent in occurrence and is not always readily obvious. At times, for example, correct speech usage may occur by good fortune under the influence of strong emotion. In general, however, the typical pattern of misspeaking prevails, and this symptom, in combination with the impairment of speech comprehension, completely explains the difficulty of conversing with such patients as well as the impression of generalized confusion which they regularly present.

The consistent simultaneous occurrence of these two symptoms, just analyzed, compels us to postulate the hypothesis already submitted in the work cited above. One must postulate that the presence of the acoustic-imagery during speech production operates as a constant unconscious monitor, and that loss of such imagery results in disruption of this monitoring process. The existence of just such an inner relationship between the acoustic memory imagery and speech movements is very strikingly demonstrated by our case. Before the patient came to autopsy, our knowledge of the problem was limited to the existence of the bilateral deafness. However, the findings relative to the left temporal lobe caused us to hypothesize a disturbance in speech expression as described above and our hypothesis was completely confirmed by the subsequent—observations.

This patient, as well as many cases reported by others, completely supports the findings leading to the major conclusions which were submitted in my work of 1874. The observation has been confirmed that the form of impairment in speech expression described above, which I named *sensory aphasia,* is a common sequel to destruction of the left first temporal lobe. We see in this what after Broca's discovery, the most important clinical finding in support of the fundamental basis of the doctrine of localization, which is now almost universally accepted. This statement can be made with confidence since our clinical findings have for the first time provided evidence that memory images of a particular sensory area can be lost due to damage to a particular location in the brain. Moreover, even at that early stage this fact led us to conclude the fundamental principles, and we accurately outlined the doctrine of memory images which now lies before us, almost fully realized. We are aware that this has provided the impetus for further experimental study of this question.

In matters of such significance, we cannot allow our proprietary rights to be violated. My monograph, *The Aphasia Symptom-Complex* (1874), was followed in 1877 by Kussmaul's book, in which he described anew the same form of speech disturbance which I had previously described under the name of sensory aphasia, without however, holding my claim as worthy even of mention. "Newly-described" is in fact no overstatement, since Kussmaul at the same time christened it anew, permitting it to go out into the world under the name of "word-deafness," without making his reader aware that it had already existed under the name of sensory aphasia. This rather questionable procedure would have had little adverse effect on the matter, had the name been as appropriate as my own. But, as can be seen from our discussion above, the term "word-deafness" describes only one part of that which we see as an indivisible, unitary picture: for in addition to their word-deafness, such patients are also always aphasic. But Kussmaul, completely misunderstanding the major issue, furthermore suppressed the facts of my localization of the disorder which was based on the findings of two autopsy studies, demonstrating that the disorder was due specifically to destruction of the first temporal gyrus. Because he himself did not have autopsy studies at hand, he dispensed with any kind of localization. To a great extent this is the reason why the question of localization stands on such precarious footing throughout his entire book. Kussmaul's contribution to clarification of this question is confined to his suggestion of the term "word-deafness". I was therefore able, in my *Lehrbuch der Gehirnkrankheiten,* to refer exclusively to my earlier publication, without leaving out anything that was essential. Kussmaul must have had ample opportunity to correct his account. Only recently he has deemed it necessary to express himself in regard to his current interpretation of the third sentence on page 52 of his book. Since he allows all the others to stand, however, I find myself finally obliged to contribute to their rectification myself.

II. WERNICKE'S MIDDLE APHASIA PERIOD

RECENT WORKS ON APHASIA

Einige neuere Arbeiten über Aphasie

Original publication in: *Fortschritte der Medizin.* Vol. 3, 1885, p. 824; Vol. 4, 1886, pp. 377, 463

Reprinted in: *Gesammelte Aufsätze und kritische Referate zur Pathologie des Nervensystems.* Berlin: Fischer, 1893, pp. 92-129.

[Wernicke's second important monograph on aphasia appeared in 1885-86, one decade following his original contribution. This essay is not primarily concerned with a critical review of the aphasia literature of the day, as its title deceptively suggests. Wernicke rather uses a brief over-view of the recent French, English, and German works as an approach to a comprehensive presentation and further elaboration of his aphasia theory.

"Recent Works," although overshadowed by the more dramatic 1874 work and the final 1906 monograph, nevertheless contains the clearest and most detailed exposition of the Wernicke aphasia doctrine.

Lichtheim's work appearing in 1885 apparently stimulated a further elaboration of the concepts first formulated in 1874. His classification was based on Wernicke's earlier three-fold division of motor, sensory, and conduction aphasia forms. The introduction by Lichtheim of a concept center into the Wernicke schema, hinted at in the earlier original monograph, formed the summit of the model and permitted the prediction of an additional aphasia form, transcortical aphasia, the seeds of which were also alluded to in the 1874 work. Moreover, Lichtheim expanded the lower tiers of the Wernicke model in his description of peripheral conduction aphasia and peripheral conduction speech deafness, later modified by Wernicke and designated as subcortical motor and sensory aphasia.

In this essay, Wernicke devotes specific attention to a discussion on the disorders of reading and writing, describing a classification of such disturbances in a system parallel to that of the aphasias in his division of subcortical, cortical, and transcortical alexia and agraphia.

In this section of the monograph a new concept, the application of temporal relationships to language mechanisms, is discussed with particular emphasis on possible processes involved in reading and writing. This idea was originated by Grashey (1885) who had published a case-study of an aphasic patient who could recall words only by means of writing. Wernicke based his notion of reading as a process of letter-spelling largely on Grashey's work. This idea, which was a product of the associationistic psychology of the time, was soon discredited. Wernicke's inclusion of a discussion of this subject in "Recent Works" is of historical interest and is not generally discussed in detail in English references.

Three concepts important to the formulation of the aphasia model are emphasized in this monograph: concept-formation. transcortical function, and inner language, i.e., the "word-concept" in Wernicke's terminology. Wernicke adapted the Lichtheim additions and incorporated them into his aphasia schema and classification system which included seven aphasia forms and parallel categories of the alexias and agraphias. Lichtheim's triangular diagram of the model was modified by broadening its summit which represented the concept center to emphasize the extensive cortical expanse involved in conceptualization.

The final aphasia schema represents a theoretical model of language and psychic function in which the basic framework alone, i.e., the motor and sensory speech centers and the known association tracts only, were assigned a neuroanatomic localization. This fact has frequently been misunderstood by some of Wernicke's critics who tended to apply too literal a neuroanatomic or "mechanistic" interpretation to his theory. This error may readily be made if interpretation of the schema is attempted without an appreciation of the characteristic Wernicke approach of integrating empirically–derived data within a deductively-formulated model.

"Recent Works" represents a comprehensive and thoughtful review of aphasia theory. Written in a direct and simple style, it reflects a more mature Wernicke than was evident in the more dramatic earlier 1874 work. It may be considered among the important monographs on aphasia produced in the decade of the 1880's and in its own right is a significant contribution to the aphasia literature.]

During the past few years a succession of new works on aphasia have appeared ed, and we shall attempt to review the most pertinent findings which have emerged from such studies. However, it will not be possible to include the mass of clinical reports which have contributed essentially nothing new. Professional interest in this subject has yielded two major points of view. The first, which is essentially psychological in orientation – at least in its present state of development – tries to analyse the aphasia symptom-complex into its component parts. In so doing, it attempts for the first time to establish a precise theory of the existence of cortical centers in the human brain whose correlative connections and functions are achieved by means of open circuits, i.e., the so-called association pathways. The second concept proposes localization of these various circuits and centers to different areas of the brain. It can be dealt with only when the reader has been prepared by a review of the clinical analyses of individual case studies and has classified them according to the centers and conduction pathways which have failed.

The Symptomatology of Aphasia

1.

The reader may find a historical review of the literature in the initial section of my essay, "The Motor Speech Pathway."

The cerebral centers under consideration are, it is true, anatomically preformed, but their functional content represents the unique acquisition of each individual, usually during childhood. The child learns to understand the speech of others and thereby develops a center for speech comprehension. He then learns to express himself aloud, thereby acquiring a center for complex motor speech patterns. Speech mimicry, which is of paramount importance in this training process, is dependent on the usage of a conduction pathway connecting these two centers in such a way that each acoustic image arouses the corresponding combination of movements. This leads to the following schema of the speech apparatus which was first submitted in my work of 1874 and which since that time has found almost universal acceptance among clinicians.

A center (a), in Figure 14, located in the central projection area of the acoustic nerve, contains the store of memory images of the speech sounds or the

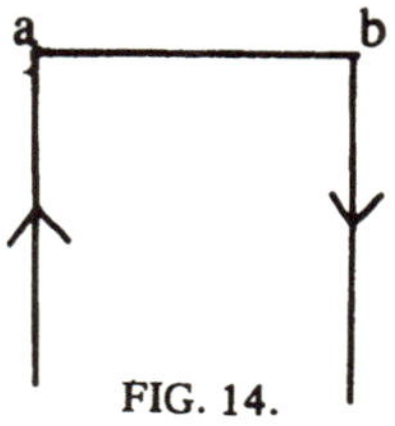

FIG. 14.

Schema of the Psychic Speech Reflex

(a): Center of acoustic speech imagery
(b): Motor speech imagery

"acoustic images." The center (b), situated in the so-called motor zone of the cortex, is likewise a depository of memory images of motor speech patterns which we may refer to as "motor speech-representation" or "motor speech images." The latter cause activation of speech movements by means of a centrifugal pathway leading to the pertinent bulbar nuclei. A centripetal tract, that of the acoustic nerve, transmits to the first center. These centers are connected by means of an association pathway (a- -b) which is utilized in mimicry of speech sounds. The destruction of center (b) causes motor aphasia, that is, loss of speech with intact speech comprehension, while destruction of center (a) results in sensory aphasia, that is, loss of speech comprehension with preservation of basic speech capacity. The disruption of the pathway (a- -b) causes word-confusion in speech, a symptom to which Kussmaul has aptly applied the term "paraphasia," and which I have designated conduction aphasia, provided that speech comprehension in center (a) and speech expression in center (b) are undamaged. Most French authorities such as D'Heilly et Chantemesse (1883), Prevost (1883), Dejerine (1884), Pitres (1884), and particularly, Charcot (1883a; 1883b), whose studies I shall return to later, have endorsed the existence of these two centers, i.e. the most essential features of this shcema. Among Italian writers, Seppilli (1884) has espoused the same point of view in his valuable work, as is also true of the American authorities Starr (1884) and Amidon (1885).

The studies of Seppilli and Amidon agree in that they both endorse the concept of sensory aphasia as a specific form and have verified its existence with case studies of their own. General acceptance of the concept of sensory aphasia as a specific form was won only with great difficulty.

In England two authors, Jackson and Broadbent, merit particular mention because of their authority. A resumé of their views as expressed in numerous publications in English periodicals is to be found in J. Ross's comprehensive textbook (1883). Ross associates himself with Broadbent in regard to the question of cerebral centers. Broadbent's concepts and my own are in fairly close agreement as far as I can see, and are only unnecessarily complicated by his assumption of two more special centers. one of which is involved in naming and the other in sentence formulation. Recently, Broadbent (1879) has reaffirmed his complicated schema, while Ross, on the other hand, abandoning it, has openly accepted my own. Jackson, however, has never at all espoused such kinds of schemas. Even in his most recent publication he lays primary emphasis on the differentiation of emotional and intellectual speech. For him, the essence of aphasia consists in the dissolution of intellectual speech with varying degrees of preservation of emotional speech. In Germany, Rosenthal (1885), Berger (1885), Kahler (1885), and particularly, Lichtheim (1884; 1885a; 1885b) have offered complete support to the schema described above, and to my knowledge of noted authorities only Westphal (1884) makes an exception, by stating in his Journal that in his view "the currently popular division of aphasia into various forms, atactic (motor), amnestic, sensory,etc., is not justified on the basis of clinical data." He thus maintains the view which he adopted in an earlier publication of 1874. Just precisely which view Kussmaul now holds is not readily apparent in his most recent facetious attack on localization theory.

As may be seen from this summary, public opinion in the major developed countries almost unanimously favors our interpretation. The few exceptions which can be found represent champions of an obsolete approach. Such unanimity, however, won only after collection of a large number of independent case studies, would seem to justify our statement that the existence of both centers, as defined above, may now be regarded as beyond all doubt.

One might even go a step further, as has already occurred in all quarters, and try to explain the reading and writing disorders so frequently observed in aphasia on the basis of two other completely analogous centers. Analogous to the speech comprehension center in the acoustic area is a center serving comprehension of written material in the visual cortical area. Analogous to the speech motor center a center for movements involved in writing. The symptoms of alexia and agraphia (to retain the old, established terminology), are explained on the basis of the failure of these centers.

The following schema, illustrated in Figure 15, may then be formulated. Let χ be the location of visual memory images of written symbols, and let β be that of graphic motor imagery. Destruction of χ would then result in alexia as an analog of sensory aphasia, while destruction of β would produce agraphia as an analog of motor aphasia. However, the hypothesis of the exist-

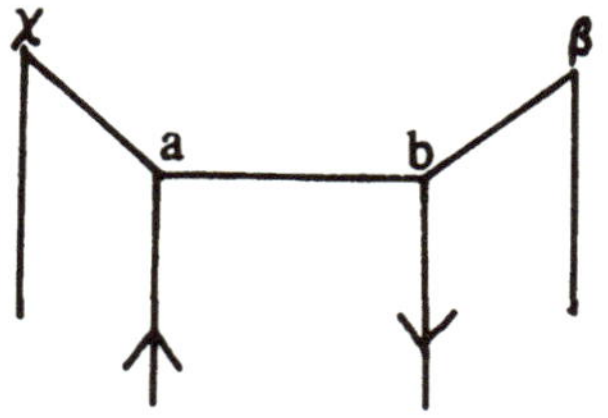

FIG. 15.

Schema of Reading and Writing

(a): Acoustic speech imagery
(χ): Visual letter imagery
(b): Motor speech imagery
(β): Graphic motor imagery

ence of such specific centers may be justified only on the basis of appropriate clinical case studies, for even if memory images of written signs are undoubtedly located in the visual cortical region, just as those of the speech sounds are contained in the acoustic area, it is nevertheless questionable, and, I believe, as yet unproven, if they always lie together and are localized at a particular point of the visual cortical region. The same is true of the graphic motor images. Undoubtedly, they are also contained somewhere in the cortical area involved in innervation of the upper extremities. However, confirmation by an adequate number of clinical case studies is necessary before their deposition in a specific area can be definitely established. I shall return later to a discussion of the curious cases which Charcot (1883a; 1883b) and Pitres (1884) use to support the existence of just such a specific center.

In my first work on aphasia I took pains to show that in such an interpretation of the speech process as has been reviewed above, we had probably found the scheme of cortical function as a whole, that memory images were the psychic elements populating the cortex in a mosaic-like arrangement as a functional development, which may very well be localized according to the regions of the nerve-endings, so that the acoustic images find their abode within the cortical terminals of the acoustic nerve; the visual images, within the cortical endings of the optic nerve; and the olfactory images in that of the olfactory nerve and so on. Likewise, the motor memory images or movement-representation could be located in the cortical sites of the motor nerve origins. For example, the images of speech movements would then be found in the Broca gyrus and those of writing within the cortical area serving arm movements, etc. Apart from that I assumed only that the discharge-sites of voluntary movements and the depository of motor images were identical. Any higher psychic process, exceeding these mere primary assumptions, could not I reasoned, be localized, but rested on the mutual interaction of these fundamental psychic elements mediated by means of their manifold connections via the association fibers. Since that time I have become even more strongly convinced, particularly on the basis of clinical studies of aphasia, that we are not justified in going beyond this elementary hypothesis.

If, on the other hand, we examine Charcot's schema of the speech process and its disorders, we detect certain superfluous assumptions which, precisely because of this, are untenable. In the process of developing speech comprehension and reading, the child acquires *une mémoire auditive* and *une mémoire visuelle* by means of the acoustic and optic nerves. The union of these two *mémoires partielles* forms the passive phase of the speech process. The active phase consists of the development of two further mémoires partielles, the partial memory for speech movements and that involved in writing movements. Each of these partial memories may be lost, thus leading to a classification of four different forms and two chief categories of aphasia:

A. Sensory Aphasia	)	Word-deafness: Involvement of the acoustic area.
Aphasie de réception	)	Word-blindness: Involvement of the visual area.
B. Motor Aphasia	)	Motor Aphasia: Involvement of speech movements.
Aphasie de transmission	)	Agraphia: Involvement of writing movements.

Each of these four types is illustrated by clinical examples. It is evident that they correspond, in a rather more schematic form, to our interpretation discussed above. But now Charcot makes a further assumption which clearly points up the superficiality of this development, although I do not doubt that it will appear to his pupils and adherents to be a revelation of the greatest profundity.

True, the movements of speech and writing are invested with their own partial memories, but on top of that they would be perceived, it is claimed, secondarily to those involved in the spoken and written word. In this way two new partial memory would be created, a *mémoire de perception des movements de la parole* and a *mémoire de perception des mouvements de l'écriture.* The loss of such would lead to production of a third group:

C. Motor sensory aphasia or *aphasie de réception secondaire,* with its two corresponding sub-classifications.

Characteristically, there is no reference to clinical examples of such a form. We shall return later to the single example of this type to be given. If I have succeeded in making myself clear up to this point, the reader may see, without need for further explanation, that these newly "discovered" centers are identical with centers *b* and *β* in Figure 15 and therefore may be considered superfluous.

Further discussion is not necessary to show that Broadbent's hypothesis of an object-naming center does not fit into our concept of cortical function. We recognize nothing but the memory images, and therefore assign functions of an alleged object-naming center directly to the acoustic, visual and motor memory images corresponding to centers a, χ, and β. The hypothesis of a sentence-formulation propositionising center would seem even more superfluous and redundant. This supposed center is apparently the chief executive agent of motor centers b and β, i.e., the cerebral hemispheres, which collectively constitute the whole organ of consciousness. The ability to think and desire to say something can occur only in association with consciousness and therefore cannot be localized.

2.

Now, before undertaking a discussion of the work of Lichtheim, that author who has been the most consistent in his support of our own theory, and who has, as I am bound to recognize, carried it further with great perspicacity, I must first explain to the reader my interpretation of the term "object-concept".

It can be readily seen that our interest in the speech mechanism, at least in the light of present knowledge, lies particularly in its role as an agent of consciousness. As was indicated at the conclusion of my last discussion, the cerebral hemispheres *in toto,* as the organ of consciousness, function as the executor of the motor speech center *b* in spontaneous speech production. Likewise, the organ of consciousness *in toto* receives the message which is first transmitted to the sensory speech center at *a,* functioning as a receiving station for acoustic messages. Therefore, it would seem that further localization within this single organ of consciousness is not the issue here. But as soon as we wish to point to a concrete example as a test of our schema, we can find other, more comforting results. For example, how might the process involved in comprehension and spontaneous expression of the word "bell" be explained? If we are to comprehend this word, the concept of a bell must be aroused within us by the acoustic message which has reached center *a.* The acoustic message must stimulate the memory images of a bell which are deposited in the cortex and located according to the sensory organs. These would then include the acoustic imagery aroused by the sound of the bell, visual imagery established by means of form and color, tactile imagery acquired by cutaneous sensation, and finally, motor imagery gained by exploratory movements of the fingers and eyes. Close association between these various memory images has been established by repeated experience of the essential features of bells. As a final result, arousal of each individual image is adequate for awakening the concept as a whole. In this way a functional unit is achieved. Such units form the concept of the object, in this case a bell. Thus when a spoken word is understood and provokes thought, these units are in a sense a second station, accessible to our own recognition, in the total activity of the hemispheres, a station which must be passed through if the spoken word is not to die away in our ears without having been understood. Moreover, our consciousness makes uses of this same station when the word "bell" is to be articulated spontaneously, i. e. as the result of what may be highly complex processes within our consciousness.

The first stage in this process then consists in the arousal of the concept of the object, "bell", and the second in the process of transmission to the pertinent motor memory images in *b*, the site involved in dispatch of the message. A schematic illustration of this process is indicated in the diagram in Figure 16, in which (B) represents the concept of the object bell. The reader may find a very similar schema in Lichtheim's work. In the same way, if we attempt

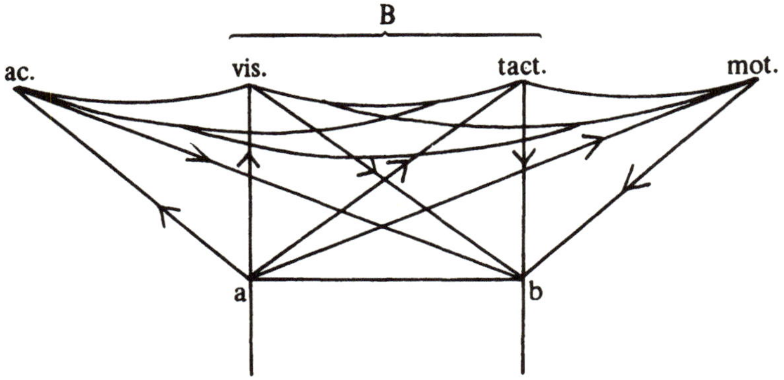

FIG. 16.

Wernicke's Composite Schema of Language and Conceptualization

(a): Acoustic speech center
(b): Motor speech center
(B): Conceptualization
(ac): Acoustic imagery
(vis): Visual imagery
(tact): Tactual imagery

to construct the concept of the word or "symbol" as the name of an object is often called such as that of the word 'bell' we find that, completely analogous to the object itself, it consists of the relevant firmly associated memory images in (a) and (b). These speculations then may suggest differentiation of speech comprehension into two stages, namely, 1) the arousal of the word and 2) arousal of the corresponding object-concept. The same process occurs in spontaneous speech, but in the reverse order, with the concept of the object emerging first, followed by that of the word.

This brief digression in regard to the word or symbol concept might seem unnecessary. However, we have an immediate need to use it. For we shall have to examine the extent to which such word-concepts are inseparable unities. Pathological research yields two lines of evidence relevant to this problem. On the one hand, if center *b* is destroyed, speech comprehension may remain completely intact; in other words, the acoustic imagery of the word is adequate for arousal of the concept of the object. If, however, center *a* is damaged, the independence of center *b* can be seen in the continued production of spontaneous speech. The latter, however, is characterized by inconsistent word-choice, with symptoms of word-transposition or paraphasia. Therefore, preservation of the word-concept is of greater significance in the active phase of the speech process than in the passive. Or, translated into terms of our schema, the association between the acoustic word image and the concrete object is firm and independent, but that between the object-concept and the pertinent motor word image is more fragile and not adequate to ensure accurate speech production. Presence of the word-concept in its entirety is necessary for production of spontanous speech. This finding, gleaned from pathological studies, is comprehensible if understood in the light of the mechanisms involved in speech acquisition. Undoubtedly the first knowledge of language which the child acquires consists of the comprehension of words, the association of acoustic images with concepts of concrete objects, while in many cases a further period of years is necessary for the development of the faculty of active speech. A preliminary stage of this last is the ability, by using the association pathway *a-b*, to imitate the speech sounds heard. On this basis I hypothesize that centrifugal innervation of the word-concept from the area (of sensory perception) of the concrete object follows a double path, namely the simple path *B-b* and the more complicated route *B-a-b*. If a portion of the latter is disrupted in any place incomplete activation of the word-concept will be reflected in the transposition of words. In this matter I differ with Lichtheim who explains these facts in another way.

According to his interpretation, arousal of the acoustic images is effected by the pathway *B-b-a*, but the influence of acoustic imagery on correct activation of speech production is first effected by the circuitous route *a-B-b*. In this interpretation Lichtheim assumes loss of the voluntary internal hearing of words experienced by patients who have sustained damage to center *b*, so that the voluntary innervation of *a* would have to pass through *b*. And, in fact, although good comprehension is evident, such patients are unable to indicate the number of syllables contained in the names of objects presented. This procedure is recommended by Lichtheim for testing the ability to voluntarily activate the acoustic imagery in aphasic patients. However, I do not regard this as decisive evidence for acceptance of his interpretation. These facts may be satisfactorily explained by recognition of the significance of pathway *B-b* and the inadequacy of path *B-a* for voluntary innervation of the word-concept itself. I believe that the later-acquired ability of analysis of words into syllables can probably occur only by means of the word-concept itself. Therefore, under certain conditions, it seems quite plausible that the pathway *B-a* may transmit centrifugally, i.e., bidirectionally, as is true of most association tracts, since voluntary mimicry is still intact in certain pathological cases demonstrating loss of spontaneous speech. And how shall the voluntary impulse reach center *b* if not by way of *B-a-b?* Later we shall offer still further applications of these preliminary observations.

If we now return to our original schema in Figure 7 and consider it in relationship to a concept center, which for the sake of simplicity we shall reduce to a point designated *B*, and if we also restrict the scope of aphasic symptoms to all such cases of speech disturbance in which the concept of the object itself is preserved, damage to the centers under question and their various conduction paths would yield seven different forms of aphasia.

Let us enumerate the causes of these, using Lichtheim's model but changing the order.

1. Damage to center *a*.
2. Disruption of the acoustic path ending in *a*.
3. Disruption of the centripetal pathway between *a* and the concept center.

Forms 1-3 constitute the group of the sensory aphasias.

4. Damage to center *b*.
5. Disruption of the motor speech pathway.
6. Disruption of the centrifugal pathway *B-b*.

Forms 4-6 constitute the group of the motor aphasias.

7. Conduction aphasia (Previously observed by us.)

For the sake of facilitating scientific understanding, I should like at this time to settle the problem of nomenclature. Lichtheim, who earlier supported use of the original terms, sensory and motor aphasia, has now abandoned them in his present work and supports application of the term aphasia to forms 4, 5, and 6 only, with the following subclassifications.

4. Nuclear aphasia.
5. Peripheral conduction aphasia.
6. Central conduction aphasia.

He would apply the name speech deafness or logo-kophosis to the forms 1-3, again including the subgroups:

1. Nuclear speech-deafness.
2. Peripheral conduction speech-deafness.
3. Central conduction speech deafness.

He proposes the term conduction paraphasia for type 7.

It is my feeling that the appropriateness of this nomenclature must certainly be questioned. It seems ill-advised to impose a new, narrower meaning on the well-established, widely accepted concept of aphasia, which already embraces all of these forms. Moreover, the application to the cortex of a term as "nuclear" – a term which should be limited to the nuclei of the cranial nerves and their analogs – seems inappropriate to me and is moreover anatomically incorrect. Finally, it seems to me misleading to draw a single symptom such as paraphasia into the nomenclature of distinct forms, since it belongs to several forms at once.

For these reasons, I would propose preservation of the older terms of motor, sensory, and conduction aphasia, and the choice of the relevant additions according to whether the cortical centers *a* and *b* themselves, or the conduction pathways on either side of them are destroyed. The adjectives *cortical* and *subcortical* have been in use for a long time, and all recent additions to the nomenclature may be included under the term *transcortical,* a new word which must be created.

The following nomenclature of aphasia may then be formulated.

1. Cortical sensory aphasia
2. Subcortical sensory aphasia
3. Transcortical sensory aphasia
4. Cortical motor aphasia
5. Subcortical motor aphasia
6. Transcortical motor aphasia
7. Conduction aphasia

Later I shall return to the objection which Lichtheim has raised in regard to preservation of the old terminology.

The critical point of Lichtheim's work lies in proof of the actual existence of his seven forms. I can only agree with that writer's comment that the general validity of my original simple schema has yet to be subjected to such a test. I am also in complete agreement with him as regards the didactic value of the schema when projected in this way.

In regard to the delineation and clinical description of the individual forms, Lichtheim considers inclusion of the associated disturbances in written language to be necessary in a study of the entire clinical picture. In my opinion, this hinders agreement on the main argument, namely, recognition of the seven different types of speech disturbance. For the present I shall disregard the area of written language and return to it later in greater detail.

1. Cortical sensory aphasia is characterized by lack of comprehension of the spoken word and inability to mimic. However, the patient is able to speak spontaneously, although vocabulary is limited and characterized by frequent word-transposition, that is, paraphasia. See Figure 17.
2. Subcortical sensory aphasia presents the same lack of comprehension of the spoken word and the same impairment in word mimicry. Spontaneous speech however is maintained, and the word-concept remains intact.

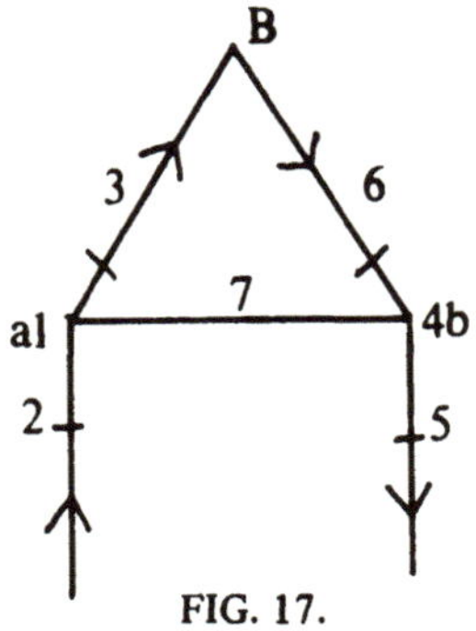

FIG. 17.

The Lichtheim Aphasia Schema.

(B): Concept center
(1): Nuclear speech deafness
(2): Peripheral conduction speech deafness
(3): Central conduction speech deafness
(4): Nuclear aphasia
(5): Peripheral conduction aphasia
(6): Central conduction aphasia
(7): Conduction paraphasia

This type of aphasia forms the basis of Lichtheim's chief argument against use of the current nomenclature, as strictly speaking it is not aphasia inasmuch as speech is totally unimpaired. However, if one regards comprehension as a part of the speech process, constituting its passive stage – a view which seems valid to me and one which is held by French authorities – and furthermore, if comprehension is regarded as a stage which can only be separated from the total process artificially then one certainly cannot challenge this use of the term aphasia. Moreover, each symptom-complex may include certain borderline cases, which can be accommodated under the nomenclature only with great difficulty. And exactly the same objection applies as I shall demonstrate, to Lichtheim's nomenclature when it is used for another form.

A second point which must be raised here is of a purely personal nature. In my controversy with Kussmaul, I have not condoned use of the term " speech-deafness" to designate that same clinical picture which I earlier had as "sensory aphasia." The usage of this term was based on the clinical material available. At that time I knew of no adequately studied case presenting isolated speech-deafness without the symptom of word-confusion or paraphasia. Nor did Kussmaul at the time have one at hand, and I regard it as greatly to Lichtheim's credit that he has examined more closely and put in the proper light such a case. Since that time I myself have had the opportunity to study a very clear-cut case of this form, which shall soon be reported in my clinic journal. Thus, I now recognize that in certain rare cases isolated speech-deafness does indeed occur: I have never doubted the theoretical possibility of its occurrence.

3. Transcortical sensory aphasia. Impairment in comprehension of the spoken word with preservation of mimicry. Symptoms of paraphasia are evident in spontaneous speech. See Figure 17. It will be agreed that the features of forms 1-3 are complete without the necessity for consideration of disorders of written language. The assumption in all cases of sensory aphasia is that common deafness is not the basis of the lack of comprehension.
4. Cortical motor aphasia. Speech comprehension is intact, but the patient presents either muteness or a vocabulary limited to a few words. Spontaneous speech and mimicry as well as the voluntary mental sounding of the word are not possible. See page 181.
5. Subcortical motor aphasia. This form is differentiated from the preceding type by the complete integrity of the word-concept. See Figure 17. The muteness is the same as that found in type 4. The patient is able to indicate the number of syllables contained in a word corresponding to an object presented to him.
6. Transcortical motor aphasia. This is the form on which the Lichtheim nomenclature founders. He interprets this type as aphasia in spite of retained ability to speak, which, however, is restricted to mimicry. There is loss of spontaneous speech but no evidence of impairment in speech comprehension.

Of these three forms of motor aphasia, only the differentiation between forms 4 and 5, i.e., cortical motor and subcortical motor aphasia, presents problems which demand a critical discussion of written language. This function, writing, to anticipate a bit, is impaired in the first form of the aphasia mentioned, cortical motor aphasia, and is intact in the second, subcortical motor aphasia. Transcortical motor aphasia, however, may be identified without this feature. The cause of muteness in motor aphasia does not lie in paralysis of the speech musculature, just as common deafness is not the basis for impaired comprehension in sensory aphasia.

7. Conduction aphasia is primarily characterized by negative symptoms. If motor or sensory aphasia is not evident, but speech is paraphasic, presenting word-transposition, one may predict a disturbance in conduction between centers *a* and *b*.[54]

I shall return later to the problem of so-called amnesic aphasia. This type is not related to the aphasia forms just reviewed, but is rather concerned with an actual memory disturbance.

3.

The complex process involved in the acquisition of reading and writing may be more readily understood if one applies its obvious analogy to speech development.

One might then say that reading consists in the activation of the word-concept by the visual written image. Conversely, the process of writing involves the activation of the corresponding graphic motor image by the word-concept.

To produce a suitable schema (Figure 18) let us use the same kind of device

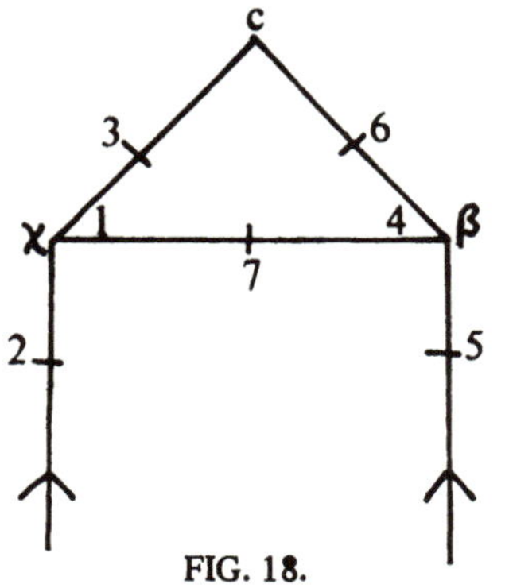

FIG. 18.

Schema of the Alexias and Agraphias

(c): Word-concept (acoustic and motor speech imagery)
(χ): Visual written image
(β): Center of motor graphic imagery
(1): Cortical alexia
(2): Subcortical alexia
(3): Transcortical alexia
(4): Cortical agraphia
(5): Subcortical agraphia
(6): Transcortical agraphia
(7): Conduction agraphia

which we used earlier to denote the concept center *B*. In other words, let us write the word-concept as $a + b = c$, where the addition sign designates integrity of the association pathway *a-b*. This then leads to the schema formulated in the diagram in Figure 18 in which χ denotes the visual written image and β the motor center of movements involved in writing. The pathway χ - β, an anolog of pathway *a-b* in the earlier schema diagrammed in Figure 17, represents the crucial pathway by means of which writing is learned. Just as the critical process involved in speech-learning is repetition of the spoken word mediated by the pathway *a-b*, so the learning of writing is acquired under the controlling influence of the visual written image. The pathway χ - β therefore has the same significance for written language as the path *a-b* for speech.

After these preliminary remarks, let us now turn to pathological case-studies of written language disorders. The theoretical possibility of seven types of disorder therefore becomes immediately evident as was also true of disturbance in speech. Let us designate these disorders by the numbers 1 through 7, labeling disturbances of the centripetal pathway as alexia and those of the centrifugal path, agraphia. This provides us with the following summary.

1. Cortical alexia
2. Subcortical alexia
3. Transcortical alexia
4. Cortical agraphia
5. Subcortical agraphia
6. Transcortical agraphia
7. Conduction agraphia

A simplification of this schema is needed at this point, for reasons which shall be presented later, before we turn to a discussion of the symptom-pictures of the seven theoretically predictable forms, which is not written without practical interest. We can only briefly indicate here that there is much which contradicts the actual existence of a pathway *c*-β and therefore the schema illustrated in the accompanying diagram in Figure 19 alone may be used as a basis for our discussion. In this way an analogy to disturbances in oral speech can be readily demonstrated, although with certain simplifications.

1. Cortical alexia. Loss of reading and writing. Disruption of the centrifugal pathway for writing at χ.
2. Subcortical alexia. Inability to read. No disturbance in writing with the exception of writing from a model.
3. Transcortical alexia. Loss of ability to read and write with preservation of the mechanical copying of printed and script material.
4. Cortical agraphia. Loss of fine motor patterns requisite to writing. Copying is not possible. No impairment in reading.
5. Subcortical agraphia. Essentially the same picture. (Further comment will be made later.)
6. Transcortical agraphia. This form is nonexistent.
7. Conduction agraphia. Reading unimpaired. Loss of writing.

If one assumes the existence of a direct pathway c-β, transcortical agraphia, form 6, would be characterized by the exclusive loss of spontaneous writing. In form 7, conduction agraphia, writing would still be possible, but paragraphia, the analog of paraphasia observed in oral speech disorders, would be present.

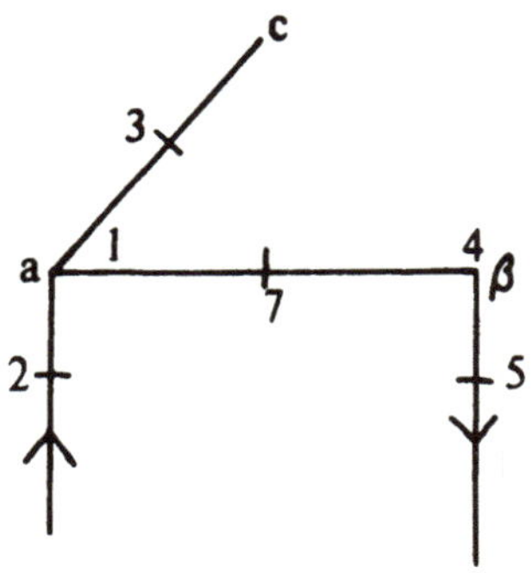

FIG. 19.

Schema of Agraphias and Alexias
(with omission of tract C - β)

(1): Cortical alexia
(2): Subcortical alexia
(3): Transcortical alexia
(4): Cortical agraphia
(5): Subcortical agraphia
[(6): Transcortical agraphia]
(7): Conduction agraphia

Therefore, the control exerted by means of visual imagery may be considered much more indispensable to the writing process than that of acoustic imagery in respect of the speech process. Writing demands greater conscious activity than speech. In the latter, distracting factors may be predominant: the influence of the acoustic image *a* is always only slight, while the writing process, on the contrary, demands at least enough concentration to produce a series of letters.

Paragraphia, which is the chief issue here, therefore probably amounts to the same as complete agraphia; with impairment in formation of the letter itself. This can be seen when attempts to write produce only scribbles and lines which depart from the correct letter form. These samples of writing also occasionally contain correctly formed letters. Such, however, are infrequent, occurring only here and there among a group of incomprehensible scribbles. If correct and completely-formed letters can be produced, and the disturbance is limited to transposition and interpretation of letters, one is dealing not with a true agraphia or paragraphia, as we interpret it, but rather with the symptom of paraphasia, which may also be revealed in writing: in a word, written paraphasia.

A second point which must be briefly touched on here concerns the building of words by the combining of individual letters. The visual memory images deposited in χ and the motor memory images at β consist of single letters of the alphabet. The word-concept, on the contrary, always includes at least one syllable, and often several syllables, and is comprehended as a series of association of letters in a specific sequence. If we should take a very simple example of a one-syllable word such as *hand*, it can be seen that only the four letters in sequence, *h-a-n-d,* are able to call up the correct meaning. This is also true of multi-digit numbers. In alexia it will therefore be possible to determine whether whole words or only individual letters can be read, i.e. recognized. Likewise, in agraphia we must see whether only letters, but not whole words, can be written, or whether whole words, too, can be produced. For both the reading and the writing of individual letters it is necessary only for the concept of the letter to be intact, and this consists of χ, β, and the area between χ and β which I need not again describe in detail.[55r]

The fact that man, however, can learn to read letters without necessarily learning to write them—one need only point to the reading of printed characters—indicates the greater autonomy of χ in contrast to that of β.

We may now complete the classification of the individual forms of alexia presented earlier within the framework of this hypothesis. In cortical alexia, the letters presented to the patient apparently cannot be recognized but appear strange and foreign, a fact which may be confirmed by the use of leading questions. Furthermore, he is unable to copy,and in so attempting does not actually write, but merely draws the letters, and even then, later recognition is not possible.

Moreover, subcortical alexia spares spontaneous writing alone, and letters presented to the patient appear unfamiliar and must be laboriously copied from the model. Copying, in fact, is not possible. Occasionally letters may be recognized during such attempts to copy, and under certain conditions may even be read, a trick which has long been observed, since it often occurs in aphasia.

In transcortical alexia, on the contrary, the letters appear to be recognized and can be copied without difficulty. Reading aloud is not possible since disruption of the path χ-c results in inability to arouse the associated acoustic image of the letter. In none of the three forms of alexia is the reading of words intact. This is readily understood, since reading of individual letters is not possible. Nevertheless, one is impressed by the striking ability demonstrated by such patients in their immediate reading of the word itself, as soon as the letters of which it is composed can be read. Therefore, it would seem that impairment of the word-concept must be postulated. A similar situation exists in the writing of letters and words. Only in impairment of the word-concept itself does it happen that the letters alone, but not the word, can be written without aid.

Our earlier discussion tacitly assumed integrity of the word-concept reviewed in the earlier description of aphasia types. It is now necessary to explore further the notion of the word-concept and the relationship between word and letter concepts.

Grashey's (1885) work in this area certainly deserves acclaim, and I would not hesitate to suggest that it may be considered the most significant contribution to the development of the doctrine of aphasia during the past decade.

In his work Grashey pursues an entirely new and very fruitful notion by postulating the temporal factor as an important consideration in formation of the spoken word, which can be likewise applied to reading and writing. All of these processes require certain temporal intervals. Aphasia may follow in certain cases in which significant reduction of memory results in difficulty in object-naming and a blocking in the arousal of concepts in the association process because of inadequate periods of memory fixation. In such cases, the memory images of the word (as that of the concept of the object itself) fade before the word is completed. The patient described by Grashey demonstrates this very phenomenon. The names of objects presented to him could be found only by the act of writing, and then only during the time they were before him. Even then the word was slowly formulated, letter by letter.

Writing thus accomplished what memory itself could not, namely visual retention of the first letter, which then did not disappear during production of the second. If the object were removed and again presented to the patient after a moment, he could not recall having seen it before. This patient therefore, demonstrates a severe disturbance in memory.

Moreover, those words which could not be held in memory which included essentially all substantives and verbs, etc., words of specific concrete meaning, could only be found in this manner, namely by the process of writing the name letter by letter.

Reading was intact with the exception of numbers, which were treated as pictures of objects. Significant impairment in writing was present but this was less than that of speech. Recovery of the aphasia coincided with that of memory and of oral speech. Because of its connection with memory disturbance, the frequently misused term of amnesic aphasia might be well applied to this type of impairment.

This completely new form of amnesic aphasia is presumably not limited to the clinical picture here presented but may manifest itself in a variety of ways. It may be defined as that form of aphasia which is not caused by destruction of centers and conducting tracts but exclusively by a closely-associated weakness in memory. That this definition which Grashey employed in summarizing his case is completely applicable to the patient, can be demonstarted by a more detailed study of the same.

The word-concept was described above as a serial association of letters. Of the two kinds of association processes, simultaneous and consecutive association, the second may be applied here, and it must be emphasized that the transience of the stimulus forms a significant factor in the process.

Let us now turn to our letter symbols and attempt to allow for this temporal factor. For example, if we divide the word-concept of the word "hand" into four intervals of time, corresponding to the letters, we may hypothesize that $c = g + g1 + g2 + g3$. The relationship to written language would then be: $g = \chi + \beta$; $g1 = \chi 1 + \beta 1$; $g2 = \chi 2 + \beta 2$; $g3 = \chi 3 + \beta 3$. This relationship is of particular importance in its assumption that we do in reality read and write by means of spelling but do not speak in this way. The symbols *g, gl, g2,* and *g3,* which combine to form the word-concept, represent specific values only as temporal intervals. In regard to speech they are fictitious values and acquire the specific meaning described above only by their connection with written language.

In reality, we do not learn to speak letters, but words. The analysis into letters is acquired later and is achieved only for the purpose of making written language more accessible. Without this assumption, Grashey's observations remain obscure, and in reality, the author himself did not completely comprehend their full import.

If the temporal factor alone were involved, then above all, the patient would immediately be able to say the letter which he had recalled. The significance of Grashey's observations however lies in this, which he himself stressed, that only by means of writing is the patient able to "find" the letter. Moreover, the significance of this particular work lies in its specific orientation which leads to such an interpretation.

It is my feeling that the following relevant facts require further interpretation. The patient is in full possession of the word-concept. However, the concept of the concrete object, which was likewise at his disposal, did not have adequate intensity over a sufficient period of time to activate the complete word-concept. Only the first phase *g* was aroused. However, the same does not apply to *g* as is true of the entire word, namely that it presumes to equal the equation $a + b$ and therefore can be orally produced.

We do not speak by means of spelling. On the contrary, *g* has a very specific value, namely $\chi + \beta$, and in this way the letter can be written and read. The writing of a word demands time, and in reality, more time than the reading or hearing of a complete word. Thus, during writing, the object-image fades and must be renewed in order to activate the second period or stage (time-interval, g2), and therefore the second letter. The entire word can then be read aloud as it commonly is, by spelling.

In reading a half-page of printed material as rapidly as possible, I have required the same time as Grashey, namely, on the average of .03 sec. per letter, and must therefore correct my earlier view that one skilled in reading may glance over entire sentences and grasp the meaning of entire words without the process of spelling. (Wernicke, 1874)

Grashey's exposition clarifies the differentiation which commonly exists in aphasics in respect to word and number reading. A number, in that it is not synthesized from letters, is considered analogous to the picture of a concrete object. In the preceding case the patient was able to succeed in finding the word to be read by writing it down, letter by letter. In addition to this circuitous method, he demonstrated another which was even more elementary. A series of numbers would be recited until the number to be read was reached. In this way it could be recalled. With the exception of numbers, reading was fluent and carried out with complete understanding. Spontaneous writing, on the contrary, was significantly impaired. Copying from a model was intact and writing to dictation was fluent. However, this could be accomplished only if the patient repeated the word to be written and in this way fixed it in memory.

Although he comprehended a sentence dictated to him, only the first or second word could be retained when writing of it was attempted. Therefore, he was able to continue only if the sentence were dictated anew. Spontaneous writing was carried out in the same manner. The patient would dictate the words to himself as he wrote, continually re-reading the sentence from the beginning, and so completing it by this laborious method.

At a certain stage in recovery, an unbiased observer noticed that the patient could retrieve a word more readily by writing than by saying it aloud. This may be readily understood in the light of the preceding discussion. A specific form of writing disturbance, i.e., amnesic agraphia, belongs to the category of amnesic aphasia.

Another point in regard to Grashey's case study is of great interest and must at least be touched on here, since the author himself has permitted it to go unnoticed. This same patient, who when first presented with a series of objects and also letters, forgot the first while dwelling on the second, but still could read fluently, comprehended all that was said to him and was able to write words to dictation. Comprehension of a word requires the retention of the sound of a number of letters, while that of a sentence requires retention of many words before the meaning can be clearly grasped. In this case the acoustic imagery can be maintained for a longer period than the visual object images, and therefore the impairment in memory lies primarily in the visual area. The severe problem presented by the patient may be a significant factor in this regard. Visual acuity in the right eye was minimal, with demonstration of a very restricted concentric residual visual field. Sight was therefore essentially limited to the macula lutea. In the left eye visual acuity was normal, but again a restricted concentric visual field was evident. In reality, only islands of vision were intact. Recovery occurred later in the left eye with the exception of one of the defects mentioned above. Moreover, this allows me the opportunity to make an observation which was alluded to above on page 187, but which I had not been able to verify at that time.

If reading and writing under all conditions are carried out by means of spelling, as Grashey has irrefutably demonstrated, then integrity of both components of the word-concept, sensory as well as motor, would seem a natural necessity. If one of the two is absent, reading as well as writing is impaired. Comprehension and also expression by means of written language would be lost. I myself earlier labored under the error that comprehension of written language is intact in cases of cortical motor aphasia. Lichtheim, in his work mentioned above, still holds this view. He tends to interpret the frequent occurrence of reading difficulty in motor aphasia on the basis of the close anatomical location of the two cerebral areas. I must admit that in the light of this new interpretation of the mechanism of written language comprehension, I am unable to imagine how preservation of the motor representation and therefore of spelling ability can be maintained in destruction of center (*b*), (Refer to footnote 55r) If spelling is lost, so likewise is reading. The same relationship holds between the acoustic center (*a*), and writing ability. Therefore, a cortical sensory aphasia can produce impairment in writing also, a view to which Lichtheim moreover after much diliberation was also finally persuaded.

At this point we must again take up a discussion of that process which plays the primary role in the acquisition of reading and writing, and which, as Grashey teaches, continually finds new applications in written language, namely, the process of spelling. If one does not speak by means of spelling, a fact which has been repeatedly stressed, one must not then mistakenly assume that each letter of the alphabet has its own acoustic image in center *a* and its own motor image in center *b*. Both in reality are artificial cultural or educational products, later-acquisitions, in contrast to the store of acoustic and motor images which correspond to those of the spoken word. Furthermore, a process which may seem extremely simple to us may in reality be a most difficult and complex task for the brain, in that it can first be accomplished by an analysis of the already existing combinations into their component parts. However, this analysis of acoustic and motor images certainly does not occur individually, with transmission along pathway *a-b* necessary for each letter, which would be a prerequisite in the process of spelling. For example, reading of the word *hand* would require the combining of its individual letters. This process would then involve transmission along the pathway *a-b* four times with the consequent artificial serial-production of letters which are closely associated with the word-concept, *hand.* In that event, it would be necessary to hypothesize a double existence for each word, first as the original component of oral speech, and secondly as a well practiced educational acquisition, namely, the serial association of specific letters.

In the reading process this cultural product first calls up the oral word which is comprehended by means of the pathway *a-B,* as also occurs in the production of oral language. The importance of the integrity of pathway *a-b* and its terminals in addition to the centripetal path from the optic nerve to χ, χ - *a*, and *a-B* can clearly be seen from this interpretation. This leads me to conclude that conduction aphasia will be accompanied by a complete alexia. Cases presenting some intact reading capacity, but whose reading as well as speech is characterized by paraphasia, may require the diagnosis of another form of aphasia.[56r] Amnesic aphasia, or a combination of cortical and transcortical sensory aphasia may presumably be involved in these rather frequent cases.

The completed schema of reading can then be formulated as indicated in Figure 20 by the unbroken lines. Mechanical reading in which comprehension

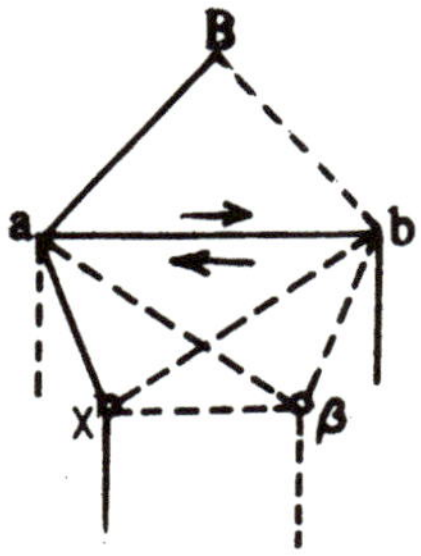

FIG. 20.

Schema of Copying

(B): Concept center
(a): Acoustic speech imagery
(b): Motor speech imagery
(χ): Visual letter imagery
(β): Graphic motor imagery

is not required, can be interpreted in the same way with the exception that the path (a-B) is not a prerequisite.

The complete schema of writing presents an even more complex process. One may differentiate:

1. Simple copying or writing from a model.
2. Writing to dictation.
3. Spontaneous writing.

1. Copying from a model, if carried out purely mechanically without comprehension of the content, requires only the tract from the eye to center χ-(χ - β) and the motor writing path proceeding from β. This however, rarely occurs in the writing of letters or documents. One might very well assume that this path is also adequate for such tasks as the copying of printed material, since the visual images of letters in both the script and printed form are close-

ly associated in χ. See Figure 18.
2. Writing to dictation without comprehension of the content is possible; this may occur if the material is a foreign language containing the same letters which occur in the mother tongue. The learning of Latin and Greek by our school children is an example of such a mechanism. This process is indicated by the unbroken lines in Figure 21. The entire path is traversed for each letter. Comprehension of dictated material requires, in addition, the centripetal path *a-B.*

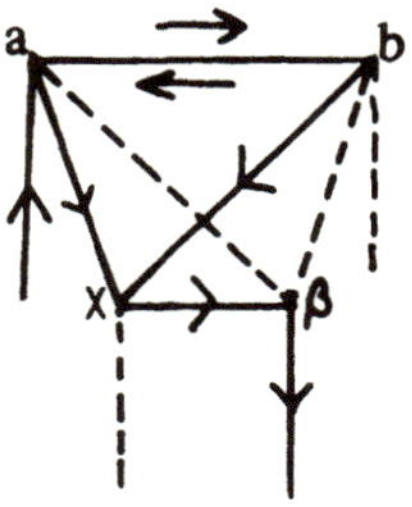

FIG. 21.

Schema of Writing to Dictation

(a): Acoustic speech imagery
(b): Motor speech imagery
(χ): Visual letter imagery
(β): Graphic motor imagery

3. The process of spontaneous writing follows essentially the same schema but is more complex because of the addition of associations between the object-concept and the word-concept. The word-concept must be reactivated for each letter. If these associations are unstable,as may be true in transcortical aphasia, writing will be paraphasic. See the accompanying diagram in Figure 22.

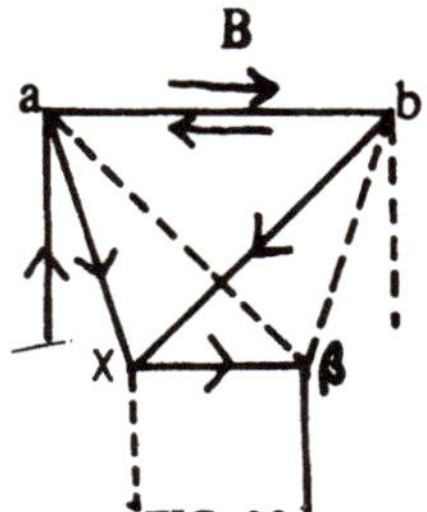

FIG. 22.

Schema of Spontaneous Writing

(B): Concept
(a): Acoustic speech imagery
(b): Motor speech imagery
(χ): Visual letter imagery
(β): Graphic motor imagery

Paraphasia is naturally more apparent in writing than in speech. In transcortical sensory aphasia one might correctly predict a very striking contrast between the mere minimal paraphasia evident in speech and the severe paraphasia demonstrated in writing. In transcortical motor aphasia, spontaneous writing, as expected, is lost. But in contrast, only a mild paraphasia would be evident in writing to dictation, if complete impairment in comprehension is not present.

The schemas presented suggest that the pathways for comprehension of written material are simpler than those involved in the process of writing itself. Reading is a more firmly established acquisition than writing and is not as readily lost. Moreover, one may consider the sum total of inner excitatory processes in reading to be reinforced by the external stimulus, and in a sense, actively strengthened by a renewal of energy. In the writing process, on the contrary, energy is expended. This might explain why Grashey's patient was more successful in spelling during the act of reading, than during writing. The greatest expenditure of energy, however, greater even than that required in the writing process, is that required by speech production which is carried out by means of spelling. This peculiar mode of speaking was necessary in Grashey's patient.

We must now undertake a review of the relationship between the various forms of aphasia and written language disturbances. In the interest of a unitary nomenclature, retention of the terms alexia and agraphia is suggested. These terms may be prefaced by the modifier "verbal" to specify them as secondary symptoms of aphasia.

1. Cortical sensory aphasia causes verbal alexia and agraphia. Mechanical copying from a model is intact.

2. Subcortical sensory aphasia. No disturbance in reading and writing is evident.

3. In transcortical sensory aphasia the word-concept is intact and fluent reading is possible. The process involved here is similar to that which frequently occurs in the reading of a foreign language containing letter-symbols identical to those of one's mother tongue, such as the Latin or Greek of our scholars. Silent as well as oral reading may proceed without comprehension of the content, and oral reading, carried out under direct control of the visual symbols, may be completely free of error. Verbal paraphasia may occur during spontaneous writing because of disruption of the pathway *a-B*. Writing to dictation is characteristically intact but is carried out with lack of comprehension of content, as might occur in the writing of Latin words which one did not understand.

4. Cortical motor aphasia produces verbal alexia and agraphia. Mechanical copying is intact.

5. Subcortical motor aphasia. Reading and writing are not impaired.

6. In transcortical motor aphasia the pathway used in oral and silent read-

ing is completely preserved, and therefore no trace of alexia is evident. Writing to dictation as well as oral mimicry are possible. On the contrary, there is loss of spontaneous writing with consequent verbal agraphia.

7. Conduction aphasia produces verbal alexia and agraphia because of the loss of spelling ability, which is caused by impairment of the word-concept. Reading and writing are possible in simple tasks which do not require spelling, such as writing one's name and the reading of numbers, which in effect are treated as object-images.

A comprehensive description of the clinical forms of aphasia, initially presented above may be completed by the inclusion of the disturbances of writing language.

This brings us to the basic question which Lichtheim also raised in his detailed study. Does clinical experience support Lichtheim's theoretical claim that individual cases in part present isolated disturbances, and in part combinations of disturbance in oral and written speech as required in our original schema, with the additions illustrating disorders of written language – a task which has occupied us in such great detail? An answer to this question requires use of the mass clinical material in so far as is possible. The availability of detailed summaries, such as that of Kussmaul, greatly simplifies this task.

A. APHASIA

1. The syndrome of cortical sensory aphasia has received such strong clinical support that it now stands as a well-established clinical picture. Lichtheim's question regarding the inclusion of disturbance in writing as an essential part of this clinical form rests to a great extent on theoretical considerations relative to the pathway involved in the writing process and may now be regarded as settled.

In the future one must take care to note the presence or absence of copying ability in pure cases of this type. This form of aphasia may show some recovery within a relatively short period of six to eight weeks, except for impairment in writing to dictation and spontaneous writing. These deficits may persist in unrecognized form for some time.

2. Subcortical sensory aphasia. Lichtheim reports an example of this form following an apoplectic attack in which speech impairment was evident in the early stages of illness. At the time of examination the patient gave the impression of one who is stone-deaf, and yet it could be demonstrated that his hearing was in reality very good. He was able to hear whistling and singing but did not recognize melodies. I am presently following a similar case who can hear and recognize melodies whistled to him and is also able to mimic whistling but who presents a loss in the hearing of higher pitches. The striking feature in Lichtheim's case, as well as my own, is the apparent permanence of the dis-

turbance. A mild improvement is observed only in the first weeks. Apparently, this picture is characteristic of this particular form.

3. Transcortical sensory aphasia. Lichtheim has reported a well-documented case-study of this form. The patient demonstrated marked recovery within a ten week period. Impairment in spontaneous writing persisted and was characterized by the interjection of incorrect words. Objects could not be named immediately with any certainty. To my knowledge, a similar case has not yet been described.

4. Cortical motor aphasia is the most frequent and familiar form. Lichtheim, following my earlier prediction, has postulated preservation of reading as the primary feature of this type, but states at the same time that many cases may frequently show a severe alexia. He cites Trousseau's well-known case in support of this hypothesis. However, his interpretation of this condition (see above) may very well no longer prove satisfactory even to him. In future studies, the ability to copy should be carefully examined. Such cases show little or no recovery.

5. Subcortical motor aphasia, with all of the characteristic accompanying features which have been described above, appears to occur relatively frequently. I am currently following a case of this type who, however, does not present a completely pure clinical picture. A similar patient (case 6) was reported in my original work on aphasia, although at that time I was unaware of its correct interpretation. This case was also complicated by a subcortical verbal agraphia, a condition which I shall discuss later. In other respects he meets all of the necessary criteria for inclusion in this category.

On the other hand, the literature contains a large number of uncomplicated cases of this type which are commonly designated as "pure cases" of atactic or Broca's aphasia. One may cite Kussmaul (1877, p. 157). The expectation of recovery in such cases is minimal.

6. Transcortical motor aphasia as a specific form has also been supported by a case study (case 7), reviewed in my first work on aphasia, where it was correctly interpreted. Kussmaul (1887, pp. 99, 193) has cited further examples in the case of Farge and those of Forbes Winslow, which unfortunately were incompletely studied. Lichtheim, on the other hand, cites a case studied in great detail by Hammond, and he himself presents a thorough description of another which agrees in all aspects with our predicted clinical picture. The patient, who at one point had essentially no speech at all, was able to mimic everything siad to him without error, and his oral reading was accurate. By the time he was ready to leave his bed, there was recovery of the ability to copy and write to dictation, as well as return of voluntary speech and writing. Initially, however, speech as well as writing was limited to the words *yes* and *no*. Later, spontaneous writing ability returned, but recovery was slower and less complete than that of speech. Speech presented essentially no significant impairment after five to six weeks, and the only marked difficulty evi-

dent was that of naming objects, which was characterized by occasional distortion of words.

7. Conduction aphasia. The few available cases of this type fit all the theoretical criteria of our schema. Cases 3 and 4, which were reviewed in my first work on aphasia (Wernicke, 1874), and which, incidentally, first motivated my formulation of this specific form, presented examples of good comprehension and a fairly large vocabulary. Paraphasia, however, was also present together with alexia and agraphia. Significant improvement in both areas occurred during the course of the illness. Disturbances in written language appeared in various forms. Chronic alexia was noted in case 3 and an isolated agraphia in case 4.

Because such variable results suggest the possibility of complications, further observation is necessary to verify the course of this form. Moreover, the first of these cases was definitely complicated by a right hemianopsia, and it is possible that the second was also so involved. Even at that time I did not diagnose case 10 of my first work as conduction aphasia. This patient's disturbance in written language did not actually represent a true alexia and agraphia, but instead, oral reading was characterized by paraphasia. (Writing was not examined.)

In the same way, I do not feel justified in including Lichtheim's first case within this particular category. The patient was able to read with complete comprehension but demonstrated the same paraphasic errors in reading as were present in spontaneous speech. Copying was intact, but severe impairment was demonstrated in writing. Only brief attempts were possible in this activity, and these were characterized by the transposition of letters. I would conjecture that the frequent cases of this type, presenting intact reading comprehension accompanied by paraphasia in oral reading and speech, may actually belong to an amnesic form of aphasia. Further information in regard to this form awaits future investigation.

B. DISTURBANCES OF WRITTEN LANGUAGE

1. Cortical alexia. During the past few months a patient with cortical alexia has been studied in my Clinic who also demonstrated agraphia and the absence of a true aphasia (Freund, 1886). This very interesting case will be reported in detail in my clinic journal, accompanied, I fear, by pathological findings. Here I shall only mention that the patient at the time presented a right hemianopsia which was later followed by constriction of the left visual fields. As a result, from the onset he was able to understand much of what he saw, and now most of that which he sees cannot be recognized, leaving him in a most confused and helpless condition.

The literature up to the present, as far as I know, does not contain examples of this type, which is not surprising in view of the great difficulties involved in examination.

One may perhaps question the significance of only one specific case. Nevertheless, the simultaneous occurrence of such symptoms would surely seem to be more than mere coincidence, and all of the predicted criteria are completely satisfied. In the introduction to my discussion. I questioned the practice of hypothesizing specific reading centers at the sites of visual cortical terminals, as well as the so-called motor centers of the arm as a center for writing. In fact I do not know of a single case which would confirm the actual existence of such a reading center. The letter and number symbols are essentially visual memory images which are deposited in the visual cortical area, i.e., the occipital lobe.[57r] They are relatively late in acquisition and may in essence be considered a product of the culture, so that one might only reluctantly invest such with the feature of hereditary predisposition. Furthermore, the presence of well-developed connections with the acoustic center by means of association paths, which very likely transmit to the occipital lobe, does not support this notion. Moreover, the letter-symbols are characteristic of most later-acquired memory images in that they have numerous and varied associations with other regions, such as the individual motor areas. Most people do not have difficulty in writing in the sand with the left foot, or with the left hand on the table, if they are permitted to use large crayons and can write in large script. It is also possible to write with the elbow, holding the arm flexed with a pencil fastened in place. This is why a specific motor writing center within the so-called arm-region cannot be recognized except in a very narrow sense. The center (χ) is identical with the cortical environs of the visual tract and is likewise bilateral. A simple right hemianopsia with disruption of connections leading to the left cortex does not abolish reading ability and cause an alexia. One may predict a cortical alexia only in the event of destruction of the visual memory images of concrete objects, and clinical experience suggests that this occurs only in the event of bilateral occipital damage. Our case is in agreement with this prediction.

2. Subcortical alexia refers to that same clinical syndrome of isolated word-blindness which has been reported in the literature during the past decase and is supported by a small number of case studies.

This form is characterized by loss of reading ability alone, with no impairment of spontaneous writing. In some cases reading ability is possible with the use of letter tracing. The letters can then be named if they are traced with the finger or if the corresponding hand movements are made. A right hemianopsia was also present in the case reviewed. This symptom also was observed in a case I recall from Westphal's clinic (1874), whom I later studied myself, as well as in a case of Charcot's (1883a, 1883b). I interpret these findings as lawful and predictable since disruption of the pathway between the eye and the visual cortical area of the left hemisphere is involved.[58r] This pathway contains the left visual tract. In one of Broadbent's cases, cited by Kussmaul (1877), the possibility of such a hemianopsia was not tested and apparently was overlooked. Case 3 (Beckmann), reported in my first work on aphasia, who presented a chronic alexia following remission of the aphasia symptoms, may also be included in this group. A right hemianopsia was also observed. Up to the present, two cases demonstrating this rare symptom-picture have passed through my hands. I was able to confirm the presence of marked difficulty in object-naming in both cases although the patients were not aphasic and recognized the objects correctly. This symptom may be explained on an anatomical basis. Recognition of objects is carried out by the right hemisphere, while the word-concept customarily has its seat in the left hemisphere. [59r]

3. Transcortical alexia might perhaps be more appropriately named subcortical verbal alexia in the light of the proposed aphasia nomenclature. See page 195. It may be recalled that this type is differentiated from the preceding forms by intact ability to copy, but meaningless interjection of letters in spontaneous writing. The form of the letter is intact. The only case which may plausibly serve as an example of this form is that of Abeele (cited in Kussmaul, 1877, p. 179). Unfortunately however, the status of spontaneous writing ability was not mentioned in this report. Because the acoustic pathway to the center (a) and pathway (χ - a) situated there have a common terminal, one may predict the occasional simultaneous appearance of subcortical alexia with a subcortical sensory aphasia. Therefore, one must be alert to the possibility of this combination in future studies. A relevant case has not yet been demonstrated.

4. Cortical agraphia. Our discussion of cortical alexia leaves no doubt that recognition of a single center for writing movements analogous to Broca's speech center is complete nonsense. The movements involved in writing essentially consist in the copying of visual letter images. This can be accomplished only after much training, and so involves more skill than the copying of other figures. If the visual memory images of letters are lost, the writing movements can no longer produce the correct letters. This is the form described on page 187.

The alternating flexion-extension finger movements may be lost together with other refined motor patterns of the right hand, which according to Duchenne, are necessary for writing. This may be observed in very circumscribed cortical damage of the so-called motor areas. I have already studied such a case of traumatic cortical damage in which the defect was about the size of a shilling. This report will soon be published. The head-wound, following trephination, is now closed, and the patient's condition has essentially stabilized. He now shows no actual paralysis and can flex and extent his hand rapidly and atrongly. Hand-grasp is normal and finger-thumb apposition is intact. However, little success is noted in production of the finer finger movements necessary for holding and guiding a pen, or in unbottoning and sewing. (The patient is a tailor.) Whatever fine movements he attempts must be carried out under the control of vision.

The patient was not able to recognize objects held in his hand while closing his eyes. For example, a sponge and key could not be differentiated, and as a result were incorrectly manipulated. No other gross sensory disturbances were noted, and there was return of the so-called muscle-sensation. The disorder was not limited to impairment of the tactile and motor-imagery of the right hand. During an early period of recovery when finger movements were still severely impaired, the patient was able to write on a blackbord and could write on paper with a pencil fastened to his fist. However, the clinical findings described seem to be consistent only with what might appropriately be designated as a cortical agraphia. According to the earlier nomenclature, one would not apply the label of agraphia to an impairment which is inconsistently present. The evidence seems to indicate that a cortical agraphia, also called motor agraphia by some writers, is not demonstrated in the case described.[60r]

Charcot's patient, who represents the most isolated and pure example cited by the various writers, is similar to mine, while that of Pitres does not belong to this category at all.

Charcot, Motor Agraphia. Pitres, Case 2. (Pitres, 1884)

In August, 1882, a 52 year old man was aware of sudden weakness of the right hand with resultant inability to write. Generalized symptoms were absent. Six months later, while attending a social gathering, he attempted to answer someone but could do so only in Russian. Comprehension of German and French, in which he had been equally proficient, was essentially unchanged, but he could no longer speak the languages. His condition gradually improved to the point where he could speak French fairly well. The loss of German, however, persisted. One day, when attempting to write, he noticed that he could not write a single word, although no paralysis was present.

In April, 1883 his condition was as follows. No impairment in speech (French) and intelligence. Oral reading in Russian, French or German was possible but the patient was not able to write in any of these languages. This was particularly evident in his mother tongue, Russian. When he was asked to give his address in Paris he answered fluently, "*Je demeure hôtel de Bade*. . etc." Attempts to write the same, however, resulted only in "*Je dem*. . . . ," The rest could be written only to dictation, and that only with great difficulty. Copying of written words was carried out without impairment. For example, he readily wrote the name Charcot in Russian, but had more difficulty in writing the same in French, and was completely unsuccessful in German. Finger movements on the right were somewhat weak, and there was a mild loss of sensation with incomplete loss of position-sense. Death occurred suddenly a few days later. An autopsy was not performed.

5. This description suggests that the problem could be called neither a subcortical nor a cortical agraphia. If it would not violate the current nomenclature, one might designate it as a paralysis of the arm usually used in writing. In cortical or subcortical aphasia, paralysis of the movements implicated in writing, with preservation of all other movements – an analog of paralysis of speech function alone – is contrary to all clinical evidence. As far as the clinical material is concerned, paralysis involving a certain extremity, thereby rendering writing impossible, is part of the common symptom-picture.

6. Transcortical agraphia was described above as an actually non-existent form. In fact, there is not a single example of clinical evidence in support of the existence of a pathway (b-β). On the other hand, this permits me an opportunity to review the importance of the pathway (b -χ) in the writing process. The centripetal path would certainly appear to be the most logical route in this process, and all available evidence contradicts the existence of a pathway (b-β). One might be justified in regarding the centrifugal path (B-b-χ) as the main path for writing in the same sense as the centripetal path (χ-a-B) is considered for reading. In that case one might designate a writing disorder caused by disruption of pathway (b-χ) as transcortical agraphia. Because this term might just as accurately be applied to a writing impairment caused by disruption of the pathway (a-χ), one should perhaps suggest a consideration of its relationship to the word-concept and its analog to subcortical verbal alexia. It might then be labeled as subcortical agraphia. This places the relationship of this form of writing disorder to subcortical aphasia in a clearer perspective. I might point to a clinical paradigm of the combination of these two functional disturbances in case 6 of my first work on aphasia. In regard to oral speech, the patient demonstrated symptoms of a subcortical motor aphasia. In written language the following notation was made. "He comprehends written language correctly and carries out simple directions presented to him in writing. Recognition of individual letters and numbers is intact. Writing ability is preserved only to the extent that accurate copying is possible. The patient is unable to write his name independently or to dictation. On the other hand, the alphabet can be written spontaneously in sequence, although many letter transpositions are evident. Numbers can be written serially without error. Script is copied correctly, and the patient is not dependent on a model of the letter in copying."

If this combination were not present, the writing impairment would appear to be much more isolated in nature. One would then essentially have an isolated agraphia. This apparently was the case in one of Jackson's patients, cited by Kussmaul (1877). This patient demonstrated a complete recovery from aphasia. When attempting to write her name the patient wrote: "Sunnil siclaa Satreni," and her address was written: "Sunese nut to mer tinn-lain."

Moreover, in case 1 of my earlier work, recovery of aphasia was followed by an isolated agraphia, which suggests that it may be classified within this category. I can see essentially no other way by which an isolated verbal agraphia might be produced.

7. Conduction agraphia. A disruption of the pathway (χ-β) may also, of course, cause an isolated agraphia. In such a case one would be dealing not with a verbal agraphia, but essentially, with an inability to consistently produce the correct letters. Production of hand movements, however, might still be intact. According to the ideas developed above in regard to center (χ) and its connections to the motor regions, complete disruption of all the numerous pathways between (χ-β) would not be expected without destruction of center (χ) itself. This type of agraphia would therefore be restricted to one limb, such as the right arm, and writing would still be possible with the left.

All of these anticipated symptoms are confirmed in the significant case of Pitres (1884). This patient may, therefore, serve as a paradigm for this form and also as proof of the accuracy of our interpretations of written language disorders. One may confidently accept integrity of center (χ) in spite of the accompanying right hemianopsia, since there was absence of impairment in reading as well as in writing with the left hand.

Pitres. Case 1 (1884)

On July 30, 1882, a 31 year old wine merchant with syphilis of ten years duration initially demonstrated moderate and then rapidly increasing generalized symptoms. For a period of one week he was partially comatose, disoriented, speechless, and presented a total right hemiplegia. Gradual improvement was noted following vigorous liniment treatment, and by the end of the year the patient was able to manage independently. Improvement continued and recovery was essentially complete by 1883. On February 5, 1884, the following status was observed. Intelligence, speech comprehension, reading ability, etc. were normal. The only complaints noted were stiffness of the right leg and complete inability to write, although movements of the right hand was intact. Visual acuity was normal. A characteristic right hemianopsia was present. Chronic rigidity of the right leg was observed, with minimal disturbance of gait, however. Foot signs were marked on the right. Knee signs were present bilaterally and particularly abnormal on the right. Dynometric testing verified the weakness of the leg. Sensation was intact. No rigidity was noted in the right arm, but there was an increase in knee reflexes. Chill-blains were evident on the right hand, which was also colder and had more color than the left. Sensation was intact except for a mild disturbance in kinesthesis. The patient was able to recognize objects held in the right hand with his eyes closed. However, such objects were reported to feel lighter than when held in the left hand. Position-sense of the right hand could not be accurately assessed, and when the patient was asked to raise both hands to the same height, the right was always raised higher. Voluntary movements of the right hand were well-executed but somewhat more slowly than on the left. The patient was able to carry out all directions with the exception of writing.

Copying of a word with the right hand, which previously could not be carried out spontaneously, was accomplished laboriously and with constant referral to the letters. The patient was able to point to single letters within whole words both in script and printed form in response to oral request. Although a word written with the left hand could be copied, independent writing was not possible. The same was true of numbers. The patient was unable to write from memory in absence of the model. He had no difficulty in copying the writing of others as well as his own. When using the right hand, the letters were merely drawn and could not be transcribed into script. Geometric figures and a man's profile were produced without difficulty with the right hand. Seven months later, essentially the same findings were demonstrated.

Additional testing revealed that the motor-imagery involved in writing was still intact. If one guided the patient's hand while he held his eyes closed during production of various letters and words, he was able to tell which word had been written in this manner. Reading was fluent in spite of the right hemianopsia. Therefore, reading apparently was carried out directly by the right hemisphere, which was also operative during writing with the left hand. It was my opinion that his was not the condition of one who had once learned to read but never to write. This was adequately demonstrated in the examination just described.

III. WERNICKE'S EARLY ESSAYS ON PSYCHIATRY

PROBLEMS OF CLINICAL PSYCHIATRY

Die Aufgaben der klinischen Psychiatrie (Original publication in: Breslauer Aertz. Ztschr. No. 13, 1887)

and

APHASIA AND MENTAL ILLNESS

Aphasie und Geisteskrankheiten (Original publication in: Verhandlung des Congresses für innere Medizin Wiesbaden, 1890).

[The two essays which follow form part of a small group of papers published between 1879 and 1892 which sketch Wernicke's preliminary concepts of psychic function and mental illness.

The first of this group, "Über das Bewusstsein" [In Regard to Consciousness], appeared in 1879 and detailed the process involved in concept formation and the three categories of consciousness: consciousness of the outer world (allopsyche), consciousness of the body (somatopsyche), and consciousness of the personality (autopsyche).

"Problems of Clinical Psychiatry," presented here in translation, together with a later essay, "Grundzüge einer psychiatrische Symptomenlehre." [Outlines of a Psychiatric Classification System], briefly sketch Wernicke's early formulation of his psychic schema and nosology. These ideas may most easily be studied in connection with the diagram illustrated in Figure 23.

In these essays psychiatric symptoms are defined as expressions of brain disease which may involve three different mechanisms, the psychosensory, intrapsychic, and psychomotor processes. Impairment of such processes, which were felt to be transcortical in nature, would find expression in hyper-, hypo-, or para-modes of dysfunction. Moreover, partial or complete impairment in any of the three spheres of consciousness might be demonstrated.

Wernicke (1892) outlined the following general classification of processes subject to dysfunction in mental illness.

Psychosensory	anesthesia parasthesia hyperesthesia
Intrapsychic	afunction parafunction hyperfunction
Psychomotor	akinesia parakinesia hyperkinesia

In the second essay included here, "Aphasia and Mental Illness," Wernicke attempts to point to the relation between psychiatric disorders and abnormal function in speech as well as other modes of behavioral expression. In fact, he later stated, "An analysis of aphasia offers a paradigm for all psychic processes which have a concrete content." (Wernicke, 1900). Disorders in speech accompanying mental illness were accordingly categorized as psychosensory, psychomotor, or intrapsychic. For example, mutism, occurring in certain psychiatric disorders, might be psychomotor and reflect a motor incapacity to speak – psychosensory, caused by abnormal sensation in parts of the speech mechanism – or intrapsychic, as a result of delusions.

Wernicke's psychic schema and classification system of mental illness was later the target of sharp criticism and debate and did not survive as did his contributions to aphasia. Liepmann later reflected that Wernicke had not intended an "actual cerebral anatomic localization of mental processes. . . but had only analyzed psychic life into such elements which might be regarded as parallel processes of the neural apparatus" (Liepmann, 1924) * Schroeder later reiterated this interpretation in his comments:

> Wernicke's familiar schema *sAZm* (Figure 23) is solely a super-structure of lines, which, presenting a mixture of anatomic and physiologic concepts in keeping with his times, was regarded by him as only a hypothetical sum of the sensory and motor projection fields, (*s* and *m*: they were intended merely to indicate and organize the sequential processes involved in psychic activity without necessarily relating them to specific cortical areas or fiber tracts (Schroeder, 1939, p. 42). *
>
> Moreover, Wernicke himself stated:
>
> I need hardly emphasize that our practical knowledge of mental illness has nothing to do with theoretic hypotheses. It is a much greater achievement. . . to separate the special disorders and to study them in detail (Schroeder, 1939, p. 42).*

This achievement, the detailed description of various entities in the area of mental illness is held by such as Jasper (1946), Schroeder (1939), Hildebrandt (1921), and others as a valued and significant contribution to the psychiatric literature.]

PROBLEMS OF CLINICAL PSYCHIATRY

Die Aufgaben der klinischen Psychiatrie

Original publication in: *Beslauer ärzt. Ztschr.* No. 13, 1887.

Reprinted in: *Gesammelte Aufsätze und kritische Referate zur Pathologie des Nervensystems.* Berlin: Fischer, 1893, pp. 146-152.

The specific clinical class of diseases described as mental illness has commonly been accepted as similar in essential points to various classes of physical illness. The symptoms of this clinical class may be acute or chronic. Certain forms may be characterized by a predictable course, including stages of onset, crisis, and recovery. Rapid improvement may occur in some types, while others characteristically present a relentless progression of symptoms. Still others may become chronic and demonstrate persisting residual defects. In short, from the physician's view-point they may be considered completely analogous to organic diseases. However, only recently has this been realized. In spite of the name "psychic" [spiritual] illness, no one of course regards them as illnesses of the spirit, least of all those who do not believe in ghosts and phantoms.

There is essentially general agreement that mental illnesses are caused by brain disease, and as such, although they are still poorly understood, represent involvement of a well-known organ. One can merely state that the specific designation of a certain area of the brain as the organ of consciousness may be regarded as strong evidence for the existence of a specific class of mental illnesses. The symptoms of this class are so characteristically related to mental functions that the brain may be considered as the organ which is typically involved. Only by recognizing such an organ, subject to disease, can one understand the existence of mental illness as an independent class which must be differentiated from other brain diseases.

As is well-known, most of the data support the hypothesis that the grey cortical mantle, covering both hemispheres, represents in its totality the hypothesized organ of consciousness. In view of the evidence that deep destruction of specific areas of the cerebral cortex is accompanied by specific types of paralysis or sensory disturbances which do not occur in mental illness, or only rarely, one must further hypothesize that only specific layers of the cortex are exclusively destined to serve as the organ of consciousness.

A review of recent findings in the area of brain physiology does not conflict with such a possible hypothesis. There is increasing confirmation of the notion which considers the cortex as a kind of sensory surface analogous to a photographic apparatus on which neural stimuli are "projected" and persist in the form of "memory images." In these layers are contained the sum total of all memory images with their lawfully-produced connections, namely, groups of ganglion cells and the nerve fibers serving in the process of "association." They form the material substrate of the organ of consciousness. Supported by these views, a clinical study undertaken to gain an understanding of mental illness has shown that mental illness may be regarded as nothing other than disease of a specific yet extensive area of the brain. Moreover, we have demonstrated that the commonly accepted hypothesis relative to brain disease may be applied to this specific group and confirms its validity.

Griesinger's differentiation of focal and diffuse generalized symptomatology has significantly advanced our knowledge of disease of the brain. The clinical picture of focal involvement may be caused by stimulation or destruction of specific cerebral areas. The nature of the disease-processes causing such stimulation or destruction may be very similar. The generalized symptoms are caused by the specific nature of the illness presented. In part, this may involve the entire physical organism (such as fever, for example), and in part, the total function of the brain, as occurs in loss of consciousness.

The relationship between these two symptom-pictures is characteristic of various brain diseases. The progressive nature of symptoms in different forms of cerebral involvement demonstrates a second important feature. One must differentiate between those illnesses which present an acute onset with gradual recession and continuing progression to eventual recovery, and others which demonstrate a predictable increase in symptoms and a more gradual progression of the disease-course. Is this situation also true of mental illness?

This question may at once be answered in the affirmative. Let us now consider the course of mental illness. Those cases demonstrating an acute and stormy onset, as far as is known now, generally present the most favorable prognosis and run a rapid course.On the contrary, those illnesses characterized by a slow, gradual onset frequently prove to be relentlessly progressive and resistant to treatment. Primary insanity, one of the few better known forms of mental illness, is a good example of this latter course, which is also found in brain disease.

An understanding of the interrelationships of focal and generalized symptomatology requires first of all an appreciation of the concept of focal symptoms which may be seen in diseases involving consciousness. To what extent is localization of varying functions in the wide-spread organization of consciousness possible, a concept which might suggest a relationship of impairment of such function to focal symptomatology?In this respect I would like to point to the following diagnostic features which may serve not only to offer unbiased evidence but which may also be useful in providing clinical examples of mental illness. One may speak of three different forms of consciousness, each having its own cerebral localization. "Consciousness of corporeality" is formed by the aggregate of memory images of one's own body-awareness, whose interconnections by association fibers are very closely-bound. "Consciousness of the outer-world" forms another type of consciousness and is made up of combinations of tightly-bound lawfully-produced associations of memory images acquired through sensory impressions from the environment which have been projected to the sensory organ. Finally, "consciousness of the personality" represents the most complicated combinations of memory images. In reality it is made up of entire complexes of such imagery associated with personal experiences of the individual and embraces the interrelationships of his corporeality to the total environment. This latter is formed to an extent by an integration of the first two types of consciousness and characterizes a point in development rarely reached by many of idiot mentality.

Just as mild involvement may impair the most complex functions, so clinical experience teaches that impairment in "consciousness of the personality" may occur in milder forms of mental disturbance (for example, pure melancholia and mania), while "consciousness of the environment" and one's own "consciousness of corporeality" remain intact. Likewise, some cases may present a primary and isolated impairment of "consciousness of corporeality," while in others, disturbance of "consciousness of the environment" may represent the chief symptom in the entire clinical picture. Furthermore, one must avoid too superficial a treatment of the subject. This might lead to the neglect of perceiving an underlying lawfulness in the production of combinations of focal symptoms arising from involvement of one area or another. Our knowledge of this problem is still in its initial stages.

Some clinical examples may be necessary at this point for orientation of the non-psychiatrist. One such example might be found in the delusions experienced by some patients who believe the body to be made of ivory or glass with consequent lack of sensation. Another patient may feel that he has no head, tongue, heart, or stomach, that he has three legs, that his head is attached to the rear, or his arms are reversed. If there is impairment of "consciousness of the environment," the patient may feel everything to be foreign or unfamiliar. He may believe himself to be in heaven or on a ship. He may not recognize people in his environment and may regard them as God, the devil, the Kaiser, a hangman, or even close relatives. Individual features may seem to undergo change while viewed by the patient. Many similar illustrations might be mentioned.

In impairment of "consciousness of the personality" the patient, in the case of melancholia, may imagine himself to be a criminal, may hold his roommate responsible for his illness, or may believe his relatives to be dead or threatened with mishap. In cases of mania the patient may feel euphoric, capable of great things, and more shrewd than before. He may be proud, obstinate, or play other roles. His condition may be generally characterized by a specific kind of suspiciousness, demonstrating feelings of persecution and the notion that others are plotting against him. In primary insanity the patient may feel himself to be of higher parentage and suspect that he was exchanged in infancy with another child. All such delusions may be classified under the focal symptoms of mental disease, since they demonstrate only a partial involvement of a component of consciousness.

In addition to the description of the three large categories mentioned above, in which consciousness as a whole is operative, further analysis of these three is still necessary. On the basis of clinical studies, it is very likely that such localization may also include important internal organs such as the stomach and heart. "Consciousness of the environment" may be divided into various areas according to the mental channels through which it is acquired. Each semester patients with progressive paralysis provide me with clinical evidence demonstrating disturbance in object-recognition through tactual avenues alone (without visual aid) to be the characteristic features of this disease. (Preservation of visual acuity: psychic blindness). The reverse may also occur, with recognition possible through visual but not tactual avenues. Therefore, one must differentiate at least two forms of consciousness, the visual and the tactual. An acoustic consciousness must also exist, since sensory aphasia is even more frequent in paralytics than the disorders just mentioned. Further classification, based on clinical study, is necessary in regard to what "consciousness of the personality" encompasses.

This review of psychic focal symptoms is still far from complete. However, I feel that for the present, at least, a framework for the major categories has been provided. Let us now explore the question of anatomic localization of such focal psychic symptoms. Three major categories of consciousness may be assigned to specific areas of the many-layered cortex. Clinical experience based on the study of aphasia indicates that the period of time necessary for development of a specific content of consciousness is essentially the same for all projection areas.

One may well ask how a blow to the head could spare the mother-tongue but erase a later-acquired foreign language from consciousness? Such experience permits one to generalize that the "consciousness of corporeality" extending from conception through intra-uterine life, and which with the exception of the sexual sphere, progresses into and is completed during childhood, is contained in one layer of the cortex. "Consciousness of the environment," on the other hand, which is completed much later, is located in the cortical layer either above or below this one. Finally, "consciousness of personality," as the latest acquisition, may claim a special layer of the association system. If these ideas prove to be true, which I myself do not question, the relationship of further subclassifications of consciousness to the projection system will become more readily apparent. So much for our most immediate problem of anatomic localization.

Mental illnesses are frequently characterized by numerous generalized symptoms. These occur for example in cases of epilepsy, apoplexy, the so-called paralytics, simpler cases of unconsciousness, deeper coma, somnalence, stupor, confusion as well as jactition with its transition to simple motor unrest. Rarer cases may show the isolated onset of fever, an abnormal pulse rate, or a decrease in body temperature. However, more often than might be thought, headache of various type and site may be present. And, finally, one may find insomnia, the counterpart of somnalence, a symptom which plays by far a greater role in this than in other brain diseases. Another series of generalized symptoms characteristically accompanies mental illnesses. These are symptoms of affect including both those which produce morbid ideas and those which result from such symptoms. The first group is characterized by fear which may vary from a mild anxiety to mortal terror which is commonly localized in the precordial region of the chest and heart. Fear and dread are modifications of such symptoms. Sometimes one may find anger varying from irritation to senseless rage, either in combination with other symptoms or in isolation. The affect of happiness is relatively rare, since it occurs consequent to a change in the content of consciousness. Moreover, the most frequent consequence is confusion expressed in various ways, such as alarm, astonishment, rapid change from crying to laughter, helplessness, instinctive resistance, and pronounced shock.

We now come to behavior patterns which may be observed as both focal and generalized disease, and one must admit that our knowledge in this area is still very incomplete. Many different forms of mental illness undoubtedly exist. However, only a fraction of these are known at present and these merely in general and vague outline.

The future task of clinical psychiatry lies in the definitive classification of the numerous and varied forms of impairment of consciousness according to focal and generalized symptoms and the formulation of specific clinical pictures of the overwhelming material available. Nevertheless, the success of such an attempt is already assured in that we have been guided to this point by a general hypothesis already confirmed in the area of brain pathology. The clinical significance of focal symptomatology is dependent upon the accompanying generalized symptoms. Moreover, psychiatric studies have definitely indicated the disappearance of pathological ideas in the presence of happy emotions. In contrast, such ideas progress into a state of rigid chronic hallucinations if positive emotional affect is lacking.

APHASIA AND MENTAL ILLNESS

Aphasie und Geisteskrankheit

Original publication in: *Verhandlungen des Congresses für innere Medizin.* Wiesbaden, 1890, p. 273

Reprinted in: *Gesammelte Aufsätze und kritische Referate zur Pathologie des Nervensystems.* Berlin: Fischer: 1893, pp. 153-160

Recently a 48 year old carpenter was discharged as improved from my Clinic following four years of mental illness. He might have been considered essentially well but for one problem, the loss of articulate speech and limitation of communication to gestures and writing. The disturbance which he continues to demonstrate may be described as motor aphasia. Although he is completely mute and unable to utter a single word, there is no paralysis of the pertinent musculature. Nor is there any question of related bulbar involvement as described by Von Leyden.

However, we know that motor aphasia may play a part in various different symptom-pictures, and therefore we shall try to determine under which category this particular case may be classified. At this point I must refer to the schema first presented by Lichtheim (1884-85) which provides us with a complete review of the anatomically-predictable pure cases of aphasia. As is known, the central speech mechanism consists essentially of two centers and their associated pathways. This mechanism includes, as indicated in Figure 23, a sensory speech center (s), the site of acoustic imagery and the terminals of the centripetal tract of the acoustic nerve, a motor center (m), which may be described as the site of motor imagery and the source of a centrifugal tract which may be designated as the motor speech tract, and finally, the path (s-m), connecting the two centers. We may also note site (B) representing a third center in the schema. Furthermore, the broken lines (s-B) indicate a centripetal and the lines (B-m) a centrifugal direction. This then leads to the following situation.

Recognition of speech sounds is mediated by center (s), but comprehension of meaning requires transmission to a supporting center (B). In this way the conduction path (s-B) assumes a specific significance. The motor center (m), from which motor innervation of the word is transmitted, is indicated on the other side of the schema. However, in spontaneous speech, this is first possible following arousal of the word-concept into consciousness, in which process center (m) is first stimulated by (B). This requires recognition of a centrifugal path (B-m). In this way (s) serves as the receiving-station and (m) as the dispatch-post of the speech message, which is read and sorted in center (B). Applying the nomenclature suggested earlier, we may then designate disruption of the centripetal pathway as sensory aphasia and that of the centrifugal path as motor aphasia. In this way various forms of these two aphasia groups may be classified and differentiated. Cortical aphasia will typically result from damage to the cortical centers (s) or (m). Disruption of their subcortical tracts may be followed by subcortical aphasia, while interruption of the pertinent paths on either sides of the centers could cause transcortical forms of aphasia.

In the case under discussion, in which a motor aphasia was unquestionably present, we must still differentiate between a cortical, subcortical, or transcortical motor aphasia. This question may be resolved if one consideres the clinical pictures already known. A cortical motor aphasia may be ruled out since our patient is able to read, although inaccurately. Moreover, spontaneous as well as writing to dictation is fluent and intelligible. The transcortical form of motor aphasia may be differentiated by loss of spontaneous speech-expression with preservation of mimicry and oral reading. Our patient demonstrates no residual ability in either area. The subcortical form of motor aphasia is characterized by preservation of reading and writing with loss of articulate speech alone. Because these symptoms are evident in this patient, he would appear to belong to this category. However, closer study disproves this assumption. First of all, reading and writing are certainly possible in this case, and one can readily communicate with him by such means. However, integrity of these two areas is in no way as complete as would be expected in subcortical motor aphasia. For example, he can no longer read or write Latin as before, and copying of the same is possible only by laborious drawing of the letters. Furthermore, certain paraphasic-like features are obvious in his writing. For example, he writes *kirne* instead of *gerne, Flasse* for *Flasche* and omits certain letters such as the sustained *ye* in place of *geh,* and *etferter* for *entfernter.* Moreover all is written in lower case letters.

Secondly, the absence of any trace of a right hemiplegia is unusual in subcortical motor aphasia, since this symptom, at least in partial form, is a general characteristic of this group. Thirdly, our patient demonstrates specific complications which are incompatible with a subcortical localization of the disorder. For example, loss of certain movement-sequences of the speech musculature, separate from those involved in speech articulation, can be observed, although a paralysis in the usual sense is not present. The patient cannot voluntarily blow through his mouth, blow out a light, and is even less able to whistle. Puffing-out of the cheeks is very difficult and can be carried out only if the nose is occluded. Neither is he able to expectorate, and sucking movements have apparently been lost. For example, when drinking is attempted the glass must be placed far within his mouth before swallowing is possible. Voluntary movement of the tongue is not possible, although it is used normally in swallowing and chewing, indicating an absence of impairment in tongue movement itself.

It seems to me that on the surface at least, one might tend to explain loss of such specific motor patterns on the basis of a subcortical lesion. On the other hand, however, the evidence is just as strong to interpret it differently, namely, as loss of articulate speech. Finally, the chief objection to an interpretation of the case as the result of a subcortical lesion lies in the characteristic manner of onset of the speech disorder. Certain case-history details are essential here for an appropriate diagnosis. The first traces of mental illness including persecutional mania, anxiety, and prior hypochondriacal complaints of various kinds occurred in September, 1885. At that time the patient spent approximately six months in bed. This was followed by a remission, and he was able to work for a few months of the years 1886 and 1887 until September, 1887. At that time the symptoms worsened considerably, and by December of the same year admission to the Clinic was necessary. The patient remained there during the second half of the year in a stuporous condition. When this subsided, he was mute and did not utter a word but tried by gesture to indicate his inability to speak. Gradual recovery of speech was noted in the latter part of January, 1889. Initially, speech was unintelligible and produced in a whisper or soft voice. The use of a sing-song tone led to the impression of constant repetition of the same sounds (verbigeration).

During February an increase in volume and intelligibility of speech was observed. However, communication was very limited, and throughout the day the patient spoke only the words, "Korensky, korensky, oh Landleben." These words could be heard from the time he arose for work, through mealtimes and up to the time of retirement in the evening. Mimicry of simple words was attempted but was not successful. By the end of February some increase in vocabulary was noticed. The patient now perseverated on the phrase, "mia Anno Kochlunski oh Landleben." By this time he was also successful in mimicking a few short words such as "Mütze," "Fritz," and "Bertha."

During the spring and summer of 1889 the patient passed through a period of auditory hallucination, and could not be examined. Following a remission of this phase, the depression lifted, and he entered a period of convalescence. At this time, however, complete muteness was observed with inability to imitate even the simplest sound. At the same time other previously mentioned motor deficits were apparent. His behavior was otherwise normal, and he worked industriously in our work-shop. Following discharge from the clinic, the patient returned to his earlier position of cabinet maker.

This case study shows beyond doubt that the motor aphasia followed a specific pattern which has long been recognized in the clinical symptomatology of mental illness. Mutism and verbigeration, which are likewise related to involvement of the central speech mechanism, were also evident.

This brings us to the fundamental issue in this problem. What is the relationship between aphasia and mental illness, and how can the origin of aphasia in mental illness as demonstrated in this case, be interpreted? I must turn once again to the schema (Figure 23) which occupied us at the beginning of this

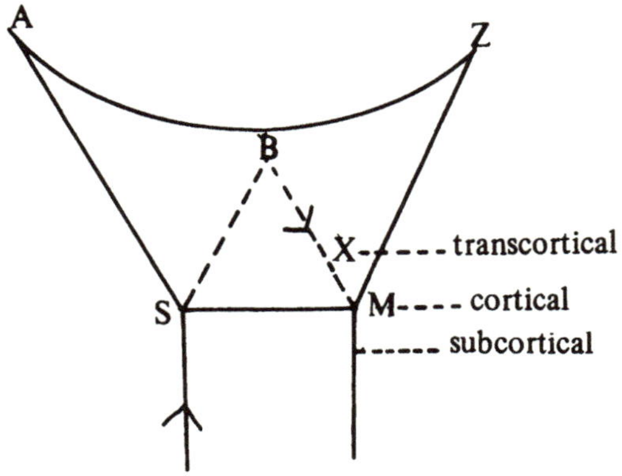

FIG. 23.

Schema of the Psychic Reflex

(s): Acoustic imagery
(m): Motor imagery
(B): Concept center
(A): Discharge–site of conceptualization
(Z): Ideational plan process

essay for a solution to this dilemna. The center (B), the concept area, serves only in a general way as the specific site from which thought-activity issues. If we try to insert this "area of concept-activity" into our schema, we are confronted with the problem of satisfactorily reaching an understanding of the psychological complexities involved in this situation. One must first determine the primary avenue through which an examination of the mentally ill may be conducted. Undoubtedly, the mode of examination necessary would involve questioning of the patient and attempting an assessment of the status of his conceptual-activity on the basis of the quality of his response. For example, we might assume that reception of the question occurs in center (s) and response by means of center (m). The response then may be interpreted as a kind of reflex movement which is directed by detour through the site of the "localization of concept-activity."

Comprehension of the question by the patient would then require arousal of the specific concepts relevant to the question. Let us designate (A) as the discharge-point of this total conceptualization. The response of the patient, however, which follows a period of deliberation, is directed from the ideational-plan-process designated by (Z). This reaches the patient by means of association, so that the pathway (A-Z) represents the association bonds which are traversed in the process of the patient's thought activity. In this modified schema, the centripetal pathway (s-B) is replaced by (s-A), and in place of the centrifugal pathway (B-m), the path (Z-m). Should the response be inappropriate in content, inaccurate, or not pertinent, we may conclude the presence of erroneous links in the association chain. If the response occurs, but sluggishly, it might be interpreted as delay and deterioration of thought processes. The outcome, as far as we are concerned, is always a function of the transcortical conductors which extend between the receiving-station on the one side, and the dispatch-post on the other. Therefore, from our point of view, mental illnesses involve the province of transcortical function, or if one would not shrink from an extension of such an idea, the province of the transcortical aphasias. But even this extension of the concept is far too narrow. The same examination procedures used to gain a sample of the patient's speech may also be used to elicit other forms of expression of movement, such as a request that a specific movement be carried out with the right hand. Our schema would then remain unchanged up to the discharge-point (A), but (Z), the ideational goal planning center, would acquire a new significance as an innervation-point of the motor imagery of the arm. An incorrect or inappropriate movement would then be interpreted in the mentally ill as an impairment of transcortical function.

Complete loss of movement may suggest a transcortical paralysis, and it is quite likely that our case of motor aphasia might be classified within this category. The objection presented earlier that our patient's clinical findings differ from those generally associated with transcortical aphasia is now no longer tenable, since the insertion of the specific comprehensive faculties (A) and (Z) indicates that the hypothesis of the transcortical paths (s-B) and (B-m) is purely schematic. Furthermore, one may assume the existence of innumerable pathways (s-A) and (Z-m), and consequently, countlessly varying pictures of transcortical aphasia.

Our patient may represent just one such possible example. The clinical picture discussed above may therefore merely serve to sketch the syndrome in somewhat greater detail. If one applies such an interpretation, the motor disturbances might appear in the same guise as the aphasias. These could then be designated as transcortical tongue paralysis, transcortical paralysis of respiration, etc.

Although an interpretation of mental illness on the basis of impairment in transcortical function may simplify the classification of our patient within the common disease nosology, we must still consider an objection which might be raised but is readily answered. Each symptom, as defined, is applicable to the area of mental illness with the exception of a very specific disease entity, progressive paralysis. Progressive paralysis is the only mental disease which may lead to cortical and subcortical focal symptoms, and this ambivalence is reflected in its accurate classification under either organic brain disease or mental illness. If our case were a paralytic, the argument presented above would have failed from the onset. The entire course of the illness and residual symptoms of mental disease contradict this. The patient is certainly not lacking in defects in the mental realm but does not present deficits which are characteristic of progressive paralysis. One look at the visual fields, which demonstrated concentric constriction, is adequate in resolving such a question for the experienced examiner. The diagnosis therefore presents no difficulty. The degree of mental anxiety necessary for such a diagnosis would not be observed in a paralytic of five years duration. Moreover, the manual skill demonstrated by the patient, the absence of tremor, etc., indicates that the question of general paresis need not be entertained.

IV. WERNICKE'S FINAL APHASIA PERIOD

THE APHASIA SYMPTOM COMPLEX

Der Aphasische Symptomenkomplex

Original publication in: Die Deutsche Klinik am Eingange des 20 Jahrhunderts Bd. 6, Abt. 1, p. 487, 1906

[Wernicke's final work on aphasia, sometimes referred to as the "Deutsche-Klinik Aphasische Symptomenkomplex" was written shortly before his death and was published posthumously in 1906.

Wernicke's final return to the subject of aphasia at this time of his life was apparently triggered by his study of a case of isolated agraphia in 1903. His interest in reading and writing disturbances in aphasia had been evident in his 1874 work which contained brain models of the processes underlying these skills. The seven-fold classification of the alexias and agraphias, discussed in the work of his middle period, "Recent Works on Aphasia", represented a further elaboration of his early thinking on this aspect of aphasia. In 1903, at a time when he was almost completely absorbed in his psychiatric writings and work, his attention was drawn to a patient under treatment in his clinic whose initial aphasia had resolved, leaving an essentially circumscribed agraphia. Wernicke's study of this patient led to the publication of a short essay "Isoliertie Agraphie," published in 1903. This paper is the only work of Wernicke's in the area of aphasia which is not included in this volume of translations, since its essential content was summarized by him in the 1906 monograph.

The 1906 Aphasia Symptom Complex may be divided into three sections. The initial part contains a review and updating of his classification system in the light of recent literature of that time. The second and major section of the work is devoted to a detailed discussion of "disorders of written language." Wernicke includes an interesting digression on word-finding impairment in this part of the paper. The final section provides a fairly detailed resume of the neuroanatomic substrate of language and the clinico-pathological correlates of aphasia.]

DISTURBANCES OF ORAL LANGUAGE

A brief case-history of an essentially isolated agraphia published earlier in 1903 serves as a preface to Wernicke's final monograph on aphasia. This rather unusual introduction hints at his underlying motive in returning to the subject of aphasia in this final period of his life, which was otherwise almost completely absorbed in the study of mental illness. That motive was the further exploration into the alexias and agraphias in the light of current findings of that period.

Before approaching his main topic however, Wernicke briefly reviews and up-dates his aphasia classification system giving particular attention to the special forms, the transcortical and subcortical aphasias.

The patient I would like to present to you today represents a remarkable kind of psychic disturbance. This 46 year old woman, the wife of a tailor, had received an education typical of her class. At any event, it was established that she had been able to read fluently and to write. She presented the symptoms of a focal lesion of the left hemisphere with a right hemiplegia associated with severe sensory impairment of the entire right side. These symptoms first developed slowly over a period of nine months, beginning with onset of weakness of the right hand following three acute attacks, the second of which was followed by a transient disturbance of speech with moderate difficulty in articulation. However, this did not impair intelligibility of expression. Although we cannot ignore the moderate anarthria, for the purpose of this investigation it may be temporarily disregarded. In respect to her mental status, the patient was attentive, rational, and apparently intellectually normal. She responded correctly to all questions, indicating that she understood what was said and could follow the train of thought in conversation. Moreover, she read fluently and also demonstrated good comprehension of what she read. Individual letters of the alphabet as well as numbers could be read accurately and without hesitation. In the same way she correctly recognized and comprehended pictures, drawings and designs. In sharp contrast, however, there was a complete loss of the ability to write. Moreover, in the course of a longer examination, which offered her additional opportunity for practice in this area, she was unable to produce anything beyond copying of the letter "a" and the numbers 2, 3, and 4 on the slate. Spontaneous writing, without benefit of dictation, continued to remain completely lost. Thus, she essentially presented a classic case of the so-called pure or isolated agraphia.

One must naturally take into consideration the fact that the right hand was not so severely paralyzed as to be generally useless. Apart from a complete tactile loss, there was definite loss of all finer movement of that hand and consequently limitation of gross motility. However, the ability to write, as is known from clinical experience, is not completely confined to the right hand. Normally, all individuals who have learned to write can accomplish this task, although clumsily, with the left hand. This is carried out more slowly and with less facility than with the right hand and, in fact, may resemble drawing because it is carried out with an entirely different technique. Nevertheless, it is legible and each word and letter can be read. Typically this awkwardness is particularly obvious only on the first attempts, and a comparatively good performance is soon achieved by practice. In our case, however, an absolute loss of the ability to write individual letter symbols, or to form syllables and words was observed. Inasmuch as gross movements of the right hand were intact, one could test writing by fastening to the right hand a block of wood with a piece of chalk attached. Placed before the blackboard with this device, the patient was able to write nothing, although she was able to support and guide the right hand with the left.

The peculiar psychic behavior of the patient in all writing attempts deserves mention. Facial gesture and posture gave the impression of one perplexed and confused. For example, she would stop and think for minutes at a time and then required persuasion to continue. After a few attempts, however, she made us understand that she was tired and could not make any further efforts.

Gentlemen, who of us would not be impressed with the apprently strong analogy between the typical, isolated psychic disturbance presented by our case and that of the frequent and well known symptom-picture of aphasia, an analogy which in fact is so obvious that our case today may serve as an introduction to the controversial question still raging in this area? The fact that the loss of ability to write in this patient was related to a localized lesion appears no more strange than the well known observation of this same occurrence in the area of speech. This may well be true if we hold to the definition which Broca, the discoverer of a localized cerebral center for human speech, applied to the type of speech disturbance resulting from damage to such a center. His patient had lost the power to produce articulate speech, the power of speech expression, which as we all know must be acquired through learning, as is also true of writing. Moreover, in our case, this isolated impairment in writing can be as little explained on the basis of paralysis of a certain group of muscles as could the loss of speech in Broca's patient. If we now acknowledge an analogy between these two disturbances, we are then forced to hypothesize the existence of a special cerebral center for writing, just as a specific center for speech has already been localized in Broca's gyrus. In fact, many authorities have already been led to these conclusions. At the pinnacle of such we find no less a man than Charcot, whom we have regarded as the intellectual leader of medicine in our neighboring country during his lifetime.

Accordingly, a deeper study of the entire symptom-complex of aphasia as well as the symptomatology of the case before us can show that we have already gone beyond the most important assumption if we accept an actual writing center. Moreover, the autopsy findings are not favorable for support of such an assumption.

We must be especially cautious in an area such as aphasia, since premature and misleading generalizations based on facts which may be correct and valid in themselves have already proven unfortunate and have resulted in censure of every attempt to support the doctrine of localization in aphasia as hopeless and utopian.

I must recall at this time that Broca's discovery (1861) occurred at a time in which the doctrine of brain pathology, represented by clinicians of such standing as Bouillaud and Andral, and that of the school of physiology, championed by Flourens, was the object of devisive conflict. The former based their views on facts which seemed to support the idea that different areas of the brain controlled different functions, while the Flourens school was inclined to explain effects on the basis of Gall's theory of phrenology, which has been justly discredited. Moreover, animal experiments which apprently had proven the lack of differentiation of function in the animal brain were used as evidence. Thus, a clinician who contested Broca's discovery found the ground well-prepared by skepticism.

Therefore, when Trousseau opposed this idea, his views gained general sympathy without much difficulty. The famous debate which occurred in the Academy of Medicine in 1864 regarding this matter proved this in a most instructive way. However, at the same time one could see that Broca's interpretation of this symptom, designated by him as aphemia, was entirely different from that of Trousseau. The pure cases of Broca's aphemia, as Broca himself had expressly emphasized, consisted only in the symptom of "impossibilité de parler" without any other further disturbance. This patient, according to Broca, had lost "la faculté d'articuler les mots", le sourvenir du procédé, qu'il faut suivre pour articuler les mots". Broca expressed himself even more clearly when he designated the process by which the child learns to speak as "par le développement d'une espèce particulière de mémoire, qui n'est pas la mémoire des mots, mais celle des mouvements nécessaires pour articuler les mots."

Now, one could not object if, in opposition to these rare cases of aphemia, Trousseau presented his own cases which demonstrated a variety of clinical pictures and used such as proof of the many striking and bewildering symptoms such patients might present. However, his cases represented an entirely different form of aphasia (than Broca's), although they belonged to the comprehensive aphasia symptom-complex as we understand it today. However, they in no way correspond to Broca's aphemia. Moreover, if the autopsy findings of many of these aphasic patients revealed no damage to Broca's gyrus, we would today interpret this as supportive rather than contradictory evidence of Broca's localization of a special speech center. The supposedly conflicting and unexpected pathological findings presented by Trousseau were related to an entirely different clinical picture. Moreover, one must also remember the numerous cases who present a picture of Broca's aphasia as an indirect focal symptom, which at that time was incorrectly interpreted and thus seemed to contradict Broca's discovery. Unfortunately, this misinterpretation resulted in focus of attention on all kinds of strange and interesting isolated signs related to the symptomatology of aphasia. Thus, that discovery which was first greeted with such anticipation and which actually served to introduce an era of further progress in the knowledge of brain function came to be viewed as unproven and was therefore neglected.

The momentous advance in brain anatomy forged by Meynert, as well as that in cerebral physiology achieved by Fritsch and Hitzig, was needed to provide a deeper understanding of the seemingly diverse clinical picture of aphasia which Trousseau presented. At the same time, it placed Broca's well-earned discovery in the proper perspective. Even at that time, the term aphemia, which attempted to describe a specific and circumscribed clinical picture, fell into obscurity.

We may recall that the hope of achieving a theory of localization of cerebral functions was fanned by Broca's discovery and thwarted by Trousseau. One might be inclined to attribute the major contribution of this effort to Fritsch and Hitzig's experimental findings, that motor points in specific areas of the brain can be stimulated. These findings permitted aphasia theory to take a new direction and to be interpreted in terms of cerebral localization. But even Hitzig's works might have remained obscure and would likely have gained few followers but for Meynert's explanations of the structure of the human and animal brain and his interpretation of the anatomic data at hand, which even at that time permitted formulation of unique concepts of cortical function. We are indebted to Meynert for the idea of a projection system as an embodiment of all sensory and motor tracts which extend between the sensory surfaces and muscles on the one hand and the cortex on the other, maintaining a physiological continuity between the two. Only by these tracts could stimulation from the body surface be projected to the sensory areas of the brain and result in transmission of motor impulses to the musculature. Meynert felt that a cross-section of the cerebral puduncles contained representation of the entire organism, which was incapable of olfaction or sight. The ganglion cells of the cortex were believed to be specific for the same elementary functions. The rich variety of modes of their connections with the suface of the body, mediated by the projection tracts, alone could differentiate their characteristic particular relationships to different cortical sites.

The anatomic evidence led Meynert to assume a division of the brain into two large regions, an anterior which was significant for motor function and a posterior, for sensory. These functions were assumed to be related to the development of memory images populating the cortex, the motor images located in the anterior, and the sensory images in the posterior region of the brain.

From this perspective, the movements aroused by Fritsch and Hitzig by means of galvanic stimulation in the anterior portions of the brain of the dog could be viewed in a new light. Such effects then did not correspond to the movements evoked by stimulation of certain peripheral nerves, but rather represented combinations of different muscle groups to specific movement patterns, as can also be observed in voluntary movement. The two ablation studies of Hitzig, published at the same time, led to an interpretation of residual disturbance in movement on the basis of the loss of motor memory images or cerebral representations-of-movements. In fact, Broca's aphemia appeared to represent just such a loss of motor memory images, and more definitively, those images of learned speech movements. The period during which the child learns to speak is the time of functional acquisition of a special kind of motor memory images, or to express it more aptly, "du développement d'une espèce particulière de mémoire, celle des mouvements nécessaires pour articuler les mots". It is obvious that Broca with the marvelous insight of the great discoverer of localization of a specific cerebral area was really referring to the very features which Meynert had attributed to the motor area of the cortex, an idea which later continued to gain more and more support.

Nevertheless, the broad variety of clinical subforms found in aphasia still remained a fact requiring further study and explanation. Such an interpretation was also anticipated by Meynert's work, since he believed he had discovered the central endings of the acoustic nerve and thus an acoustic speech field in the gyral walls, a peculiar structure of the claustrum and the surrounding areas of the island, which according to his interpretation, was composed entirely of association cells. Although the anatomic evidence, that is, the tracing of the course of the acoustic nerve to the island was not confirmed at this time, the implications of the significance of the acoustic nerve and the island for speech functions nevertheless drew attention to this relationship, which previously had been neglected..

It is therefore evident that Meynert's works had already satisfied all the requirements for realization of a penetrating interpretation of aphasia. My work, *The Aphasia Symptom Complex,* which appeared in 1874, merely contained a further development of Meynert's concepts and their special relation to human speech. In the anterior region of the brain we find a *motor speech center,* Broca's gyrus, which we have designated as the site for motor speech imagery or speech-movement-representation, the discharge-point of the speech impulse. In the posterior area we assume the presence of a *sensory speech center,* the site of acoustic memory images of speech and the terminal point of the acoustic nerve. At this site, memory images of the speech sounds heard in childhood are stored up, and mimicry of such sounds is gradually learned. In this way speech is acquired by each human being. The connecting fiber masses, the "association tracts" coursing between sensory and motor speech centers, mediate this act of mimicry and thus the learning of speech. General knowledge of anatomy suggests the impression of the entire first primordial gyrus overlapping the entire island as a single unity. I have hypothesized the sensory speech center to be located in the first temporal gyrus and the postulated association tract regarded by Meynert as an organ of association processes, a fiber system which converges in the island cortex, its deepest layers losing itself in the claustrum. By a happy chance, this hypothesis of a sensory speech center in the first temporal gyrus was soon confirmed by two autopsy studies. In both cases the posterior half of the longitudinal extension of the first temporal gyrus and a directly adjoining area of the second temporal gyrus were damaged by focal softening. The differentiation of three different clinical forms of aphasia was a logical consequence of this finding. These included the *motor* and *sensory* types as well as a third clinical form which I have described as *conduction* aphasia. The motor form had already been satisfactorily described by Broca, and indeed represented his own clinical form of aphemia. Sensory aphasia was characterized by the inability to comprehend speech sounds which could be heard but not comprehended and the relative preservation of articulate speech expression. The accompanying symptom, the word-confusion, (Kussmaul's *paraphasia*) was explained by assuming that the acoustic memory images provided a monitoring influence on the speech act. The existence of the clinical entity of conduction aphasia appeared to be supported by cases of paraphasia with intact ability to speak, together with preservation of speech comprehension.

This work of 1874 provided an explanation for the apparent contradiction raised by Trousseau's classic presentation, which had denied all attempts to localize speech. The claim of Broca's gyrus as the one and only speech center was thus abandoned and replaced by the correct assumption of its specific function as a motor speech center. This removed the skepticism which had frustrated any further attempts at localization. In fact, this period of skepticism came to a close with the appearance of Kussmaul's book, which continues to hold merit from the standpoint of clinical symptomatology. Moreover, the application of Meynert's interpretation of an area of brain pathology, which until then had presented particular difficulties and was not readily accessible to study, opened the possibility for further study of the mysteries of the brain, an expectation which has not remained unrealized.

In comparison, the association of the clinical picture of sensory aphasia with localization in the first temporal gyrus and an adjoining strip of the second temporal gyrus has enjoyed fairly rapid recognition. Kahler and Pick, followed shortly by Lichtheim, as well as various French, Italian, and English authorities, have essentially supported this idea, and one may assume today that the clinical picture and pathological findings of this specific type of aphasia have been as firmly established by further evidence as has the entity of Broca's motor aphasia. I feel it particularly my duty to emphasize the fact that the chief symptom of sensory aphasia, the loss of speech comprehension in association with preservation of speech capacity, had been previously correctly recognized by two earlier authorities, Bastian (1864) and Schmidt (1871). Their studies, however had not associated these speech symptoms to a specific cerebral site; therefore one cannot help but marvel at the great acuity which these men demonstrated in correctly recognizing the actual condition without having the benefit and support of Meynert's ideas at hand.

As I have already indicated, the essential point of this line of reasoning lies in the confirmation of both contrasting clinical pictures of motor and sensory aphasia within the scope of the total aphasia symptom-complex, as well as confirmation of localization of these two contrasting pictures to two entirely different areas of the brain. A historical review in this regard will yield little that is new and therefore seems unnecessary. An essential and very important step forward, however, has been made in this direction by achieving a clearer understanding of the possible relationships of the opposite functions of the two centers. We may then make the following statements in regard to the point of view we hold at this time.

The *sensory speech center,* containing the central acoustic nerve endings, provides the anatomic substrate for the images of spoken sounds, the "sound images" of Helmholz, in the ganglion cells of the cortex, the "cortical units" of H. Sachs.

These elements are involved in mediating "word-sound-identification" (Liepmann) the recognition or "identification" of the sound perceptions making up the word. This function must be definitely differentiated from "word-meaning-comprehension." In order to really appreciate the importance of this distinction one might call attention to the way in which one's mother tongue or any foreign language is learned. In most children"word-sound-identification" and "word-meaning-comprehension develop considerably earlier than the ability to articulate speech. Because of this, the sensory speech center achieves a certain independence of the motor speech center, which as we shall soon see, is much more dependent in this respect. Nevertheless, we would be justified in recognizing individual differences in this acquisition, since there undoubtedly are children in whom "word-sound-identification" progresses at the same rate as articulatory capacity. What the child learns in speech development has nothing to do with the kind of training involved in forming the sounds of written language. Rather, the acquisition of complex words occurs through the repeated practice and use of the acoustic word image together with the motor speech image.

The possession of these two very closely bound memory images is that which the French call "inner speech," thereby indicating its psychic nature which may be viewed as a certain kind of memory as Broca regarded it, as has been discussed above. Later we shall see that a close association of these interrelated images constitutes the nature of the concept. Therefore, I have proposed the term "word-concept" for this association and regard the development of such word-concepts as the most important process in the acquisition of speech. Dejerine has accepted this view and uses the expression "notion du mot." Caro's term "speech concept of the word" also appears to me a very apt choice. It would seem that the integrity of both components of the word-concept, the sensory as well as the motor, are essential for correct speech usage.

Now, although we may feel relatively certain of the mode by which speech is acquired, one may still question whether the same tract continues to be utilized for transmission of the speech impulse involved in speech movements as was originally used in the act of mimicry during the learning of speech. A number of authorities regard this as so self-understood, to mention only Kussmaul and Bastian, that they do not even wish to enter into a discussion about it. In spite of this, clinical experience would seem to strongly dispute this assumption. This is particularly apparent in experience with sensory aphasia following damage to the sensory speech center. We would then need to assume that the chief speech impulse from the entire area of the cerebral cortex acts directly on the word-concept. If the word-concept is silenced as a result of damage to the sensory speech center, the impulse must then be mediated by the speech motor images, with the result that articulate speech remains essentially preserved and is disturbed only in so far that there is impairment in the regulating influence of the sensory speech center which safeguards the selection of the correct motor images.

These preliminary explanations should remove any difficulties in reaching an understanding of the clinical picture of **sensory aphasia.** One may summarize the essential symptoms of this entity in this way.

1. There is loss of word-sound perception and, since the concept of word-meaning-comprehension is based on the process of hearing, the meaning of

the spoken word would therefore also be lost. Nevertheless, the disorder is purely acoustic, and the examiner may be easily deceived because word-meaning-comprehension may be readily accomplished by means of signs, a look, or gestures. However, if adequate precautions are observed in this respect, one can readily establish that essentially no speech sounds are comprehended by the patient. Moreover, the use of signs and gestures indicates that some reception is still possible, and that hearing is either intact, or any impairment which may be present is only partial. Therefore, the loss of hearing can in no way explain the disturbance in word-sound-comprehension. As is well known, word-sound-comprehension may be commonly well-preserved in cases of severe peripheral deafness.

2. Articulate speech is intact and, for the most part, such patients are strikingly verbose, perhaps as a result of the frequent misunderstanding to which they are exposed. Although they generally have a fairly extensive fund of words at their disposal and utilize apparently appropriate sentence construction, errors in the choice of expression and the unconscious use of incorrect or transposed words are frequently evident. Language expression improves under the influence of strong emotion, and in fact, entire sentences may be produced without error. Frequently, errors of word-substitution or distortion are made in the naming of objects. Indeed, the distortion words in spontaneous speech may degenerate into complete unintelligibility commonly referred to as *jargon aphasia.* When attempting to answer questions, these patients never repeat or mimic words which they have heard. The loss of word-sound-identification obviously makes the repetition of such words impossible.

3. At this time we shall not take up the problem of written language, since this cultural achievement is not yet common to all men, and therefore often cannot aid in interpretation of the symptom-complex. Later, we shall see that written language is dependent on the integrity of inner speech, which we have labeled the word-concept. This is always severely disturbed in sensory aphasia.

In the majority of cases, sensory aphasia is caused by occlusion of the vessels and therefore is characterized by an acute onset. The symptoms of the attack are commonly mild and at times may be completely lacking. Moreover, there may be no signs of a unilateral paralysis. Opinions in regard to prognosis are divided. On the basis of his observation, Dejerine has concluded that the condition is generally permanent. However, the majority of authorities maintain an opposite view, which based on my experience, I also must support and feel that a comparatively rapid remission of the disturbance is the rule. In fact, marked evidence of the disorder is noted in the initial weeks only, and this, except for recurrence of the original episode, is followed by gradual remission over the course of some months. This is consequent to the formation of new memory images of the word-sounds mediated by hearing, which is intact. However, the sound images which are not utilized in daily conversation because of lack of opportunity, continue to be lost. Thus, I have repeatedly been able to detect traces of earlier involvement in that the unfamiliar words such as "spine," "bend-of-the-knee," "armpit," etc. can no longer be comprehended. Moreover, the ability to correctly name objects presented continues to remain impaired. However, as is also the case in recovery of written language, this observation has not been confirmed by an adequate number of case studies.

The picture of **motor aphasia,** the aphemia of Broca is not less easy to describe. In keeping with our preceding train of thought, the following primary symptoms of the clinical syndrome are clearly evident.

1. There is loss of the ability to articulate speech. The patient has lost the process, the mechanism which must be utilized in producing speech sounds. Moreover, he is essentially mute except for use of a small number of residual phrases. In some typical cases even this is not possible, and the ability to speak is restricted to production of certain unintelligible sounds repeated again and again. Frequently, the only speech at the patient's command may consist of essentially meaningless syllables, a few words or phrases, and in the most severely involved cases, merely a curse or some similar emotional utterance.

This residual speech, which is always limited to repetition of the same few utterances, does not represent propositional language, and such responses do not specify the appropriate object but rather may simply be the only word available to the patient which is used as a response to all attempts to elicit speech. Under exceptional circumstances, an essentially mute patient may produce a rather appropriate expression, usually an interjection, but later will not be capable of repeating this. Moreover, it is sometimes observed that words or phrases produced during sleep are later no longer at his disposal. In general, however, the ability to speak is entirely lost. This loss is not related to a paralysis of specific muscles, since examination of such muscles excludes the possibility of bulbar paralysis.

On the other hand, symptoms of a partial hemiplegia or hemiparesis, with unilateral weakness of the inferior facial-lingual area or the right hypoglossus, may be demonstrated. A common clinical sign of the latter is deviation of the tongue to the right upon protrusion. Clinical experience has strongly confirmed the appearance of such paralytic symptoms in association with essentially unimpaired articulation. Such symptoms may therefore merely represent supplementary signs.

WERNICKE NOW BRIEFLY ALLUDES TO THE PROBLEM OF APRAXIA, A CONDITION WHICH HAD NEWLY BECOME THE FOCUS OF ATTENTION AS A RESULT OF LIEPMANN'S RECENT WORK ON THE SUBJECT.

In contrast, however, specific disturbances in movements are so frequently seen that we cannot avoid interpreting such as analogs of the speech disorder. This involves the inability to carry out many other complex movements involving the same muscle groups. For example, many such patients typically cannot protrude the tongue upon command, puff out the cheeks, show their teeth, or even open their mouths without protruding the tongue, etc. The unsuccessful attempts to carry out such actions, which before this were common everyday movements, clearly reveals the loss of ability to organize the execution of such movements. Such movements lack, as Broca has aptly put it, "le souvenir du procédé qu'il faut suivre." Such symptoms are frequently observed only in the initial acute stages of the illness.

2. For the most part, speech comprehension is essentially intact; at least the common examination methods used with such patients would lead one to this assumption. Some responses may also be attributed to impairment in movement similar to that just described. Such patients, for example, generally follow directions correctly and point to objects named. Moreover, comprehension of questions, if one may judge from facial expression, appears to be intact.

One may still be able to elicit a certain loss in speech comprehension for complex sequences of words and speech requiring a more refined discrimination. This has definitely been proven in numerous cases by Dejerine. Nevertheless, the marked contrast in the ability to comprehend, revealed by the two aphasia forms, is so striking that it continues to be one of the primary differentiating signs. Moreover, the sensory disturbance may completely remit after a time, as long as attention span and environmental conditions are favorable. I now no longer hold the view that speech comprehension remains completely intact in a pure motor aphasia. I base this on the fact, discussed above, that the development of word-concepts must be considered a most important stage in the learning of speech. In examination and diagnosis of the patient, one must of course take into consideration the fact that marked individual differences may exist in this respect.

3. One may apply what has been stated relative to sensory aphasia to written language. If this skill had been earlier acquired by the individual, it would be lost as well as articulate language.

Motor aphasia, as is true of sensory, frequently occurs acutely and commonly together with other symptoms of the apoplectic attack and a more or less marked right hemiplegia.

Prognosis for recovery is generally unfavorable, unless the disorder represents merely a transient focal symptom, as occurs in embolic episodes which may be shortly compensated for by establishment of collateral circulation. Another example of this might be an aphasia occurring as an indirect focal symptom in which the motor aphasia merely represents the effect of a lesion in the neighborhood of Broca's gyrus. This occurrence is fairly common. Occasionally, motor aphasia may reflect an indirect focal symptom in association with a left hemiplegia, if unusually severe symptoms of the attack are present. Although recovery of the motor aphasia may occur without the occasional possible exceptions mentioned above, symptoms of a very specific type of speech disturbance may still frequently be evident. For example, I have observed a patient who after a period of intensive teaching was able to speak with fair intelligibility in a manner similar to that of the deafmute. Nevertheless, his speech was extremely effortful and slow, and the speech movements were accompanied by marked facial grimacing. In my experience this typical and readily recognized loss of control of the "procédé qu'il faut suivre pour articuler", is a chronic symptom even in the less severe cases. Mimicry continues to show the same impairment as spontaneous speech. Nevertheless, recent reports by Dejerine and Thomas indicate that even cases of long standing, (fifteen years following the attack!) respond successfully to systematic teaching methods such as those used with the deaf (i.e., visual methods). This may occur even in a relatively short period such as six weeks! I shall later return to this point, which is of theoretic interest. In relatively few cases the motor aphasia may not be as severe as indicated above, or after a certain period of time, some residual speech production may be observed.

In such cases it is possible with effort to elicit mimicry of some simple words, but little success is noted in producing longer and more difficult words composed of complex syllable combinations. These attempts may be characterized by gross distortions such as the substitution of /u/ for /i/. In some cases, instead of repeating the word requested, the patient may simply say his own name, however, dissimilar it may be to the word attempted.

In cases demonstrating significant residual speech, very dissimilar motor images may be substituted and interchanged when speech is attempted. Such patients may also produce interjections such as "Oh, Lord" when they are not appropriate. Although I admit that such symptoms do indeed occur, nevertheless, I do not feel that the clinical picture of partial motor aphasia is a common occurrence. Therefore, the contrast between sensory and motor aphasia is sharply apparent even to a novice.

In regard to **conduction aphasia**, the third clinical form which I have attempted to differentiate in the diverse aphasia symptom-complex, observations are still so sparse and contradictory that formulation of a unified empirically-based clinical picture is not possible at this time. I originally was inclined to classify under this form the majority of cases which belonged neither to the symptom-picture of Broca's aphasia nor that of sensory aphasia, since they presented only word-interchanging in association with intact word comprehension. This attempt foundered on an underestimation of the numerous possible alternative possibilities and therefore could not be upheld. Yet, certain criteria must be met for inclusion in this category. Most important of these are inability to mimic and disintegration or loss of the word-concept, the clinical signs of which I must go into later. According to the ideas developed above, this form of aphasia results from disruption of the tract which is involved in mimicry of the sounds of words heard. Completely satisfactory case-studies meeting both of these criteria have not yet been observed.

Therefore, I shall restrict myself to a few important comments. If, under certain conditions, the acoustic image of the word alone is adequate to insure comprehension, and this, as we have shown above, may occur in comprehension of the majority of commonly-used words, and if, on the other hand, words can be spoken spontaneously without the need for arousal of the acoustic images of the same, then, in the event of interruption of the association tract between sensory and motor speech centers, there is still the possibility that words whose meaning can be grasped may also be mimicked to command. However, this kind of mimicry may not be produced with the same perfection that was achieved at the period of childhood when this tract was used for speech acquisition. Thus, speech may in part be correctly mimicked and in part it may be paraphasic. If the latter occurs, the patient may be aware of his error and may attempt to correct it. The ability to mimic immediately at the first attempt, i.e., echolalia, may be considered proof of the preservation of this very old tract. This echolalia is purely automatic. It is not produced in response to command and often follows at the very moment the words are spoken. The ability to mimic sequences of words and phrases unawares without comprehension, as occurs when hearing words of a foreign tongue, may also be proof of integrity of this tract. If this type of mimicry is exclusively lost, in contrast to preservation of speech comprehension and speech expression characterized by paraphasia, of which the patient, however, is unaware, I then feel the criteria of a paradigm of this form to be satisfied, at least in regard to the clinical aspects. However, I would not hesitate to admit that the available autopsy findings which primarily reveal isolated or predominant destruction of the island do not properly serve to support the concept of conduction aphasia as postulated by me.

On the other hand, if the hypothesis of a sensory as well as a motor speech center has been confirmed by anatomic findings in addition to clinical data, as I have indeed demonstrated, it would logically seem to follow that the comprehensive aphasia symptom-complex must certainly contain still other more narrowly circumscribed clinical subforms. Lichtheim was first to clearly recognize this logical principle and has accurately drawn the pertinent deduction. In the rare cases, and the pure cases are always rare, the white substance containing the projection fibers to both centers alone is disrupted, leaving the centers, themselves intact. If the connection between both centers should remain intact, a condition which only rarely occurs, a new clinical form would emerge, which is somewhat similar to that described above. The chief symptom demonstrated in this event would be that of loss of word-sound-comprehension or that of articulate speech; but the differentiating symptom would be represented by preservation of inner speech, i.e., integrity of the "word-concept". In fact, the corresponding clinical picture in the motor area is not so seldomly encountered, particularly if a hemiplegia occurs at the same time. From an anatomic point of view, the term *subcortical motor* or *subcortical sensory aphasia* would be justified for both of these clinical types. In clinical practice the terms commonly used are *pure word-muteness* and *pure word-deafness.*

Pure word-muteness can be differentiated from the cortical form by the presence of damage to Broca's gyrus which results in a type of word-muteness.

This form is characterized by the integrity of inner speech or the word-concept in spite of futile speech attempts, even if this can be detected only by preservation of speech melody or inflection. This is particularly apparent if production of some sounds is still possible. Attempts to mimic never result in words completely dissimilar from that attempted, as occurs in cortical motor aphasia. Comprehension of the spoken word is intact even for more complex commands. The final feature of this form can be seen in the lack of impairment in written speech and writing. Writing can be carried out with no evidence of disturbance. In fact, in spite of the right hemiplegia, the latter can be accomplished, although awkwardly, with the left hand. The patient is capable only of the mechanical ability of translating the word-concept into sounds. The same situation prevails in pure word-deafness. In this case also, the entire inner speech apparatus, both cortical centers and their mutual interconnections are intact and therefore also the word-concept. Spontaneous speech is produced with complete accuracy and is free of word-transpositions. Likewise, written expression is undisturbed, as is reading. Only the understanding of the sounds of words is impaired, in spite of confirmed preservation of adequate hearing acuity.

Let us now look more closely at these two clinical pictures which we have finally come to recognize. They deserve study not only from the standpoint of academic interest, but also in view of the lively battle of opinions which led to their recognition and correct interpretation. There are the disturbances of pure word-muteness and pure word-deafness which encounter no controversy from the standpoint of interpretation. The former has long been established as a clinical entity. In his period Trousseau already recognized the rare occurrence of aphasic mutes who still maintained the ability to read and write. The rare cases for a long time were regarded as the most pure examples of motor aphasia, since, according to Charcot, a special center exists for reading and writing. It was primarily Dejerine's contribution, by supplying the necessary pathologic evidence, that he, in opposition to Charcot's opinion placed such cases in their correct perspective and gained the general recognition of a subcortical form of motor aphasia.

Authorities are essentially in agreement regarding the anatomic site of the lesion, that is the subcortical disruption of the corona radiata fibers radiating from Broca's gyrus. Only the white matter of Broca's gyrus or its juncture in the centrum ovale can come under question in this regard. If the projection fibers located below, within the brain stem itself, should be involved, the picture of motor aphasia would no longer prevail but rather an articulatory disturbance with impairment in the intelligibility of word sequences, apparently as a result of disruption of fibers whose location is still not precisely established. The frequent cases of right hemiplegia caused by focal involvement of the striate bodies or the internal capsule is typically not accompanied by a motor aphasia. Or if present, such a disturbance is only transient, and must be regarded as an indirect focal symptom. I shall later return to a discussion of the facts which earlier led me to postulate a special motor speech path coursing without interruption from Broca's gyrus, by passing the internal capsule, to the nuclei of the cranial nerves in the medulla which are involved in speech. Here I shall limit myself to the mere mention of the question regarding exclusive unilateral innervation of the bulbar apparatus in speech production. This point shall require further study later on, but now it would lead us too far afield. The integrity of the word-concept leads to recognition of this form in those also who are unable to read or write. Lichtheim attempted to assess the patient's inner knowledge of the number of syllables contained in a word which could not be orally expressed because of the speech impairment. For example, he would carry out this method in naming of pictures in the following way. The patient was asked to press the examiner's hand as many times as there were syllables in the word he was attempting to say. An objection to this method, however, was the fact that the uneducated were also uncertain of the number of syllables contained in a word. For this reason the ability to count the numbers of syllables of words was considered a prerequisite for integrity of inner speech (Fränkel and Onuf). It would seem to me to be a more reliable approach to guess the intended words from the rhythm of the incompletely articulated sounds which are left over. One would rely on the same aid if one were to attempt to prove the preservation of "inner speech" in advanced cases of progressive bulbar paralysis.

A somewhat more detailed study of *pure word-deafness* or *subcortical sensory aphasia* must now be reviewed. It is generally recognized that the above-described clinical picture in its complete and pure form does not actually occur so very rarely. The objections which are raised in opposition to postulation of this syndrome refer to the unilaterality and the subcortical site of the postulated lesions and, moreover, to the assumed possibility of a peripheral origin of the clinical picture as a result of damage to the terminals of the cochlear nerve in the labyrinth of the organ of hearing. In regard to the question of unilaterality of function I shall return in greater detail later. However, as has been discussed above, it is unquestionably and, specifically, located in the left hemisphere. In regard to the motor speech center, we may refer to the principle of economy of effort, which is generally acknowledged at this time, in order to understand that the process of speech acquisition, since it is related to symmetrically functioning musculature, is directed indeed by a single hemisphere. We have postulated anatomically similar conditions in the relationship of the projection system to the cortex for both acoustic nerves, and particularly of such a type that each hemisphere contains a central projection field for both auditory nerves. However, in this regard it is difficult to believe that the sensory projection active in this process is limited only to the left hemisphere. Thus, the memory images of speech which are heard, and so the center for word-comprehension, would be found only on that side. However, the facts revealed in cortical sensory aphasia permit no other interpretation. If we are satisfied with the principle of economy of effort, which has been plausible up to the present time, one may also keep in mind that recent experiments have revealed that the acoustic imagery, and indeed the most primitive tonal perception, from the outset is combined with a motor component. Thus, the principle of economy of effort, or to state it more specifically, an economy of motor neural performance, also operates in the acquisition of acoustic memory images. At any rate, acceptance of the unilateral localization of the center of word-sound-comprehension permits the consideration of a possible unilateral disruption of the projection fibers extending to that area and thus a blocking of the entrance to the center of word-sound-comprehension. However, the integrity of the same projection field in the other hemisphere allows correct perception and interpretation of the remaining tones and noises.

A few anatomic remarks may be justified here. The clinically unquestioned union of the auditory nerves with both hemispheres must find its anatomic substrate in a semi-decussation of the auditory nerves. The site under consideration here is the posterior area of the medulla. Moreover, the posterior quadrigeminal bodies and the medial geniculate body represent primary hearing centers (analogous to the primary center of vision in the anterior quadrigeminal bodies and the lateral geniculate bodies). Thus, the posterior arm of the quadrigeminal bodies, particularly the stem of the medial geniculate body is a part of the tract under consideration, which issues from the first temporal gyrus. It is quite likely that, apart from the peduncle of the medial geniculate body, i.e., the posterior arm of the quadrigeminal bodies there exists a special quadrigeminal component of the temporal lobe which belongs, at any rate, to the central acoustic tract. This could lie only very close to the area just mentioned. It is certain that in this portion of the corona radiation of the temporal lobe representation of both acoustic nerves is contained. That a unilateral lesion in this area of the visual radiation of the temporal lobe could result in the picture of pure word-deafness as a permanent symptom has been demonstrated by Liepmann's case, which is free of objection.

S. Freund has advanced the hypothesis of pure word-deafness as a result of peripheral involvement of the acoustic nerve in the labyrinth. In support of this concept he refers to a patient from my clinic, whom however, he did not represent accurately, in that the symptoms of brain disease which had been reported in the journal article were ignored. (Liepmann, 1898). His two cases provide even less proof of his hypothesis. Nevertheless, Freund has made a valuable contribution demonstrating the necessity for use of an exacting and specialized battery of tests in such cases.

WERNICKE NOW REFERS TO CASE STUDIES RELATED TO THIS GENERAL PROBLEM. AMONG SUCH STUDIES BEZOLD'S WORK ON HEARING WAS UTILIZED IN WERNICKE'S FINAL INTERPRETATION OF THE MECHANISMS INVOLVED IN SENSORY APHASIA.

Bezold (1895; 1896) has found evidence that the majority of acoustic fibers are not involved in comprehension of speech sounds. Moreover, he states "of the entire tone-scale only a small interval from b 'to g" inclusive, i.e., a large sixth-interval, is absolutely necessary for perception of sounds involved in speech comprehension". Liepmann (1898) has stated that at the most, an octave either above or below this interval may be involved in comprehension of human speech. In regard to the case from my clinic, which has been confirmed by Freund, an examination of the entire continuous series of tones was needed. This testing has since been completed and revealed that the required two tonal octaves were perceived by this patient. This examination was also given to the patient from my clinic. These autopsy findings were later reported by Liepmann, thus demonstrating the necessary evidence.

Thus, we see that human hearing embraces a series of tones extending over eight octaves. Should only two octaves at the most be absolutely necessary for speech comprehension and the radiation of the acoustic nerves in the cochlea be the same throughout, we would be led to hypothesize that only about a fourth or fifth of the projection fibers of the acoustic tract terminate in the sensory speech center. Perhaps this may explain the relatively limited extent of the sensory speech center, since according to the numerous pathological findings at hand, this center does not extend beyond the posterior third of half of the first temporal gyrus and the neighboring area of the second temporal gyrus. However, this does not negate the fact that the rest of the temporal lobe also provides terminal points for the acoustic nerves, which has veen verified on anatomic and physiological grounds.

On the basis of these new findings, I am forced to conclude that the sensory speech center coincides with the sites of the cortical endings of those projection fibers mediating the tonal pitches from b 'to g". This would lead to the hypothesis that the left temporal lobe, in cases of subcortical sensory aphasia, must in reality always be deaf to the perception of these specific tonal pitches, if its function could be studied in isolation, which of course is not possible. In other words, the fact that a word-deafness and not an actual partial deafness for specific pitches commonly results from a unilateral lesion may be explained only by the fact that a significant portion of the auditory tract also can be found in the right hemisphere, in this way mediating the perception of the same tones.

Moreover, this hypothesis explains the possibility mentioned above of acquisition of new acoustic word memory images, thus compensating for the disturbance. Should the right temporal lobe later suffer damage, a permanent sensory aphasia would follow, which no longer could be compensated for, as one of the earliest studies on this subject, that of O. Berger, has demonstrated.

An extension of our hypothesis would lead to the assumption that cases of sensory aphasia consequent to bilateral temporal lobe involvement may result in true deafness in the area of the above mentioned tonal pitches.

The immediate future shall show whether this explanation shall actually be realized. Up until the present these particular types of investigation, which we admit are not easily carried out, have not been undertaken in the area of cortical sensory aphasia, at least in the systematic manner which is necessary.

On the contrary, one can now understand that in extensive bilateral involvement of the temporal lobe, the picture of speech deafness is masked by the generalized deafness. In this event, the most immediate terminals of the majority of acoustic nerves are destroyed, and therewith the possibility for production of a central cortical deafness arises. A. Pick has reported two cases of this type. These cases presented such a severe degree of deafness that the essentially complete loss of word comprehension could in fact be explained on that basis, particularly if one takes into account the fact that only a very severe deafness on a peripheral basis can lead to complete impairment in word comprehension. In no event do they demonstrate the cortical signs of subcortical sensory aphasia or a pure word-deafness to be based on cortical damage involving both temporal lobes. A third case of Pick's who in addition to the severe deafness also presented the essential characteristics of pure word-deafness, may certainly be interpreted as presenting a combination of both disorders, which is also consistent with the pathologic findings.

WERNICKE NOW TAKES UP A REVIEW OF THE TRANSCORTICAL APHASIAS, CLINICAL FORMS FIRST SPECIFICALLY INTRODUCED BY LICHTHEIM AND LATER AMPLIFIED BY WERNICKE IN HIS PUBLICATION "RECENT WORKS ON APHASIA."

Up to the present time we have primarily been interested in these forms of aphasia which have either gained general recognition in respect to their anatomic and clinical aspects, such as the cortical, sensory and motor aphasias, or those which are generally recognized as specialized clinical types, such as the subcortical forms of aphasia. However, I would like to discuss an area which is completely controversial and which still requires confirmation by further observation as well as by evidence from the anatomic findings.

On a purely logical basis, one may not ignore the possibility of the existence of a transcortical motor as well as a transcortical sensory aphasia. Such aphasia forms would be hypothesized on the basis of interruption of the tracts which provide the connections between both postulated speech centers and the so-called concept regions, which in the final analysis must be regarded as including most areas of the cerebral cortex. The designation of these two clinical varieties is justified in that there is no lack of clinical examples corresponding with the theoretically constructed picture. Although I put a great deal of weight on Dejerine's impressions, he interprets such a purely theoretic construction.

I still cannot acknowledge the objections submitted by Pick as valid. I shall soon return to this point. However, let us first attempt to develop the primary signs of the clinical picture in a theoretic manner, as we have previously attempted.

First of all, we must clarify what we understand by the term "concept of the object" or the "*concrete concept*" of Ziehen, for, as has already been emphasized, the concept of the object must first be aroused from the sensory speech or word sound center before comprehension of the word can be accomplished. As a result, the term "*concept center*" has been used; this would essentially be identical with our "*center of word-meaning-comprehension.*" Now, it is certainly self-understood that postulation of such a center is merely imaginary and only serves as a schematic simplification. In reality, such processes involve areas which are located in various parts of the cortex, as the following interpretation reveals. If we turn once again to the point of view advanced by Meynert, discussed at the introduction of this monograph, which specified various sensory areas, we may be able to understand the concept of concrete objects as a function of various different projection fields of the cortex. For example, the concept of a rose is composed of a "tactile memory image" – "an image of touch", in the central projection field of the somesthetic cortex. It is also composed of a visual memory image located in the visual projection field of the cortex. The continuous repetition of similar sensory impressions results in such a firm association between those different memory images that the mere stimulation of one sensory avenue by means of the object is adequate to call up the concept of the object. In some cases, many memory images of different sensory areas and in others only a few will correspond to a single concept. However, by the very nature of the object, a firmly associated constellation of such memory images which form the anatomic substrate of each concept is established. This sum total of closely associated memory images must "be aroused into consciousness" for perception not merely of the sounds of the corresponding words but also for comprehension of their meaning. Following our anatomic mode of interpretation, we also postulate for this process the existence of anatomic tracts, fibers, connections, or association tracts between the sensory speech center of word-sound-comprehension and those projection fields which participate in the formation of the concept. We may call these tracts transcortical, since they course from the most immediate cortical endings of the acoustic nerve, in contrast to the well-recognized subcortical neural tracts. Therefore, they can be disrupted by a focal lesion close to the merging of the fibers at their terminals in the sensory speech center.*

A very similar process must take place if the word "rose", for example, is spoken spontaneously, that is, as a result of internal cerebral processes. In this event, the concept must arrive first, and from it, the impulse must course to the motor images corresponding to the word "rose" in the cortex of Broca's gyrus. This also requires the involvement of the analogous "transcortical" tracts which again must be regarded as a converging radiation of fibers. Such a concept also has acoustic components, for example, in the ringing of a bell or the barking of a dog. The accompanying schema represents these connections between a center of the so-called "concrete concept" and the two speech centers (Figure 17).

These ideas then lead naturally to a very clear definition of the symptom-picture of *transcortical sensory aphasia.* This syndrome is characterized by loss of word-meaning-comprehension in association with preservation of word-sound-comprehension. The sounds of speech in themselves are adequately understood as is demonstrated by the intact ability to mimic, although the related concept is not awakened. The active component of speech is preserved to some extent and is disturbed only in this respect that what is spoken cannot be comprehended, and therefore its accuracy can no longer be tested. In such cases, there may be only slight indications of paraphasia with a mixture of inaccurate or transposed words or syllables. Mimicry may be intact for entire sentences or may be limited only to the ability to repeat the last words of an utterance in association with more or less retained attention; moreover, such mimicry may at times be completely without errors and at other times with interjected paraphasic transpositions. Such mimicry at times occurs in response to commands, and at times is more involuntary, apparently related to the form of question asked. At other times it is produced compulsively and essentially reflexly. In the latter case, this mimicry is designated as echolalia,

* The definition suggested here which regards concrete concepts as specific constellations of associated memory images is based on only the most absolutely necessary assumptions.

One such an assumption, which incidentally in my opinion would seem to be superfluous is the hypothesis of the necessity of special association centers between memory images located in the various projection fields to carry out the processes of association.

Flechsig believes that he has demonstrated the existence of such association centers or "coagitation centers", as he calls them. They are characterized by the absence of any projection fibers or fibers of the corona radiata. In the meanwhile it has been demonstarted that such fibers of the corona radiata extend to all coagitation centers. I feel that only one cortical area offers a proper anatomic substrate for that kind of center; that region is the island with its claustrum which has already been designated by Meynert as an association organ.

a symptom which is primarily associated with loss of the sensorium or a generalized intellectual disturbance. Repetition of a question, although its meaning is not comprehended, is characteristic of this form.

The counterpart of this picture in the motor area is *transcortical motor aphasia,* consisting of impairment or a very severe reduction in spontaneous speech, although mimicry is fluently carried out without error, and comprehension of speech is not disturbed. The residual speech does not consist of the few constantly recurring words and syllables so typical of cortical motor aphasia but, rather, is characterized by occasional expressions of anger, discontent, and helplessness; in other words, such residual speech is stimulated by emotion. The vocabulary, as can be tested by mimicry, is unlimited and consists of automatic so-called serial speech utterances such as recitation of the Lord's prayer or the multiplication table which may be produced fluently upon request or when the initial word of the series is given to the patient (Heilbronner, 1900). In this form, the simplest communication, the telling of a story or expression of an opinion, is not possible by means of speech. In most severe cases questions may be answered only by means of gesture, although at times simple isolated responses may be possible. Articulation is essentially intact.

These are the clinical types. The picture could be completed by a description of the characteristic signs of written language corresponding to various levels of educational achievement of the patient. Such symptoms in written language also reveal the two contrasting aspects of speech, the perceptive and expressive. In transcortical sensory aphasia, reading is accomplished without comprehension. However, because the word concept is intact, no impairment is apparent. At other times some paraphasia may be evident. In transcortical motor aphasia spontaneous writing is not possible, in contrast, writing to dictation is carried out at times without error and at other times only with various paraphasic transpositions. Nevertheless, the patient reads with complete comprehension and only paraphasic errors are evident in reading aloud.

The disturbance in reading in the first case may be compared to the reading of a foreign language which cannot be understood but which contains the same familiar sounds. Moreover, the disturbance in writing to dictation is similar in that writing is fairly successful, although not completely without error. Spontaneous writing, on the contrary, naturally reflects a severe paraphasic disturbance of expressive speech; in fact such paraphasic transpositions may result in complete unintelligibility.

One may note that the course of our discussion has led from relatively simple and well-established facts to a consideration of even more complex and controversial clinical pictures. The interpretations of such pictures leave far behind the observations gathered by Trousseau and Kussmaul, which at that time seemed strange and completely incomprehensible. A more detailed study of the disturbances of written language may enable us to clarify a few related points which may be merely tentatively postulated in order to complete the clinical sketches. Before we go further, however, it would be helpful to review the schema depicting the essential characteristics of the various aphasia forms which I have previously described. I shall refer to Lichtheim, who related my two separate speech centers, the motor and the sensory, to a hypothetical concept center, and who was first to provide a complete framework permitting the schematic preduction of all aphasic symptoms. In the accompanying schema (Figure 22) the letter (B) designates the concept center, namely, the pertinent memory images of concrete images localized in various places which, as we have seen above, as a result of their firm functional associations, merge into a psychological unity, the concept of the concrete object. The sensory speech center is designated by the letter (a), while (b) represents the motor speech center.

The tract (a-b) represents the association tract which serves mimicry of speech sounds. The tracts (a-B) and (b-B) refer to such association tracts which serve to connect the concept of the concrete object with both speech centers. The centripetal and centrifugal tracts, i.e., the sensory and motor pathways, course into the centers (a) and (b). These are components of the projection system. The sensory speech path carries at least the specific tonal pitches referred to above, corresponding to fibers of the acoustic nerve, while the motor speech tracts contains those fibers flowing into the internal capsule belonging to the nuclei of the nerves involved in speech production. The fact that the transcortical forms of aphasia occur only under specific conditions and in great isolation, as well as the reasons underlying this circumstance, is readily apparent from the schema. Thus, the tracts (a-B) as well as (b-B) are essentially radiating bundles which have only their end-points (a) and (b) in common. Representative cases can therefore be produced only by interruption of both of these tracts by means of a single focal lesion, close to the two centers, (a) and (b). If one would use numbers to designate different parts of the schema, one would find that the numbers 1-3 represent the sensory forms, while 4-6 designate the motor forms of aphasia. Therefore, depending upon their relationship to the cortical centers (a) and (b), we may differentiate subcortical, cortical, and transcortical forms.

With the exception of the 7th form, that of conduction aphasia, one would have to concede with Lichtheim that the mere existence of different individual cases of aphasia derived from the schema provide evidence that the facts predicted by the schema in reality actually do occur. I can produce definite proof only for the cortical and subcortical forms 1, 2, 4 and 5, while the transcortical forms 3, and 6 may be accorded only a certain degree of probability. Nevertheless, the simultaneous appearance of such characteristic symptoms as are presented in the transcortical forms is difficult to explain on the basis of mere accident.

One may be somewhat justified in objecting to the nomenclature I have chosen, particularly in respect to the transcortical forms, since I still find the anatomic evidence in support of this form inadequate. However, in favor of this classification I may state that I know of no other which would be more suitable in view of the particular peculiarities these types present. The situation is much different in the subcortical forms for which the terms pure word-deafness and pure word-muteness are well-chosen. Nevertheless, I see no reason to avoid anatomically-derived terms in cases where I am convinced that the findings justify their use. There are theoretic considerations which favor continued use of the term transcortical which I allude to at the conclusion of this lecture.

The question of localization in respect to the pathologic-anatomical findings, will demand our special consideration. However, at this time I must not neglect to draw attention to certain authoritative points of view. One of these ideas, the rare occurrence of pure cases, has already been emphasized and has been repeatedly mentioned by me on the basis of general clinical experience. Thus, it would be unlikely to expect the same constellation of symptoms in each case of aphasia as are found in the pure forms. The second point of view is not less important and is related to the possibility of a combination of various different clinical pictures corresponding to their anatomic findings. Two such combinations must particularly be mentioned which appear to represent a total aphasia with loss of speech comprehension as well as the power of expressive speech, i.e., a sensory in addition to a motor aphasia, which, moreover, can be further differentiated by the different levels of preservation of the word-concept or so-called inner-speech. The more frequently seen symptom-picture is related to loss of inner speech, thus corresponding to a sum of the cortical types described above. It is consistently accompanied by hemiplegia. The other forms, in which inner speech proves to be more or less intact, are much more rarely observed and correspond to a summation of the two transcortical aphasia forms. This combination may also occur without hemiplegia. Moreover, a look at the schema will show us that occurrence of combinations of subcortical and transcortical forms, whether they be motor or sensory, may be influenced by the anatomic conditions and are more readily produced as isolated forms by focal lesions in Broca's or the first temporal gyri. We shall later undertake a discussion of other combinations which should be considered as natural groupings and which occur more frequently in our detailed analysis of written language.

The material regarding clinical data presented up to this point permits us to return to a more critical review of our case of pure aphasia. If this patient should present proof for the existence of a motor writing center, analogous to that of Broca's area, the same type of circumscribed impairment must be demonstrated, i.e., *le souvenir du procédé qu'il faut suivre pour écrire les mots.* However, inner speech, the word-concept, must remain intact, for we do not write merely words, but series of letters of the alphabet which correspond to the word, and which, in combination, require integrity of the word-concept.

However, this primary prerequisite is not met in our patient. She is able to designate neither the number of syllables contained in a word, nor can she build words when individual letter-blocks are supplied. This is not possible even if she is presented with the letter-blocks *d, n,* and *u*, and requested to form the word *and*, [Germ. *und*]. This behavior, moreover, is consistent with her. Clinical experience teaches that agraphia, in the sense that it has been understood up to the present, i.e., if it is limited to one hand, is exclusively observed in association with and caused by certain disturbances of inner speech. Stated more precisely, it involves a disturbance of the control which the "word-concept" exerts on the purposeful selection of letters which form the word and is essentially, a transcortical function.

THE NEXT SECTION CONTAINS TWO SUB-PARTS. THE FIRST, WERNICKE'S REVIEW OF THE ALEXIAS AND AGRAPHIAS, ESSENTIALLY REPRESENTS THE HEART OF THE MONOGRAPH. IT SUMMARIZES MUCH OF THE MATERIAL FOUND IN THE AUTHOR'S ESSAY ON ISOLATED AGRAPHIA PUBLISHED IN 1903. THE SECOND SUB-PART PROVIDES AN EXCELLENT RESUME OF WERNICKE'S INTERPRETATION OF THE NEUROANATOMIC CORRELATES OF LANGUAGE AND THE APHASIAS.

DISTURBANCES OF WRITTEN LANGUAGE AND THE GENERAL PATHOLOGY OF SPEECH DISTURBANCE

The fact that *disturbances of written language,* a subject which we shall now review, have their own unique significance and do not occur only in association with or as part of an aphasic disorder has been demonstrated by the observation of certain rare cases of such disturbances. An example of this may be found in the case of an apparently isolated agraphia, a review of which has provided an introduction to this discussion.

In contrast, isolated alexia without significant involvement of speech has been frequently observed in the past. In fact, it would be tempting to assume the existence of a special cortical center for written language which is completely independent of speech functions, or rather, one which is analogous to the actual motor and sensory speech centers. The former might then be designated as the site of motor imagery involved in writing, and the latter as the site of the visual memory images of words.

We have acknowledged Charcot to be the most venturesome and daring representative of this interpretation, which essentially applies the schema of spoken language to written language. Nevertheless, the indefensibility of this grossly schematic mode of interpretation has become more and more apparent and can now boast only a few adherents. Indeed, the only surviving idea of this concept is the wide acceptance of a special and essentially unilateral visual speech center in the angular gyrus of the inferior parietal lobe, although even this is rejected by Von Monakow.

If we wish to accurately evaluate the importance of written language to oral speech, we must consider first of all that it is a relatively late acquisition and is not commonly used by all men as is oral speech production. Moreover, because its content varies in different people, the cerebral mechanisms involved in its production cannot readily be analyzed, as is true of oral language.

The translation of hieroglyphics, for example, requires a different form of cerebral mechanism than the alphabet form of writing, commonly used by peoples of a higher level of cultural development. The importance of alphabet letters in written language function becomes strikingly evident if one realizes that the act of reading generally takes place by means of spelling. This principle now seems self-evident, and yet it was not generally accepted until Grashey presented his findings. Grashey and Goldscheider in particular, however, have found that this rule does not invariably hold, since one can correctly comprehend a four letter word at a glance by means of synthesis. This is especially true of very familiar words which can be recognized without synthesis of the individual letters to form a word. Thus, allowing for individual differences, we all have at our command a certain number of either printed or written visual memory images, the most familiar of which is one's own signature. We shall encounter another problem in analyzing this process in the course of our discussion. However, it may be said that for most types of reading material, the act of reading occurs by means of letter-spelling, and, therefore, we accept the existence of memory images for letters only, and not for entire words. The fact that reading does occur by means of spelling can be seen from the process in which the written images of a word is produced by adding letter-to-letter. What we thereby produce is the same variety of letter combinations which can be found in the act of reading by means of spelling. This leads to the conclusion that, apart from the exceptions mentioned above, a direct relationship between the concept of an object and written language must be rejected. This point is so important that we must now explore it in greater detail.

The means by which inner thought is translated into spoken and written language is still obscure. One must remember that this process occurs by means of acoustic imagery in many individuals. However, the assumption of mediation of this mechanism by written imagery in event of the absence of acoustic imagery would seem to be absurd in the light of the above discussion, since we do not possess visual images of words but only of letters of the alphabet. At least, all phenomena evident in the process of reading and writing can be explained by this very simple hypothesis. If one would go beyond the simplest and most essential assumption, who can tell how far afield one might be led in the area of brain pathology? The twenty-five letters of the alphabet in themselves surely do not make up the material of thought. Nevertheless, the differentiation of three different forms of thought, by which individuals are classified as motor, auditive, and visual types, an idea which is maintained by many psychologists and some pathologists, of whom I must mention Bastian in particular, is based on this hypothesis. Charcot was the father of this idea. As is known, he reported a case who spoke, at least in part, by means of reading the internal written images of words. Far be it from me to dispute his observation, although I have never seen anything similar. However, I do not believe that such cases represent the general rule and therefore consider them as exceptions. The possibility that such exceptions do in fact exist, which has already been proven in the case of deafmutes, does not contradict my interpretations—or at least only in so far that specialized training may bring about an unusual organization of cerebral mechanisms, Deafmutes of normal intelligence undoubtedly learn written language without dependence of the spoken word. For them, combinations of letters making up the single word are learned as a whole, and the analysis into letters is a later acquisition. This can occur by use of educational techniques analogous to the breakdown of the sound of a word into the sounds of individual letters. It is true that some individuals think primarily in word-sounds, (It is self understood that this would not occur with sounds of the individual letters of the alphabet). Deafmutes might then be assumed to think in the corresponding visual combination of letters, each of which is similarly associated with the analogous object-concept by means of the transcortical tracts. In deafmutes the question may also be a matter of use of visual word images in contrast to the images of individual alphabet letters. This type of individual requires a special study in itself and must therefore be neglected in our discussion here. In all other individuals the storage of transient letter combinations as special memory images of words would seem to be a superfluous performance of the brain, since the corresponding images of the sounds of words are already present. We may assume then that such storage of words does not typically take place. The studies of rare cases reported by Rieger and Sommer are very relevant in this respect. These authors report cases which present permanent loss of certain segments of written language such as the unavailability of specific letters of the alphabet for use in writing, in association with no evidence of speech disturbance and preservation of the corresponding letter sounds. In Rieger's famous case, three German and seven letters of the Latin alphabet in lower case letters and fourteen capitals were unavailable to the patient. Moreover, the same letters were lacking in both languages. These two cases are particularly significant in that only minimal signs of aphasia were demonstrated. They therefore represent the most isolated disturbance of written language reported up to this time.

Sommer, who has published one of these cases and who has followed

Rieger's model of examination very carefully, concluded the existence of an indirect relationship between the concept of the object and the motor images involved in writing. In fact, in Grashey's case he held this interpretation to be absolutely essential. In interpretation of that case he went a step further than those who support the existence of a special independent writing center and who, at least in part, (Dejerine, for example) reject a motor writing center. The essentially critical tendency of his supposedly unbiased point-of-view is therefore clear. In reality, the manner by which Grashey's patient succeeded in finding words strongly supports the idea that visual word synthesis occurs by a combining of the elements thereof, i.e., the images of the individual alphabet letters. This is particularly true in the light of the interpretations offered in a study of this case by Sommer (1894) himself and Wolff (1897).

As is known, Grashey's patient presented the peculiar symptom that only by writing was he able to find the word for the objects presented visually or through some sensory channel. Without this device he was usually unable to recall the word. However, he was able to say the word aloud only if he had completed writing it. If this were not possible, the writing of mere fragments of the word was useless in connecting it with the object. Portions thereof, even letters in combination, evoked no connection with the object which was seen or felt.

Grashey's case is an example of the various possibilities of training the brain under special conditions. In this patient, recalling the word by means of direct contact with the object was not possible. We shall later discuss this kind of disturbance. To compensate for this disorder the patient utilized the device of writing. However, in contrast to deafmutes, he would need to proceed in this purpose by spelling the word. The writing movements which he performed in this act were first of all the result of intensively evoked visual memory images of the letters in which the motor components, the 'directional concepts' were the primary elements, as we shall later see.

I agree with Sommer on one point. The problem in Grashey's case cannot be attributed to a loss in attention or the impairment of memory for recent impressions. Nevertheless, the significance of this case for interpretation of the relationship of written language to oral speech has not been decreased by later investigations, but rather has been strengthened.

Therefore written language is dependent on spoken language and can be disturbed whenever the word-concept or inner speech is impaired. Written language, however, may be considered intact if the word-concept or inner speech is preserved, which indeed is the major prerequisite for preservation of the act of writing.

The preservation of an alphabet language is therefore a primary sign of subcortical motor aphasia or pure word-muteness and, analogously, the same is true also of subcortical sensory aphasia or pure word-deafmutes. In transcortical disturbances of spoken language, the integrity of the word-concept is demonstrated in the preservation of the purely mechanical processes of reading and writing. Reading aloud, writing to dictation, and copying are intact. The symptom-picture of written language has not yet been verified in all of its details, nevertheless, one may make the general statement that disturbances of written language essentially reflect those of spoken language in that spontaneous writing is lost as well as oral speech and spontaneous writing ability. In oral reading, as well as in writing to dictation, paraphasic symptoms, confusion of terms, and transpositions are evident to the same extent as they are observed in mimicry. This particularly holds for transcortical sensory aphasia, with the exception of an increase in paraphasic symptoms in writing. This process continues to be very difficult. In describing such cases the common expressions "paralexia" and "paragraphia" should be avoided, and one might better refer to such symptoms as paraphasic disturbances of reading and writing.

In regard to transcortical motor aphasia, it can readily be seen that the loss of spontaneity which characterizes oral production must affect attempts to write to dictation, since, with individual varation, this activity requires the participation of the writer. "Word-finding" in relation to the act of spontaneous speech is the characteristic function of the path (b-b) and in writing, involves the further task of finding letters of the alphabet, since according to our interpretation, the sounds of individual letters belong to the word-concept.

WERNICKE CONTINUES WITH A DESCRIPTION OF THE CORTICAL AGRAPHIAS AND ALEXIAS WHICH HAD BEEN DISCUSSED EARLIER IN DETAIL IN "RECENT WORKS ON APHASIA". IN THIS REVIEW THE MORE SEVERE DISTURBANCES OF READING AND WRITING SECONDARY TO CORTICAL INVOLVEMENT IN CONTRAST TO THE LESSER IMPAIRMENT ENCOUNTERED IN THE SUBCORTICAL AND TRANSCORTICAL SYNDROMES, ARE EXPLORED. WERNICKE'S FOCUS ON THE SIGNIFICANCE OF THE WORD-CONCEPT, OR INNER SPEECH IN RECOVERY OF WRITTEN LANGUAGE IS AGAIN UNDERLINED.

Written language, as has already been mentioned, is most severely involved in the cortical forms of aphasia, in which the word-concept itself undergoes severe damage. Cortical motor aphasia, as a direct focal involvement, is usually associated with a permanent alexia and agraphia. The letters, however, continue to be recognized as visual images and can still be graphically produced. (This is proven by preservation of the ability to copy and translate symbols into different graphic forms.)

Recovery of the receptive act of reading is more favorable in the intact and healthy brain than the expressive performance of writing. Later, we shall discuss the reasons for this finding. The sequence of recovery in cortical motor aphasia has been studied by Thomas and Roux under Dejerine's direction. The reverse sequence of learning to read was evident in the fact that at first entire words, then syllables, and finally, the individual letters making up a word could be read consistently. However, for a period of years an isolated or at least predominant agraphia might retain in addition to the muteness. This represents an agraphia marked by intact ability to copy from a model as well as the ability to translate from one form of letter to another, as was presented by our case study which introduced this essay.

In general, writing recovers to the same extent as articulate speech, and in fact, recovery of writing to dictation occurs more slowly than spontaneous written formulation (Dejerine). The preservation of the word-concept indeed seems to be the chief requisite for such recovery. This concurs with Dejerine but is in opposition to Von Monakow's view. Moreover, on the basis of my experience, I cannot confirm Von Monakow's observations that written expression in motor aphasia can be carried out more readily than speech. This observation may refer to cases of predominantly subcortical motor aphasia. Furthermore, I feel that the clinical picture of cortical motor aphasia is too broadly interpreted by Von Monakow, since he recognizes a partial aphasia in a much broader sense than I. Of course, exceptions to the rule must always be recognized—the case of Banti deserves particular attention in this connection—in which the ability to write as well as reading comprehension remain intact. Von Monakow holds that such cases sustain only partial damage to Broca's gyrus. More shall be said in this regard when the subject of autopsy findings is discussed.

It is generally recognized that cortical sensory aphasia is always accompanied by a severe disturbance in writing. During the recovery of oral language the ability to read returns before that of writing. In brief, common experience indicates that the agraphia continues as the most severe permanant residual impairment. This agrees with our impression that the acoustic component of the word-concept maintains its important influence from the time of its acquisition. Perhaps the purely anatomic situation is not without importance in this respect, since the posterior upper end of the superior temporal gyrus is very close to the important association tract involved in the motor act of writing.

Beyond this, there unfortunately is a lack of useful clinical material for confirmation of the progression of symptoms in disorders of writing during the possible recovery of disturbances of oral language.

In assessing the dependence of written to oral language, it is important to understand the clinical symptoms of alexia, agraphia, paralexia, and paragraphia in a double sense, in order to determine whether they represent sequelae to disturbance of the word-concept or exist alone without such involvement. The former may be designated as the 'verbal' form of the disorder, and the latter as the 'literal'.

The isolated disturbances of written language which are observed in association with preservation of the word-concept or inner language are related, moreover, to the production of the particular form of the alphabet letters. Literal agraphia consists in the patients's inability to produce this form from a model. The case presented above is a specific example of this type. Literal alexia is characterized by the unique impairment in recognition of letters, and, as a result, that of words. As we shall soon see, a specific kind of alexia and agraphia may result from disruption of tracts which serve as the substrate for association of the psychic elements involved in connection between the word-concept and the alphabet letters.

WERNICKE NOW TAKES UP A DISCUSSION OF THE SCHEMA AND NEUROANATOMIC SUBSTRATE OF THE WRITING PROCESS, AS IT WAS FIRST DETAILED IN "RECENT WORKS ON APHASIA".

A review of all forms of disorders of written language, analyzed on the basis of our schema, as has been done for oral language disturbances, would take us too far afield and would not be germane to our purposes here. Our main objective is the provision of a form which such a schema might follow in order to accommodate most of the clinical features. Generally speaking, such a schema would correspond to that sketched for oral language above, if one would replace the concept center (B) with the word-concept (C), the motor speech center with the written motor image (β), and the site of the acoustic images with the visual memory images of letters, (α). In our schema the direct pathway (B-b) has been well-established. However, it is very improbable that a corresponding tract for written language (c-β) actually exists, and such a path is therefore only hypothetical. The schema thus is essentially simpler than that for oral speech. The detour over the site of visual imagery (c), through which the stimulus always travels in the writing process, would seem to be cumbersome. Perhaps, use of this route may reflect the common mode of instruction used in learning to write. I think it not unlikely that a change of method in this respect might well influence the clinical significance of this tract. Thus, our older citizens almost without exception have first learned to read letters of the alphabet and then later have learned to write the same. Nowadays, however, the two are learned at the same time, so that instead of learning to read first, and then to write, children, by means of writing, learn to read. The motor component thus assumes a certain significance in recall of the individual letter.

The difference between the printed and script form of letters reveals that the motor component of the written motor image is not absolutely necessary for recognition of the letter. Therefore, the motor image of the written letter cannot be regarded as an essential characteristic of the same.

I do not wish to be misunderstood in my use of the term "written motor image" (representation) [Schreibbewegungsvorstellung]. This expression merely signifies the use of motor representation in Meynert's original meaning i.e., the source of discharge of the movements involved in writing, which is different from the innervation of the muscles which are involved. Thus, a certain memory of the process involved in writing is recognized and cannot be disputed. Neither can one deny the existence of localization of this particular kind of memory in the left arm in those who are right-handed. However, this cerebral localization would be the same as that representative of all refined movement of the right hand, and does not imply that a special site is reserved for this purpose, as is necessary for the motor speech images. . . . "*L'écriture n'est qu'une des formes de mobilité de la main*" (Dejerine).

The same movements in the left-handed would be represented in the right arm region, and if one would write in the sand with the left foot, representation would be found in the right cerebral leg area.

These are the directional-concepts (Richtungsvorstellungen), the significance of which Storch has emphasized. They provide the components which guide the limbs in all motor acts, including that of writing, except for the fact that we possess a special storehouse which contains the visual memory images of letters and the completed schema of the content of these directional-images which operates in the writing process. Thus, there are individuals who can write with their tongues. The necessity for existence of a special motor writing center (at the foot of the second frontal gyrus), as Exner advocates, appears improbable, apart from the fact that it is based on a completely uncritical application of very questionable clinical material, and up to the present, lacks anatomic-pathological confirmation. A loss of these motor images, analogous to Broca's aphasia, would thus have to be assumed in all cases of paralysis of the right hand, as a result of a left-sided cortical lesion. The generalized inability to use the right hand also precludes writing with this hand, while integrity of movement in the left allows use of this hand in writing and proves the preservation of the necessary directional images. Such a unilateral agraphia could in no way be evoked in Broca's aphasia. This also holds for the case of Pitres, whose involvement was presumed not to be cortical, and who, in spite of return of the finer movements of the right hand, presented a permanent and exclusively right-handed agraphia. I shall return later to a discussion of the significance of this extraordinary and instructive case.

Most authorities have not yet agreed on the question of a so-called visual word center. which, as we have seen, is really a visual center of letters. From a purely practical standpoint, the issues still open to question may be ignored, and, as far as localization is concerned, one may be satisfied with the importance of a circumscribed unilateral lesion in the inferior parietal lobe as the site of generalized aphasia. On the basis of his statistical studies, Naunyn has called attention to the importance of this particular site. The findings which are most important for us here indicate the presence of a unilateral lesion, situated in the depths of the white matter of the parietal lobe, which produces a combination of right hemianopsia with an isolated writing blindness or alexia as a chronic residual. If the involvement is more extensive and involves the cortex of this area, the alexia is commonly accompanied by an agraphia. (Dejerine).

If these facts can be considered as analogs of the processes involved in oral language and are inserted into our schema, the cortex of the cerebral area might be regarded as the site of the visual memory images of letters and pure writing blindness, or subcortical alexia, as an analog of sensory aphasia. It is self-understood that further confirmation of these observations is necessary before we accept this interpretation without qualification.

Even on a theoretic basis, everything we know about the nature of visual memory would oppose a strictly circumscribed and unilateral localization of the memory images of letters. Moreover, recent studies have demonstrated the motor component to be an integral element of the memory imagery which cannot be arbitrarily separated from it. Storch has applied the apt term "directional images" to such visual memory images. These "directional-images" have interconnections with all motor projection fields, but they are revealed in their most specific form in the visual oculomotor projection fields. In differentiation from the actual visual field, (Lichtfeld of Sachs) this area includes the convex surface of the occipital lobe and the angular gyrus of the inferior perietal lobe. Such directional images are located in the so-called middle third of the central gyri, and in so far that they represent the arm and hand, coincide with the graphic motor images of writing.

Now the visual memory images of letters, as well as those of numbers, are two-dimensional and are differentiated from images of all other objects in that they possess only a visual form, while the images of concrete objects, in contrast, possess countless forms (Storch, 1902). Nevertheless, the limited numbers of such letter images and their frequent use, based on the principle of deeply-traced cerebral paths, suggests that they represent a firmly established and readily aroused store of memory images. They are, therefore, without associations, except for a well-worn and thus readily available tract which is particularly closely connected to the unilateral speech region, and, as we may assume, primarily with the acoustic speech center.

However, these three characteristics which differentiate them from all other visual memory images do not allow us to assume a special cerebral localization for this process. If that were true, one would have to assume the area of clearest vision, or the most specific and differentiated oculomotor directional imagery to be found in a specific site of the cortex. This has not yet been proven. Only one characteristic is significant, i.e., its exclusive connection with the temporal lobe. This factor must be considered in support of the unilaterality of localization of memory images. I shall return to this subject later. If we study the process involved in the functional acquisition of memory images of letters, the left hemisphere does not appear to have any priority. In fact, the form of the visual fields in a typical hemianopsia would lead one to conclude that the immediately surrounding area of the point of fixation is always bilateral and served by each optic tract. The image of a letter characteristically falls exclusively in the area of central vision, and, therefore, a memory image may arise in either hemisphere. If the letter happens to be rather large, one can still see it at a glance, as occurs when looking at any large object, but the central visual area would still be exclusively involved in the act.

One might, therefore, try to confirm the unilaterality of localization of the visual memory images of letters by testing for a possible difference of recognition of such images in the peripheral portions of the visual fields to determine whether reading occurs by use of the right or left visual fields. However, this evidence founders on the condition that only the largest letters are read entirely at the point of fixation, and beyond that one cannot recognize letters as such at all. One might say that central visual acuity rapidly deteriorates from the fixation point. Just how rapidly is obvious, since no difference between left and right visual fields can be found in recognition of letters.

However, far more important than these academic questions, is the actual evidence gleaned from the area of brain pathology. Above all, the common combination of isolated writing blindness with a right hemianopsia would not likely be interpreted as a functional disruption of the subcortical tracts representing hemianopsia. That is, the functional disruption of the left optic tract representing subcortical paths would be interpreted as the cause of the writing blindness, just as that of the acoustic tract ending in the left temporal lobe would be considered a cause of subcortical sensory alexia. Reading is disturbed very severely by the hemianopsia itself, that is, by loss of a broad overview of the sequence of letters or words. The individual letters, however, as well as those following in sequence, can be recognized as long as a severe disturbance in attention does not interfere with this, as occurred in a case of Redlich's. It is interesting that this finding may be observed during the period of acute onset of the hemianopsia, and one need not therefore assume that the loss of reading was primarily caused by the hemianopsia. In all of these cases we must assume the participation of the right hemisphere in reading. On the other hand, the left hemisphere must be regarded as blind to a certain extent as a result of involvement of the left optical tract. If now, in spite of this, the recognition of letters and a series of letters is not impaired, the cortical endings of the optic tract must be assumed to be located in the right hemisphere, which permits this function. This interpretation is so persuasive and provides such a strong argument against the unilaterality of localization of the so-called visual word center in the left hemisphere, that the adherents of this doctrine, Dejerine and Bastian, cannot ignore it. They try to strengthen their argument by the fact that the corpus callosum, which extends from the visual projection field in the cortex of the right hemisphere to the analogous cortical field on the opposite side, permits entry to the left visual word center.

They therefore differentiate between a general visual center and a specialized visual word center. The former is felt to be bilateral and the latter unilateral and located on the left side. In the same way, they differentiate between a general hearing center in both temporal lobes and a unilateral specialized center for comprehension of the spoken word.

I regard this entire interpretation as incorrect because it contradicts Meynert's basic premise and attributes functions to the callosal fibers which can be accomplished by simple transmission along fiber tracts of either the optic or acoustic tracts from their cortical projection fields to the opposite hemisphere. If this were the case, the hemianopsia in a unilateral tract lesion would be compensated for by the other hemisphere and would not be demonstrated. Finally, one might refer to the clinical evidence of studies of psychic-blindness which often occurs in association with writing blindness or literal alexia.

Therefore, if the pathological evidence contradicts a unilateral and strictly circumscribed localization of a visual word center, a special study is needed to explain the appearance of such unilaterality by the association fibers mediating connections between the visual memory image of the letters and the unilaterally located speech center and, specifically, its acoustic component. Two possibilities may be suggested to explain this. One, which has also been accepted by Monakow, holds that an interruption of the crossed visual acoustic commissure (Bastian) i.e., the association fibers between the left temporal lobe and the right optic oculomotor projection fields, is produced by a focal lesion in the white matter of the angular gyrus, separate from the visual radiation. The visual memory images of the left hemisphere in that case would be blacked out by the disruption of the visual radiation (hemianopsia). The visual memory images of the right hemisphere would be mediated by the right optic tract which is still active, but is not able to be used for reading, since the necessary associated acoustic word component of the letters mediated by the commissure just mentioned, can no longer be aroused. Translated into our interpretation, there is a loss of word-finding ability for the individual letters, and as a result, reading by means of spelling is no longer possible. Reading, therefore, is restricted to a few words, which we have learned to recognize as individual exceptions to the rule of reading by spelling. The striking difficulty in word-finding of objects presented, which is noted in the majority of cases of isolated word-blindness, is commonly attributed to involvement of the association tract leading to the left temporal lobe. This is inaccurate, as we shall soon see. Moreover, one must explain the observation that only such letters which can be seen are not identified, while all other visualized objects, in contrast, can be correctly recognized. In fact, we have seen that connections other than those to the acoustic projection field do not actually exist for letters of the alphabet. One may then raise the question. In word-blindness so caused, can the form of the letter itself continue to be recognized and copying remain unimpaired, as well as the ability to recognize the various forms of a letter and the translation of one form to another? The purely optic-visual component would therefore remain undisturbed.

However, this prediction does not apply to some of the cases observed so far. These patients are not able to really copy the letter but merely attempt to draw it, in a manner of speaking. Moreover, this is carried out only with very careful and laborious dependence on the model. Whoever has observed patients of this kind laboriously draw each letter whether it be in print or script, would have difficulty in attributing the cause of this disturbance to an interruption in the crossed-visual-acoustic commissure.

Above all, it must be mentioned that the visual memory images of letters represent groups of directional imagery which are significant because they are associated with the corresponding word-concepts of the letters. The sounds of the letters are word-concepts i.e., firm associations between a certain acoustic image and a speech motor image, which are connected to the visual memory images only by the association tract described above. Moreover, the latter deteriorate into meaningless lines if these connections are absent. This explains the inability to relate the identity of a printed letter to one produced in script form or a Latin with a German letter, whenever the internal reverberation of the sound mediating the connection no longer exists. Therefore, the question still remains whether the purely visual component of the letter, cut off from that of the acoustic, can permit continued recognition of the letter.

If we attempt to apply this first possibility to our schema, we find that it corresponds to a combination of subcortical and transcortical symptoms. The unilateral tract involvement would result in production of the subcortical symptoms, while those of a transcortical nature would be related to the interruption of the crossed-optic-acoustic commissure. The alexia might then be explained on the basis of disruption of only one of the two tracts (c-d), the crossed and the uncrossed. The other tract would be useless because of disruption of its subcortical fibers. In contrast, the uncrossed tract (c-d) is completely adequate to support the act of writing as previously.

The second possibility attributes priority to the left visual oculomotor projection field as indispensable for the act of reading, in contrast to the first hypothesis in which the left projection field appears to be essentially blind. This supports the hypothesis consistent with the principle of economy of energy in that only the visual memory images of letters on the left are connected by a deeply traced path to the acoustic projection field, and assumes the existence of the uncrossed acoustic-optic path (c-d). This leads to the further assumption that the connections between (c) and (d) which are established in reading always detour over the left visual oculo-motor projection field. Moreover, if as a result of right hemianopsia, reading can be mediated only by the right hemisphere, the interruption of communication causing the alexia can be then sought in the commissure between the two visual oculo-motor projection fields, and particularly the oculo-motor projection fields, a hypothesis which in general agrees with that of Bastian and Dejerine. The difference would be that not the sites of perception but rather localization of the memory images should be regarded as connected by the callosal fibers. I have discussed this possibility in detail elsewhere. To apply this to our schema,the disruption in this case would not primarily involve the path (c-d). However, in respect to (χ) it would hold significance subcortically, first of all because of the fiber tract located on the same side but also because of the disconnection of the visual memory images which can still be visualized on the right side. The act of writing which primarily involves the left center (χ) would still be preserved because of the integrity of the path (c-χ-β).

It is obvious, therefore, that the question of unilaterality of a visual word, or more accurately, letter center is very important for the entire doctrine of localization. If it is rejected—which in my opinion must happen—the door is opened for investigation of a pathology of the callosum in causing a subcortical alexia or a pure word blindness.

I will not conceal the fact that our case reviewed at the introduction of this paper, who presented an apparently isolated literal agraphia, could not be more easily explained than by turning to the theory of unilaterality of the center (χ). The tract (χ-β) would then be disrupted on one side and isolated transcortically from (χ). This would also be possible if one assumed the existence of two tracts, one on the same side and one coursing to the opposite arm region inasmuch as they have the same discharge point in (χ). Nevertheless, this seemingly natural and most obvious explanation is contradicted by other cases. The case presenting fairly intelligible speech in association with inability to write or even draw the most simple designs argues against the assumption of a special center for alphabet letters which is located within the area of visual memory imagery.

The clinical picture of pure word-blindness, more aptly called letter-blindness, discussed above, or subcortical alexia, the term I have suggested earlier, has already been confirmed by a significant number of cases. Redlich (1895) has found no less than twenty-seven cases in the literature, and pathological data certainly is not lacking. The chief symptom of this highly individual syndrome may be described in a review of a patient who presents a very typical picture of the problem.

The patient, a 62 year old plasterer, clearly demonstrated that he correctly understood and answered all of my questions. He presented himself as intelligent and revealed no speech disturbance at all. We requested him to write what was dictated to him. This he accomplished accurately and in fluent script. Numbers could also be written to dictation without error. A letter written to his married daughter at my request was generally correct and readily understood, although some errors in spelling and difficulty in alignment of letters as well as unintentional interruptions and repetitions were demonstrated. Had he been well-schooled and literary, the letter might well have been without error. However, if the man was asked to read what he had written, the amazing symptom would be obvious that he was completely unable to read a word, letter, or even a number.

The same syndrome is observed in all similar cases if they represent complete and severe examples of this disorder. Such cases may differ only in regard to numbers which frequently can be read correctly. The patient himself convinces one that the problem is not essentially related to a visual disturbance since he states that he is able to visualize every thing very well. Moreover, he can copy letters and words although these cannot be recognized. However, such copying is carried out by drawing the letters line by line, as if they were completely unfamiliar designs. Moreover, our patient cannot comprehend written material, while analogous patients by circuitous methods are able to decipher what has been written, although slowly and laboriously. Furthermore, the patient's visual acuity was definitely adequate for recognition of letters. Nevertheless, one cannot say that the patient was completely without some kind of visual disturbance. This was revealed by the peculiar head posture assumed when writing was attempted, the overlapping of words on each others, and the misalignment of sentences on the page. This was due to the presence of a right hemianopsia, commonly characterized by a vertical cutoff of the visual half-fields, leaving only a narrow margin of intact vision on the right. Visual acuity was bilaterally at least one-half of normal, and the eye-grounds within normal limits. The difficulty revealed in reading in most cases is manifested only in the inability to read rapidly, since it is no longer possible to grasp a large sequence of letters at one time. In our case, however, there was complete lack of ability to recognize individual letters. Moreover, the presentation of various objects to the patient convinced one that vision was adequate and all objects could be accurately recognized. This symptom, the difficulty in recalling the name of an object, is frequently seen in similar cases and usually to a greater extent than that demonstrated in our patient, who presented this problem only occasionally. When this occurred, he would substitute a word or use a circuitous expression; when the word he was seeking was suggested, he would gladly accept it as correct. In other cases, such as one which I observed some twenty-five years ago at the Charite Hospital, there was complete inability to produce the sought-for word. This was the only symptom of an aphasic nature demonstrated by our patient. In spontaneous speech he had no difficulty finding words even for objects which were actually visualized. When this symptom is severe, such as in the cases already mentioned, which I have observed earlier, some difficulty in word-finding for concrete objects is often also present in spontaneous speech, although not to the same extent as is observed in naming of directly-presented objects.

Earlier in the patient's illness another symptom was demonstrated which was of even greater significance than the gross difficulty in word-finding. For a long period of time the patient was unable to correctly recognize objects which he, however, could visualize with adequate clarity, thus presenting the well-known problem of psychic-blindness. Moreover, this combination is not just coincidence, but is frequently seen in cases of so-called pure word-blindness. From the course of recovery of our case, one may assume this to be an extension of the alexic disturbance, a secondary effect and indirect focal symptom of the lesion causing the alexia. In respect to the combination of these two symptoms, experience shows that psychic blindness is commonly accompanied by word-blindess, but in contrast, an isolated writing or word-blindness may frequently occur without psychic-blindness. Thus, in the case I observed some time earlier, psychic blindness was not particularly in evidence. In our case it is significant to note that during the time he was suffering from a psychic blindness, he was also unable to recognize objects through the sense of touch. The psychic blindness thus revealed an asymbolia, which is the most severe of all sensory types of disturbance attributed to focal involvement. The course of recovery in our patient, as well as that of similar cases leads one to conclude that we are dealing with a generally chronic condition, although one may perhaps expect a certain degree of improvement. Although no symptoms of hemiplegia are evident at this time, such were present a half year earlier, but completely remitted within two to three weeks. This course of recovery may be interpreted on the basis of an embolic process. The most striking aspects of the symptom-complex now demonstrated is the patient's inability to read the newspaper in his usual way. This symptom may well be attributed to an embolism and the consequent cerebral softening (Storch, 1896). Later, I shall return to the question of the hypothesized localization of the focal lesion in this disturbance.

In addition to the typical symptom-picture presented by our case, there are doubtlessly still other types of isolated reading disorders, such as that of dyslexia first described by Berlin. (1883). This disturbance is characterized by difficulty in reading which is first apparent only to the patient but which rapidly increases to complete inability to read. After a brief rest period this loss is followed by recovery of reading but with rapidly increasing signs of fatigue. Particularly striking is the disinclination to read (shunning of reading: Bruns). One cannot help but assume a functional disorder either of the same or very similar localization such as occurs in pure word blindness, and therefore the suspicion of an organic basis of some type must be kept in mind. Berlin has called attention to the unfavorable prognosis for remission of such symptoms which usually have a sudden onset. Hemianopsia may be present but is not a consistent component of the problem as it is in alexia. Most cases terminate after a few years in more severe brain disease. Atheromatous and luetic involvement of the cerebral arteries have repeatedly been confirmed in such patients.

As we have seen, isolated word-blindness is connected with a combination of various conditions, and particularly the disruption of a subcortical tract and the preservation of one which is transcortical in nature. On the basis of the established site of the focal lesion in the deep white matter of the angular gyrus which is necessary to produce the typical symptoms, we may conclude that the intact pathway must be closer to the cortical surface than that which has been disrupted. Thus Dejerine's assumption of a separate center of visual word memory images, mentioned above is based on the findings that destruction in addition to a literal alexia, also produces a literal agraphia and therefore a complete loss of written language. Moreover, if in addition to the damage to the deep white matter, destruction of the cortex of this area later occurs, agraphia may be added to the previous symptoms of pure word blindness: This combined agraphia and alexia is thus caused, to translate it into terms of our schema, by a disruption of the tract (c-χ). This is the same tract which, as we have seen, is necessary for every form of written language. It is formed, as I have previous described in detail, of two entirely different tracts, the anatomy of which we must still review. The situation is such that the effect of their common disruption may result in an exclusive disturbance of written language without involvement of oral language, which up to now has been rarely observed. We shall see that only the two already mentioned cases of Rieger and Sommer provide fairly good examples of this. Nevertheless, it would be a rather common finding if the cortex of the angular gyrus actually were a visual word center, as Dejerine maintains.

Certainly, on the basis of Dejerine's ideas regarding the extent of the speech center, it is obvious that he feels that the optic word center, so named by him, exerts the same influence on oral language as does the acoustic word center. This view, as described above, we cannot accept, since in normal individuals visual images exist only for letters and not words.

As has already been mentioned, we have found the simultaneous occurrence of literal alexia and agraphia without essential involvement of oral language reported only in the two cases of Rieger and Sommer. These case, however, are so significant that we must describe them in some detail. Rieger's case, which apart from this provides an unbiased mode in a most difficult area of investigation, deserves the greatest attention. This patient could no longer use three letters of the German alphabet, namely, *p*, *x*, and *y*, as well as seven Latin letters, which included, in addition to the three just mentioned, *d*, *h*, *k*, and *v*. Of capitals letters in both Latin and German alphabets. fourteen letters were missing. In addition to those just mentioned, except for D, these included B, E, F, M, N, R, T, and W, with the result that only eleven letters were preserved. This disturbance involved both the printed and script form of the letters. In naming of these letters in response to direct visual presentation, the patient reacted as if to foreign objects. Moreover, if he were given a choice and asked, for example, if a letter were a B or E, he would shake his head and say that he didn't know. In contrast, letters which were preserved could be immediately identified, named, and written. The same situation prevailed relative to words which were constructed of letters which he knew. He was completely unable to spontaneously write letters which he could not identify or name. Such letters had to be laboriously copied from a model as if they were completely unknown designs. The patient was able to write to dictation and copy those same letters which were available to him, although this was carried out for the most part without comprehension. Spontaneous written expression, however, was completely impossible, and reading material could not be comprehended. Spontaneous speech, in contrast, was not strikingly impaired, except for occasional difficulty in finding words, particularly the substantives. In respect to numbers, only 0, 1, 2, and 3 were intact. Apart from this comparatively circumscribed disturbance, the patient also presented a generalized disorder in the area of speech, namely difficulty in word-finding for objects which were brought to his attention and required visual or tactile perception. He also revealed a loss of the ability to maintain attention in all sensory spheres, and this disturbance was not less severe than that demonstrated in Grashey's famous case, later studied by Sommer and Wolff. Moreover, the impairment in drawing demonstrated by an individual who previously had been a skilled sculptor is significant. Furthermore the patient was no longer able to produce so-called serial speech utterances; however, there was no impairment in intelligence in the narrower practical sense of the word. For our purposes, however, it is important to note that word-finding for visualized objects was successful, although responses were abnormally delayed. Moreover, better response was observed in object-naming if letters were placed under the object. Such naming required only one-half the time as that needed to name the object itself. This condition, according to Rieger's explicit description, continued unchanged for a period of two and one-half years. This patient had sustained a severe skull fracture in a railroad accident. At first the disorder was not evident, or at least not to the degree which was obvious later. The symptoms first appeared to develop one half-year after the accident.

Sommer's case also demonstrated a similar chronic loss in the use and recognition of specific letters and a partial literal alexia and agraphia, as a result of a stroke. Recognition of a number of other letters was variable and unstable. Moreover, the patient was not able to build and thus read words composed of the letters which were still preserved, which would thereby demonstrate presence of a complete alexia also. An even more complicated situation was noted relative to his writing ability which was in part better preserved than reading and was similar to that found in cases of subcortical alexia. However, for practical purposes, the patient was also agraphic. It is interesting to note that the patient was unable to read and write for a period of a year and half after the stroke. Furthermore, in the early period following his attack, he was unable to find words. The right hemiplegia improved after a period of fourteen days. During the time he was studied, a right hemianopsia was revealed. Apart from the disturbance in reading and writing and the very rare difficulty in word-finding, the patient behaved essentially normally and rationally. Thus, we may assume that the disturbance in oral language was even less noticeable than that of Rieger's case. Necropsy studies in both cases are not yet available.

One might attempt to explain the characteristic partial loss of such specific isolated disturbances of written language by the fact that the less frequently occurring letters such as *x* and *y* are more mildly disturbed in all kinds of reading disorder than the others which are used frequently. Nevertheless, in both cases one finds that the disorder is not by any means restricted to the more seldomly occurring letters, but also to those which are very common. Moreover, the constancy of the disorder would seem to rule out functional factors. One cannot find anything analogous in the entire area of speech disturbances secondary to focal cerebral involvement, except that of a case of mental illness who also presented a motor-sensory aphasia and whose vocabulary consisted only of a certain specific words (Heilbronner, 1897; 1900). In fact, as occurs in the mentally ill, we might assume presence of a similar degenerative process which involves only certain selected association tracts and performance–in the first case as a result of cerebral convulsions, and in the second, following a stroke. Apparently the tract involved is the hypothesized pathway (c-χ).

The case presented at the beginning of this discussion would seem to support the existence of a pure isolated agraphia. This type of case is very unusual and rare because the postulated damage is evidently comparatively circumscribed. Nevertheless, an exhaustive study revealed that the patient was not entirely without a disturbance of inner speech or the word-concept. Moreover, one must assume the probability of a disturbance in oral speech earlier in the course of recovery, which later had essentially resolved. The reduction in spontaneous expression, which was very marked at the time of initial examination and continued to be severe two years later, contrasted sharply with the intelligent and rational behavior of the patient in other ways. This may justify the diagnosis of a moderate transcortical motor aphasia. I refer to my publication of this case in another journal, where it is clear that the few essentially pure cases of agraphia which I have abstracted from the literature consistently present the same complications. This fact leads me to conclude with Dejerine that a pure literal agraphia, or motor agraphia to use Pitre's term, in essence does not occur. Nevertheless, one may note that the characteristic symptoms of this case cannot be explained only on the basis of disturbance of the word-concept, but rather that, apart from this, the most conspicuous aspect of the disorder lies in the literal or, one might say, motor character of the agraphia. The same is also true of the few analogous cases which I have been able to find. The relative preservation of reading indicates that our case undoubtedly possesses intact memory images of letters. However, unlike the normal individual, the translation of such images into the movements of writing, which were still intact per se, was no longer possible. If one applies this to our schema, one would find interruption of the pathway (χ-β). This tract, as is evident from my previous discussion, is bilateral, and the significant aspect of our case, as well as the few other analogous cases, is the bilateral loss of function of these tracts.

In our case, one might raise the question of symmetric lesions in both hemispheres, with somewhat less extensive damage on the right. This would be consistent with the transient appearance of left-sided symptoms and should be kept in mind. And yet, similar cases present exclusively left-sided symptoms of focal involvement which cannot be explained on the assumption of symmetric lesions. One is then forced to conclude that disturbance of the word-concept or a generalized involvement may also have an effect on cerebral performances and, under certain conditions, may exert some influence on the writing process. Thus, apart from the direct damage to the unilateral tract, function of the other may also be impaired. In our case, apparently the barely noticeable transcortical disturbance of oral language was enough to prevent innervation of the intact pathway on one side, needed to carry out the difficult task of writing. When this occurs, as a general rule we must take into consideration the disruption of the postulated unilateral tracts. In reality, we find an excellent example in Pitres' case mentioned previously, which in spite of the unilateral involvement, revealed a pure motor agraphia. This case presented an earlier agraphia similar to ours, but this remitted and persisted in the right hand alone, although recovery of mobility of the hand for other actions occurred. A right hemianopsia was present, although visual acuity was good. The patient originally also presented a right hemiplegia with severe generalized symptoms. One might rightfully question the use of the term agraphia for such cases of unilateral writing disturbance. Undoubtedly, this could be attributed to unilateral disruption of the tract (χ-β) in our schema. A careful examination of Liepmann's case of unilateral apraxia also shows the same signs of an isolated agraphia involving the right hand, except that this was masked by the total picture of a unilateral apraxia. The patient could write with the left hand but used mirror-writing. This example is helpful in understanding the significance of the tract (χ-β) on the right. Mirror-writing or abduction script, to use Liepmann's term, represents a cogent example of the purely mechanical mode by which the memory images of letters are translated into motor action. This process is acquired at a volitional level in most individuals only by use of the left tract and may be explained on the basis of the principle of economy of effort. General clinical experience also indicates the presence of unconscious symmetrical movements of opposite body-parts in company with such actions. This act involves not only the anterior motor horn cells of the spinal cord but also the more complex processes of the cerebrum.

This assumption is based on what has been called conclusion by analogy. However, if the same innervation of the right cerebral arm center, mediated by the memory images of letters located on the right side, is transmitted by the tract (χ-β) on the right—just as in normal writing the impulse is transmitted from the cerebral arm center over the tract (χ-β) on the left—mirror-writing or abduction script must result. This pathway may be involved in the execution of writing movements of the left hand in such a way that, instead of the symmetric oppositely-located directional images, the corresponding images implicated in writing with the right hand are aroused. This is essentially an act of drawing or painting, not previously practiced. This act, in contrast to the adventitious innervation in the opposite direction, involves a far more difficult cerebral process than that of mirror-writing, which is mediated by a path already somewhat worn. Subjectively, some conscious effort is necessary to achieve this performance. As we understand it, a motor aphasia, mild though it may be, can interfere with the correct process of writing which is transmitted by this tract through a decrease of the source of the stream of innervation necessary for completion of the task. However, what is not so readily understood is the fact that our patient never demonstrated even a sign of mirror-writing. One must therefore be suspicious of a possible circumscribed symmetrical focal involvement of a right hemisphere. Moreover, the conditions under which mirror-writing occurs are still obscure. In association with a right hemiplegia, either with or without speech disturbance, this symptom is sometimes observed, while at others, under apparently the same conditions, it may be completely absent. Furthermore, this symptom of mirror-writing may often be found in mentally deficient individuals with or without signs of unilateral cerebral atrophy, especially in children presenting mental deficiency. If normal children, exposed to exactly the same elementary training, are asked to write with the left hand, mirror-writing is present but is generally accurate, revealing no sign of agraphia. Rieger's case, reported by Wolff, seems to present a case of pure cortical agraphia. The complete central blindness caused by bilateral destruction of visual projection fields also commonly results in cortical alexia.

I shall later return to the question of the location of the hypothesized pathway (χ-β). We shall see that a specific localization of the same may be fairly certainly determined. In this way, an isolated agraphia as a focal symptom may become an important sign of diagnosing the site of the lesion in the same way that an isolated alexia has come to be regarded as a focal clinical symptom of damage to the angular gyrus. Moreover, the fact that an anatomic substrate for such a clinical picture exists has already been emphasized.

One must concede that a theoretic basis for such a hypothesis is not lacking. The principle of conservation of energy would seem to support a unilateral localization. Moreover, the peculiar characteristics which distinguish the memory images of letters from all other visual memory images, a subject to which I shall return later, would seem to speak for a correspondingly specific localization. Finally, the significance of this view-point is enhanced by its acceptance by such authorities as Bastian, Dejerine, and Pick. Nevertheless, one cannot accept it without relinquishing the essential relationships involved and being untrue to the basic principles which Meynert taught with such renowned success. Nor has Von Monakow excluded these possibilities. He protested the existence of an actual visual word center and held instead that visual memory images of letters were localized bilaterally. I, myself, had earlier taken this stand and had opposed the notion of any universal localized site of visual word memory images. However, an inaccurate interpretation of evidence may threaten the progress of localization doctrine, as we have seen happen in the case of Broca's aphemia. Therefore, I feel compelled to relate in some detail the indefensibility of the hypothesis of an alleged visual word center in the cortex of the angular gyrus.

The patient of Wolff-Grashey favored the visual sensory channel in preference to all other sensory areas in that only the object which was seen, and not merely felt or heard, allowed the patient to find the word in writing. Only certain uni-sensory tactile concepts such as the wind, warmth, and cold, or those related to the acoustic channel, such as thunder or the music of the polka and waltz, proved to be exceptions to this. The fact that concepts which were predominantly tactile in nature—such as smoothness, roughness, and sharpness, etc., participated with visual perception in aiding word-finding indicates the significance of visual memory images in the process of word-finding in this particular patient.

Wolff's study has at least demonstrated that the different concepts should not be regarded as complexes of individual components or memory images which are essentially equivalent. In contrast, a single sensory area may provide the primary influencing element, while the remaining are of secondary importance. However, the fact that the visual sensory channel exerts the major influence on word-finding, as Wolff assumes on the basis of his case, is highly improbable and is contradicted by Rieger's case.However, if we assume the visual area in Wolff's case to be better preserved than the other projection fields, we can well understand this extraordinary and not previously observed finding that the patient recalled words by the round-about method of first producing them in writing.

In the above-mentioned case of Rieger and Sommer, the disturbance in word-finding was of such a nature that there was loss only for specific letters, while the rest were still intact. This would lead to the logical conclusion that the corresponding letter-concepts were lost. More frequently, however, one encounters the situation of instability of word-finding for letters, with lack of consistent restriction of the impairment to specific letters only. At times such individuals without hesitation may be able to read words containing letters which previously caused great difficulty. At a certain stage in the recovery process our case of an isolated agraphia presented an example of this. An even more severe disturbance in the reading of letters was observed in a case of Bastian. This patient could not name individual letters correctly, and, as a result of a severe paraphasia, could not correctly read entire words aloud, although he was able to comprehend what he read. I specifically mention this type of problem because, more than any other form, it provides a very convincing argument against our hypothesis that reading occurs by means of spelling. However, such cases may be explained by two common clinical facts. One is the difficulty in executing sequences of individual acts acquired by practice whenever complete attention is focused on the individual component of the act. The simplest example of such is the act of going down the stairs without attention to the individual steps. The attention focused on the individual act, which here would refer to naming of the individual letters, is thus detrimental to carrying out the total act. This leads us to conclude that the total act is more readily carried out than its individual components in isolation. One may find a similar experience in cases of pure word-blindness who are able to speak without hesitation and without paraphasia, but when confronted with objects, are unable to find the name of such or do so only with great difficulty. In this case, concentrated attention on the task may be the detrimental factor hindering success. As far as I can see, Bleuler has presented similar considerations in his differentiation of the more automatic and well-known association processes. The second common clinical finding which appears appropriate to compensate individual defects of this nature, notwithstanding the process of reading by means of spelling, is the well-known case of carrying out all impressive processes by means of secondary identification. The most relevant example of this is recognition of objects by tactile means only, in spite of a confirmed marked sensory disturbance. The fact that this process may be related to suggestion and also normally plays a role in the reading of hand-writing is also commonly known to all of us.

The impressive aspect of Grashey's case, moreover, does not lie entirely in the form of his aphasic disturbance. Rather, it must be sought in the particular devices used to hide the characteristic aphasic symptom of word-finding difficulty for visualized objects.

THE SHORT DIGRESSION ON WORD-FINDING IMPAIRMENT WHICH FOLLOWS CALLS ATTENTION TO AN ASPECT OF APHASIA NOT DISCUSSED IN ANY PARTICULAR DETAIL BY WERNICKE PREVIOUSLY.

We have seen how this device supports the fact that our written language is essentially a language of letters of the alphabet. The difficulty in word-finding, however, has always been regarded as a significant aphasic symptom and very early was presented by Trousseau as a form which contrasted with that of the aphasia of Broca. Therefore, Pitres' (1898) contribution serves a practical purpose when he combined all cases presenting this symptom, either in isolation or as the predominant feature within the total classification system, under the term amnestic aphasia.

However, we cannot concede more than an acknowledgement of the practical need for such a category but, in contrast, must stress the variability among such cases which present this common feature. The majority of cases of isolated word-blindness belong to this group, as does the extraordinary case of Grashey. Finally, even the earlier-mentioned case of Rieger may be included under this category. The last two cases both demonstrate an almost complete loss of attention. However, this symptom alone cannot represent the cause of word-finding difficulty, since it is also observed in some cases of pure word-blindness who also present difficulty in word-finding. However, the etiology of this problem differs completely in the great majority of cases demonstrating this difficulty, in that they involve the type of aphasia in which a certain compensation in oral language occurs.

Pitres found involvement of the lower parietal lobe in eight of ten cases he collected, a finding which is not inconsistent with the statistical results of Naunyn, who frequently found lesions in the inferior parietal and occipital areas of his cases of so-called "amnesic aphasia."

Of all forms of disturbance in oral language, predominance of word-finding difficulty is most rarely evident in the course of recovery of the motor form of aphasia. This would support Pitres' feeling that Broca's gyrus is usually not involved in such cases of word-finding disturbance. However, one cannot help but be impressed with the great variation among the patients themselves. This may be related either to the great variability in cerebral localization or variations in localization of disturbance of function. Pitres, who maintains the existence of the commonly recognized disturbance in oral and written language, also emphasizes the infrequency of pure cases in his sample. His criteria include absence of disturbance in comprehension, reading, and writing in association with an isolated involvement in word-finding.

Moreover, the significance of a decrease in attention in such cases did not escape him. He points to the well-known observation that a patient with impaired word-finding, in spite of continued correction, experiences the same difficulty in finding a word, regardless of whether the word, which he readily recognizes after it is presented, is given to him in its entirety or he is offered merely its initial sound as a cue. If Pitres would attempt to explain the loss of reading comprehension on the basis of a memory disturbance, Grashey's case, demonstrating intact reading capacity with externally reduced attention, would speak against this. It is very interesting that Pitres does not unconditionally implicate the inferior parietal lobe as the only site involved in this disorder but rather recognizes that excitation of the spoken word center in the act of word-finding involves neurones which are spread throughout the cortex and which may be regarded as carriers of psychic functions. Thus, there is no specific consistent site of the lesion, and the symptoms may be caused by an interruption of connections between different centers involved in word-building as well as neighboring sites which are involved in higher psychic processes.

"Amnesic aphasia" therefore represents solely a disturbance of the associative binding of the concept with the word itself in speech expression.

From a practical standpoint, recognition of amnesic aphasia requires differentiation between cases who demonstrate only a reduction in word-finding and those who also present paraphasia. The latter is often the most frequent residual symptom in the recovery of disturbances of spoken language and for our purpose shall be disregarded. Apart from this symptom, the word-finding difficulty is demonstrated most vividly in naming of objects seen (and perhaps also those which are heard or felt). This may be revealed by errors in finding the specific word, particularly substantives.

To cover up the disorder the patient frequently resorts to use of circumlocutions or substitute expressions such as "you know". The use of distorted or inappropriate expressions falls in the area of paraphasia.

Difficulty in word-finding also occurs in the daily life of normals. In more severe forms of the disturbance, difficulty is observed in naming of objects. Rieger, in this respect, has very appropriately remarked that in normals this affects only proper names of limited significance such as "Magnolia." "As soon, however, as one fails to recall a name such as 'tree', we are dealing undoubtedly with brain damage." It is also well-known that the extent of this problem may vary with the patient's mood. Rieger, to my knowledge, has also been first to draw attention to the fact that each individual who is not in complete mastery of a foreign language usually may have more difficulty in recalling words in that language which, however, can be comprehended without difficulty. However, should the same situation prevail in his mother tongue, it would fall under the category of amnesic aphasia. Under the same conditions, an increase in the disorder would be confirmed as soon as naming of objects directly presented is involved. Generally speaking, this is more difficult than finding the word in the course of conversation. Perhaps the major contributory factor to this is the problem of increased awareness in the former situation.

Pitres has shown that the "systematic aphasia" of polyglots demonstrates a stage of recovery in which word-finding for a foreign language is completely lacking while comprehension has already recovered; thus it represents a stage in the recovery of amnesic aphasia.

Following this train of thought, it becomes clear that difficulty in word-finding is nothing else than a special form of transcortical motor aphasia. In other words, it represents a functional disturbance which involves the pathway (B-b) in our schema.

In Rieger's case as well as that of Wolff-Grashey, this functional disorder consists in a delay in the process of word-finding which, nevertheless, is finally successfully completed. In other cases, however, word-finding attempts may not succeed, or such success is partly related to chance. This does not occur in patients who are actually suffering from this disorder.

We now are led to the assumption that a disturbance in area (B), which is involved in carrying out complex psychological processes, may be the cause of difficulty in word-finding. This assumption is supported by Rieger's case, who, apart from the disturbance in the ability to use letters, also presented a marked loss in conceptualization. This patient revealed a loss of the concepts involved in discrimination of playing cards, use of coins, postage stamps, and the like, since comprehension of the latter could not be awakened by any means as was true also of any numbers exceeding the digit 3. Moreover, concepts were also lacking for algebraic symbols, musical notes for piano playing, and punctuation marks. An analogy to a decrease in the number of concepts may be found only in residual symptoms of mental illness. This reminds one primarily of the findings in Rieger's case of aphasia following mental illness, which was described by me and later by Heilbronner. This case presented a partial motor and sensory aphasia with a limited residual vocabulary for which the corresponding concepts were lacking. However, the clinical findings compel one to assume a mild reduction in the arousal of concepts as well as the individual components (memory images) of such concepts, since the delay in the pr ocess of recognition of objects can be understood physiologically only as a diminution in the excitation of a certain sensory channel. The same retardation may be demonstrated in relation to the comprehension of words associated with the concepts. The difference in preservation of word-comprehension and word-finding which may contradict an impairment in the concept itself is not absolute; both processes are slowed and one merely more than the other. If one is dealing with objects which are directly presented to the patient visually or by the tactile sense etc., one may establish the time required for conceptual recognition and at the same time ascertain word-finding difficulty to be the chief factor in the delayed response.

However, at the same time it is apparent that the concept itself and not its component memory images must arouse recall of the word. The symptoms demonstrated by the Wolff-Grashey case is also consistent with the evidence that only the concept *in toto* and not its component sub-concepts may arouse the word. The unisensory concept alone, mentioned above, presents a self-understood exception. The difference between sensory and motor performance in the apparently preserved word-sense-comprehension and the difficulty in word-finding is, in fact, very marked here, but integrity of the concept itself is by far not proven. If, for example, Wolff's patient, would respond to the question "Is this sheet of paper blue?" by answering "That could be" or "I don't know," it would be obvious that an impairment in word-meaning-comprehension of the words 'page' and 'blue' would be present. In other words, one would be able to point to a disturbance in the concepts relative to the receptive aspect of the speech process. Should the situation be such that a certain amount of excitation of the entire association complex which we call the concept is necessary to transmit the correct word-concept or the right word-motor image (Wortbewegungsvorstellung) over the path (B-b), we would also understand the influence which the sensory perception may under certain conditions have on the process of word-finding. The corresponding concepts in this way achieve a certain measure of intensity. The significance of this influence may be dependent on the value of the corresponding individual concepts comprising the total concept. If one refers to the schema in Figure 16 one can clearly see the significance of the remark mentioned above that not less than four of the same sensory streams of innervation must combine in order to discharge the correct word-concept.

Now we can understand why the disturbance in word-finding is such a frequent symptom following focal cerebral involvement also causing some type of sensory disturbance. Of the many pathways which come together in (b) only one or the other need be damaged to decrease the amount of innervation of the total concept because of damage to one of its component concepts. This in turn leads to the word-finding difficulty.

It might not be superfluous to mention that word-sound-comprehension neither in the case of Grashey-Wolff nor in that of Rieger was impaired, since both patients were able to mimic without hesitation.

Generally, one might speak of a transcortical motor aphasia only if the involvement of word-finding has resulted in the complete loss of spontaneous speech or approaches this degree of severity. If one contrasts this with disturbance in the area of amnestic aphasia (Pitres), one is presented not only with the symptoms of focal involvement of the brain, but also the suspicion of a disturbance of thought or intellect, as we have seen in comparison with the mentally ill. Rieger has carefully outlined the type of examination needed for testing such cases. No doubt such investigations may show the presence of some kind of intellectual deficit in most cases of this type. Whatever focal symptoms are found in addition to such possible deficits may then be of secondary importance in pointing to the area of general involvement which has caused the overall loss of cerebral function. Heilbronner has indicated that one can often demonstrate symptoms without any trace of focal cerebral involvement as a result of senile cerebral atrophy which may fall under the general category of a transcortical motor or sensory aphasia. Such cases may also reveal some signs of psychic blindness or asymbolia, which are generally based on disturbance of secondary identification, as is also true of the mentally ill. A more detailed consideration of such symptoms at this time is prohibited by the wealth and importance of the available data which would require very special consideration and treatment. However, I cannot avoid referring to the most recent progress in the area differentiating mental illness and cerebral focal involvement, since it has a very intimate relationship to our specific subject of word-finding. This is the masterly-developed and described picture of unilateral apraxia by Liepmann. Just as an unusual chance occurrence resulted in the typical clinical picture of transcortical motor aphasia, so by the same kind of chance accident the sites of cerebral lesions in Liepmann's case were such that the transcortical tracts controlling movements of one side of the body were transected. Because the patient sustained a subcortical motor aphasia and thus was deprived of the ability to speak, a test of intelligence could be undertaken only by means of the patient's motor actions. Such testing revealed a very severe psychic type of impairment, and in fact, a severe mental deficiency, if one evaluated reactions carried out with the right extremities only. However, a comparatively high level of intelligence was found to exist if one tested only by means of response carried out by the left extremities. The pathologic findings of this much-discussed case, which have not yet been published, confirmed the hypothesized focal cerebral disease.

I shall refrain from going into a detailed-discussion regarding the examination of aphasics of various forms, since this seems to me to be unnecessary here. In the course of this discussion all of the leading points of view in this matter have already been emphasized. However, two symptoms deserve careful mention and consideration. One is the marked ready fatigue of this patient, necessitating interruption of the testing with resumption after short periods pf rest. If no regard is given to this point, one might easily accept conflicting findings at different times. The second possible source of error is the symptom of perseveration (Neisser). This consists of the tendency to repeat an action or response made earlier, in spite of the fact that the patient may be aware of the incorrectness of the response. Patients often express their annoyance regarding this and clearly show that they did not intend to produce that particular last response. In other words, there appears to be some unconscious compelling force at the basis of this. This symptom makes study of such an aphasic patient difficult, and one is often required to pause or in some way shift the patient's attention into a different direction, in order to obtain a new and correct response. As A. Pick has demonstrated, this disturbance may be exaggerated to the point of pseudo-apraxia.

I cannot conclude this essentially clinical portion of my discussion on symptomatology without exploring in some detail the problem of unilaterality of the cerebral center of oral speech discussed above. My entire thesis regarding the unilaterality of these so-called centers has been based on clinically established findings. Indeed, the hypothesis of the left hemisphere as the only seat of speech function was in fact based on such a clinical finding. This was felt to be so significant that it led to the first attempt to localize speech (Marc Dax, 1836). I have referred only to the left hemisphere in this respect, but I must later explain the exceptions that exist regarding exclusive left hemisphere speech localization. In this matter, there are two major groups of facts which are somewhat interrelated. One category of exceptions refers to speech disturbances in the left-handed. In almost all cases such disorders are caused by involvement of the right hemisphere since a corresponding relationship exists between location of the right-sided lesions and their consequent symptomatology as prevails in focal involvement of the left hemisphere. At present we do not know why in the majority of individuals, predominant right handedness, favoring of the right hand in activities requiring great strength or skill, is accompanied by the functional development of a left cortical speech center. That such unilateral predisposition serves a useful purpose, however, is definitely supported by the principle of conservation of energy. Further analysis of this problem would lead us to a clinical study of P. Oppenheim's case, who presented a predominantly sensory aphasia caused by a tumor associated with a left hemiplegia. A review of the history reveals that the patient had not been left-handed since early childhood, but following an injury to the right hand at the age of 17, was forced to use his left hand and thereafter had become left-handed. The pathologic findings demonstrated the assumed tumor to be in the right hemisphere. This clinical study leads to two conclusions: 1) At a later age the right hemisphere may be able to take over the function of speech originally laid down in the left hemisphere. 2) The left hemisphere may lose the speech function it previously had developed, if use of the left hand replaces that of the right. I do not know of a similar case which so convincingly supports our hypothesis that localization of the speech center is a functional acquisition of each individual.

The other category of exceptions of localization of speech on the left refers to pathologic studies in childhood. According to the stage of the child's development, focal lesions of the left hemisphere at times may be accompanied by speech disorders which may be either mild or severe. Recovery of speech, however, occurs relatively soon even if later evidence reveals complete destruction of the speech centers of the left. In childhood, apparently, the transfer of left-sided brain function to the right occurs quite readily. Under such conditions one need not develop left-handness for localization of speech to be transferred to the right side. Thus, lesions of the left hemisphere may not show (speech) symptoms in right-handers as long as the pathologic findings are carried out later on in life. Furthermore, recent lesions of the right hemisphere may cause aphasia, although the patient is not left-handed. As one can see, the principle of the development of such centers based purely on individual variables may lead to a series of possibilities which are difficult to interpret and may erroneously appear to be exceptions to the rule of left-sided speech localization. Inadequacy of the case history is one such source of error. One cannot particularly rule out the many alternatives which may exist in different cases if at one time only the left speech center is in control and at another, the right, or in some cases, bilateral speech function may prevail. One may also assess the function of the other hemisphere to be preserved or severely compromised. In the latter case, prognosis for transfer of function is not favorable. Experience generally shows that the sensory speech center is more resistant to damage than the motor. More correctly, we may differentiate an impressive and expressive act of the speech process in this connection. The conditions regarding transfer of speech representation to the other hemisphere in circumscribed or predominantly destructive brain disease, such as hemorrhage and cerebral softening, are much clearer. In such cases, the possibility of recovery by means of development of a new center may be strongly influenced by the generalized symptoms of the stroke. A more severe attack, without one-sided focal symptoms of the brain, may result in generalized damage with easy fatigue, decreased attention span, and emotional instability. Because clinical experience teaches that the accompanying symptoms in motor aphasia are usually severe, while in sensory aphasia and pure word-blindness they are generally minimal or not at all marked, we can appreciate the well-known rule favoring recovery of sensory speech function, and the significance of pure alexia as a focal symptom may be put in a clear light.

One other experience is related to the question of unilaterality of the speech center which in my opinion indicates that the motor, or more correctly, the expressive component of the speech process is not always and exclusively unilateral in nature. As is known, the indirect focal symptoms of the acute focal cerebral lesions of the brain following a frank stroke is generally limited to the involved hemisphere. This leads to the perhaps frequent expectation of a more or less marked motor aphasia following a severe stroke and left hemiplegia. This symptom, however, lasts only for a few days, contradicting the possibility that one is dealing with a case of left-handedness in which the aphasia may continue for a longer period as an indirect focal symptom. This symptom may only be explained by the hypothesis that prior to the stroke, the right hemisphere also participated to a certain extent in the innervation process of activer speech production. If the lesion involving the right hemisphere induced indirect impairment of the left hemisphere, then those very functions which relied on participation by the right hemisphere would mostlreadily also be affected. Whether this indicates a chronic destruction of the left Broca gyrus as a result of the trauma of the stroke, or merely represents a passing functional disturbance, may readily be established by the further course of the clinical picture. Thus, we have a safe criterion for the destruction of Broca's gyrus as a result of a stroke in the symptom called syllable-stumbling. This is commonly held to be a reliable sign of general paresis, and therefore is called a paralytic speech disturbance. One finds this same disturbance of syllable-stumbling in the majority of patients who have once sustained a motor aphasia, but merely as an indirect or transient focal symptom of the left hemisphere.

Although these facts appear to be little known, I can support them on the basis of repeated clinical experience and would like to draw particular attention to their significance in differential diagnosis of general paresis.

THE FINAL SECTION OF THE MONOGRAPH IS DEVOTED TO THE CONTROVERSIAL SUBJECT OF THE NEUROANATOMIC LOCALIZATION OF LANGUAGE AND APHASIC SYMPTOMS. THIS REPRESENTS WERNICKE'S MOST DETAILED REVIEW OF THIS ISSUE.

We now have reached the point where we must undertake a description of the anatomic boundaries of the speech area of the brain, which according to Dejerine, might be called the *zone de la langue,* on the basis of the clinical findings discussed above. I believe that I can best do this by referring to the illustrations found in the works of Von Monakow and Dejerine (Figures 24 and 25). In the illustrations of both of these works the darkly-shaded portions designate the well-established centers. The shaded areas specifically refer to the speech region. A comparison of the two illustrations, in this respect, reveals a nice agreement, if one considers the independence of the two studies. One can see that, with the exception of the most anterior extensions and the inferior part connecting the two central gyri, the entire first primordial gyrus, that is, that area contained within the Sylvian fossa region, may be counted as the speech area. The part corresponding to Broca's gyrus in the frontal lobe is the motor speech center; that area lying in the temporal lobe, below the Sylvian fissure, is the sensory speech center; the portion above the posterior end of the Sylvian fissure, the so-called supramarginal gyrus, is counted by both authors as part of the speech region, without however, assigning it a specific role. Both authors, moreover,agree that the area above Broca's gyrus, the so-called foot of the second frontal gyrus, should not be included as part of the speech region, although Exner, Charcot, Pitres, and recently Ziehen designate this area as the motor writing center. Moreover, both authors also agree that the portion of the gyrus bordering on the first primordial gyrus in the inferior parietal lobe, in which its longitudinal posterior extension acts as an anastamosing bridge connecting with the second primordial gyrus, may still be counted as part of the speech area. This posterior portion of the speech region, extending in a horizontal direction, is the angular gyrus, the *pli courbe* of the French authorities. Dejerine's inclusion of the neighboring portion of the second temporal gyrus as part of the speech zone, while it is not expressly indicated in Von Monakow's illustrations, seems to me to agree more precisely with most of the findings. Within the grey-tinted speech region in Monakow's illustration we find two more darkly shaded areas, while Dejerine delineates three such sharply defined areas. Both authors agree in designating those two areas which correspond to the more narrowly defined sensory and motor speech centers. Only Dejerine characteristically includes a third center in the narrow sense, namely the area of the angular gyrus, which he designates as a center of the visual memory images of the word. I have previously described in detail just in which sense this may be understood. Von Monakow does not recognize such a special visual word center. These two illustrations

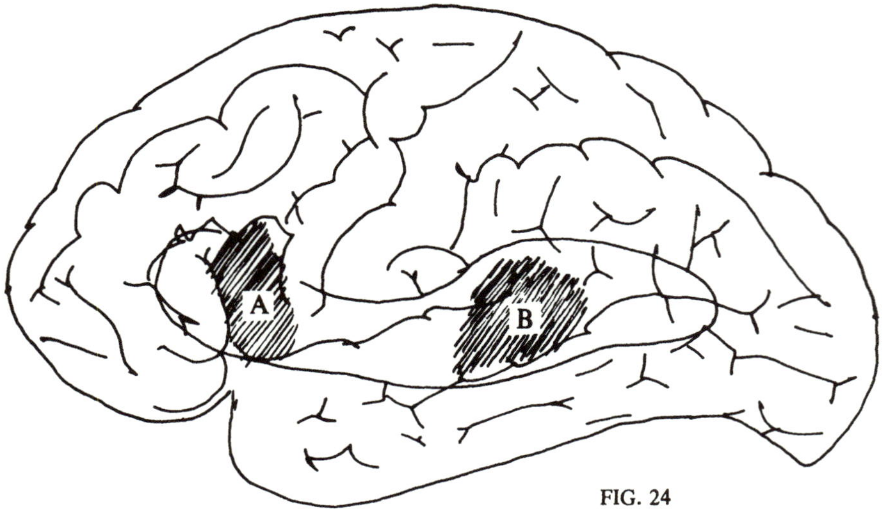

FIG. 24

Speech Centers (Von Monakow)

A. Broca's gyrus
B. Sensory Speech Center

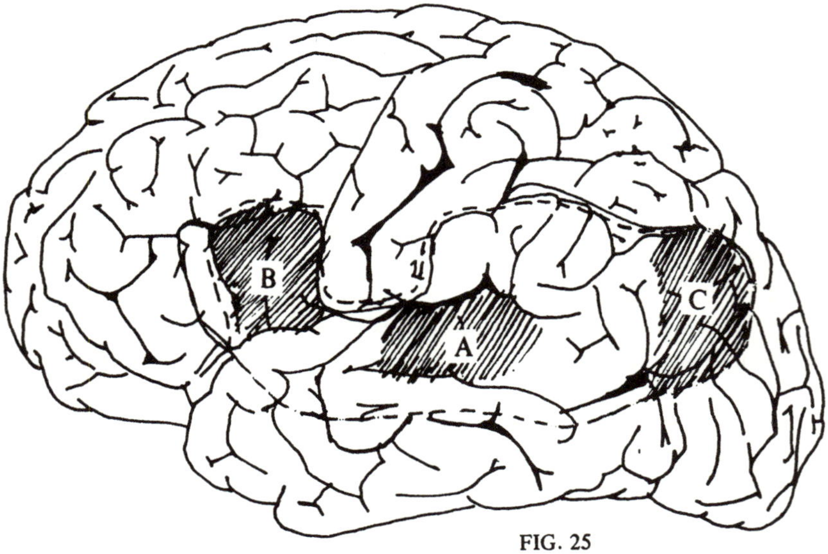

FIG. 25

Speech Centers (Dejerine)

A: Sensory speech zone
B: Motor Speech zone
C: Center of visual memory images of the word

clearly show that the speech region not only includes the two centers which up to now have been narrowly differentiated, but also takes in the neighboring regions of the cerebral convexity. Nevertheless, they present only a portion of the entire speech area, since these two authors, together with most authorities, agree that the island lying in the depths of the Sylvian fossa and the overlapping portions of the first primordial gyrus must also be included. In order to understand this, one must explore the Sylvian fissure and separate the surrounding gyri belonging to the primordial gyrus mentioned: The island thus presents itself as a three-cornered structure with fan-shaped gyri lying in the depths of the cortical area. It is differentiated from the overlapping cortical substance by three deeply grooved sulci. These are the anterior, the superior, and the inferior sulci according to Burdach's designation. At the top corner of the merging of the inferior and superior sulci a deep fissure, overlapped by the marginal gyrus and the first temporal gyrus, extends posteriorly in the direction of the superior sulcus, so that in the unfolded brain it reaches almost the transverse plane of the angular gyrus. The accompanying illustration, Figure 26, taken from Henle's anatomy text gives us a notion of these relationships.

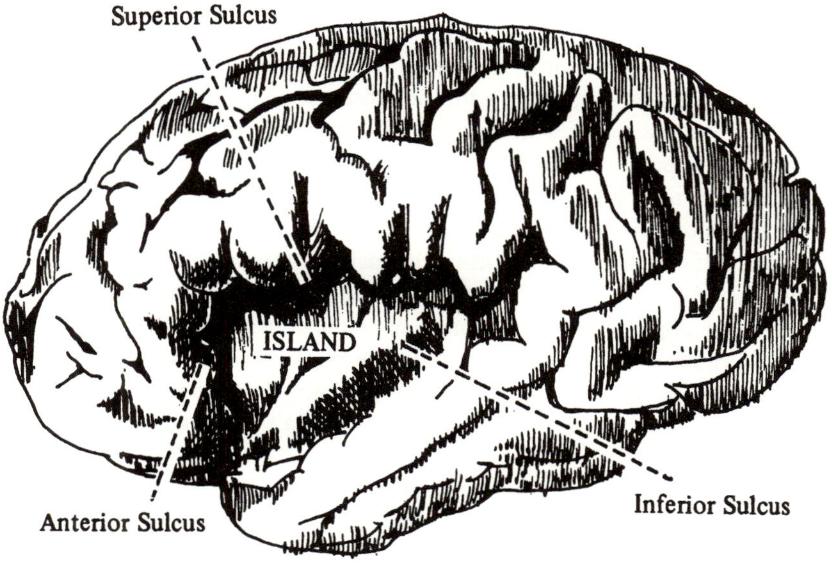

FIG. 26

The Island Region (Henle)

The island is assumed to be significant for speech function in that it forms a focal point for the union of the association tracts connecting the two speech centers and whatever other regions may be related to speech function. In fact, the detailed anatomy of the island permits no other interpretation than that this area represents an actual association center. This is based not only on the fact that the three deep sulci which divide the island reveal a rich development of well-known fibrae propriae, or the arcuate lamina of Arnold, at the base, but the cortex of the island at this site also presents a specialized kind of structure. As is known, the extension of the island cortex corresponds to the outer wall of the largest ganglion of the brain, the lenticular nucleus. Between the lenticular nucleus and the island cortex one can find two layers of white substance. That lamina which lies close to the lenticular nucleus presents a very thin inner layer, the external capsule; the other, the capsule extrema belongs to the island-cortex and consists of a firmer layer adhering to the island cortex. Between the capsula externa and capsula extrema, however, we find a structure of grey substance entirely unlike that found elsewhere in the brain, namely, the claustrum. This ganglion, which is fan-shaped, broadens toward the top as the island cortex, but diminishes in its longitudinal extent. As Meynert has already demonstrated, as it diminishes, its peripherally-directed processes merge within the first primordial gyrus. It consists exclusively of the spindle or association cells, which Meynert has differentiated. According to that authority, this is nothing other than a specially developed cortical layer, deeply situated within the brain which faces the layer of white matter. In fact, it merges sporadically in the island cortex as the so-called foot of the island, that is, the lower union point of the radiating island gyri, just as with the substance of the amygdalate nucleus. In addition to the cortex with its claustrum, two important association bundles are important for the anatomy of the speech area. One of these, is the fasciculus uncinatus, penetrated by the broad foot of the claustrum, dividing it into numerous layers giving the appearance of a union of cells and fibers. If one deflects the cortex, the main portion of this association bundle may be found at the foot of the island and somewhat within. Here one can best appreciate its hook-shape, reminding one of the arcuate lamina. From this mid-portion, the bundle splits, diverging into the frontal and temporal lobes, whose shortest connection it represents. Portions thereof also extend into the third frontal gyrus, including Broca's gyrus, and into the speech area of the first temporal lobe.

While the uncinate fasciculus appears to be the shortest connection between the portions of the frontal and temporal lobes facing each other, there is a second bundle, the arcuate fasciculus, which is not actually a special bundle but part of the general system of the sagittal association fibers of the convex cerebral surfaces. The ganglia cells are not included in this bundle. The anatomic conditions of the brain are such that the appearance of a special bundle of this type can most readily exist at the point where the foot of the corona radiata passes from the internal capsule, that is, above and external to the lateral edge of the lateral ventricle, somewhat over the superior edge of the lenticular nucleus. As it also courses through the substance bordering on the Sylvian fossa of the temporal and parietal lobes, one may be able to visualize it in a hardened brain if the cortex of the superior space with its fibrae propriae is deflected. One can then be certain that a special bundle penetrates into the deep white matter of the marginal gyrus up to the first temporal gyrus and in an arch surrounding the posterior branches of the Sylvian fissure. That portion of the arch-like bundle, coursing in the former sagittal direction, lies medial to the thus previously described line and is generally compressed into a narrow space on the one side by the deep interparietal sulcus, and the posterior branches of the superior Burdach sulcus on the other. In this region the arch-bundle no doubt is joined by fibers originating from the marginal gyrus and the posterior third of the first temporal gyrus. The white matter of the inferior parietal lobe consists to a great extent of these comparatively narrowly-compressed fibers. One may note that the course of the anterior part of the arcuate fasciculus in part lies in the roof of the lateral ventricles above the lenticular nucleus.and a sagitally-directed continuation of this tract courses in the parietal and occipital lobes. At one point in the previously mentioned sulci, the bundle is compressed by the above mentioned furrows and the posterior end of the deep parallel or first temporal sulcus. It therefore is readily seen that the white matter of the lower part of the parietal lobe presents a comparatively narrow space for passage of a large portion of the association fibers of the arcuate fasciculus, and thus a large segment of the same may be damaged at this point by one lesion. I shall limit myself to those anatomic remarks which shall primarily show that this peculiarity of the lower parietal lobe, that is the angular gyrus, must contain a very important passage way to the speech area. Apart from this, as one moves inwardly toward the ventricle, divided longitudinal layers can be found. That which is most external is the inferior longitudinal bundle, the next, the so-called visual radiation, and finally, the tapetum of the corpus callosum; all three of these bundles combine to form the sagittal medullary layer of the occipital lobe. The narrow space containing such important and different types of tracts can readily present the appearance of a center, and this accounts for the hypothesis of such a center by Dejerine, which in my opinion is in error. One might certainly recommend Dejerine's *Anatomie des centres nerveux* as well as my own *Atlas* of brain sections to anyone who might be interested in the finer details of the anatomy of this area. The illustration shown here (Figure 27) is taken from the work of Von Monakow and shows a horizontal section through the left cerebral hemisphere at the top of the first temporal gyrus, the third frontal gyrus, and the splenium of the corpus callosum. The three obliquely shaded areas on the convexity show the sites of

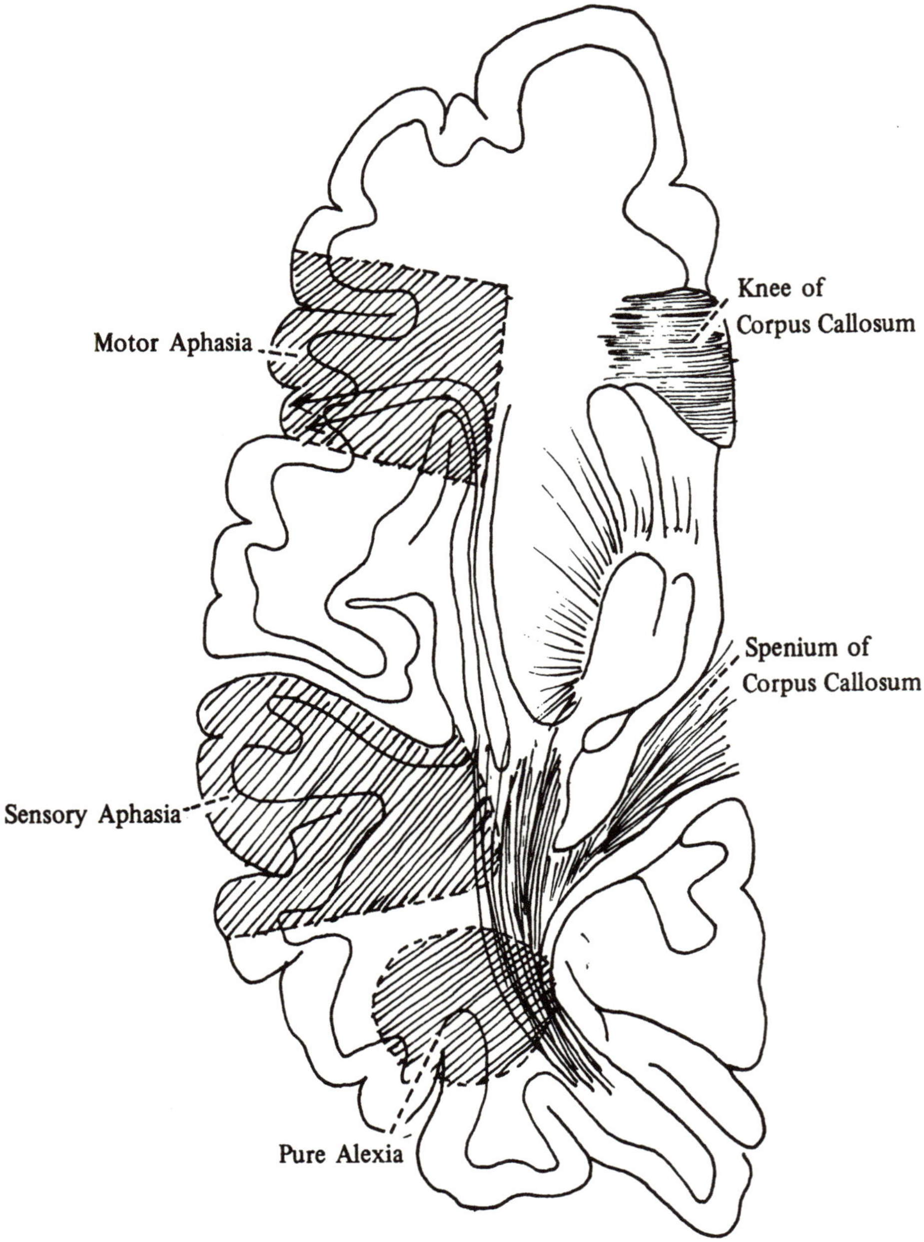

FIG. 27.

Horizontal Section (L) Hemisphere (Von Monakow)

the lesions in motor and sensory aphasia and in pure alexia. In contrast to the oblique shading in the illustration one may note the longitudinally shaded areas which designate the fiber masses comprising the three fiber bundles. Thus, in the schematic illustration one can see the above-mentioned sagittal white matter of the occipital lobe, which is a hardened preparation, is sharply differentiated from the white matter of the temporal lobe and inferior parietal lobe, as indicated in the illustration. As can be seen from the circular shaded area in the inferior part of the parietal lobe, Von Monakow regarded the disruption of these three fibers as a prerequisite for the occurrence of pure alexia which, according to this interpretation, was caused by destruction of the connections associating the sensory speech center with the two posterior occipital lobes.

As I have indicated above, I agree with Von Monakow's point of view in this that I cannot regard Dejerine's hypothesis of a unilateral center for the written word images in the angular gyrus cortex to be a proven fact. Dejerine's observations do not prove this conclusion but merely indicate that destruction of this area as a rule severely impairs written language, the effects of which vary dependent upon the depth of the lesion, i.e., whether the deep or superficial layers of the angular gyrus cortex are involved. In the first case, pure alexia would result, while in the second, alexia would be accompanied by agraphia. The cortex of the angular gyrus, nevertheless, in both cases may be completely uninvolved. The anatomic conditions permit one to conclude that disruption of all the connections between the speech center and both occipital lobes may be easily accomplished because they form a compact bundle in the lower parietal lobe. It shall be the task of the immediate future to apply the pertinent pathological findings in this direction. The following anatomical tracts are relevant in this situation and shall be briefly reviewed here. The first is the sagittal layer of white matter of the occipital lobe with its three separate layers. Of these, disruption of the middle bundle, the so-called "visual radiation" offers the most characteristic clinical symptom, namely, the accompanying hemianopsia. The innermost layer, the so-called tapetum, originates from the splenium of the corpus callosum and contains at least two known tracts, namely, a connection between the two temporal lobes and a connection of the temporal lobe with the opposite occipital lobe, the forceps tapetum tract of H. Sachs. It also appears to be well-established that this latter tract, which corresponds to Bastian's crossed optic-acoustic commissure, passes into the splenium of the corpus callosum. The outer most layer, as the fasciculus longitudinalis inferior, mediates a rich connection between the temporal lobe and the occipital lobe on the same side and so may also contain the same sided optic acoustic commissure of Bastian. According to recent studies by Probst, it contains exclusively the corona radiata fibers coursing to the optic thalamus, which, however, I cannot verify. Only in regard to the upper half of its highest branches can this be conceded. As far as the rest is concerned, one may only be certain of its importance as an association tract between the temporal and occipital lobes. This sagittal layer of white matter with its three component parts is located not only within the inferior parietal lobe but also within the sensory center in the posterior third of the first temporal gyrus. Second, the white matter of the angular gyrus does not only lie external to but also above the sagittal layer of white matter. It contains a diffuse and generally undifferentiated mass of white matter divided into at least two major components i.e., the callosal fibers stemming from the splenium which originate in the forceps major penetrate the sagittal white matter forming a fiber bundle, and that part of the arch-bundle or fasciculus arcuatus described above. This is formed of all tracts which connect the motor cerebral region with the occipital and lower parietal regions on the same side and provides the shortest connection between the sensory speech center and the lower parietal or occipital lobe. The considerations which I have presented above make it highly probable that the syndrome of pure alexia is caused by destruction of the sagittal white matter with preservation of the tract coursing through the white matter of the angular gyrus.

The pathologic findings in pure word-blindness with hemianopsia do not reveal just one focal lesion, as is evident in Von Monakow's illustration, but rather more frequently a number of lesions, which interrupt the optic radiation at the point of its origin in the occipital lobe, and moreover, portions of the corpus callosum. One segment of the splenium of the callosum merits particular mention, since the same artery, the posterior cerebral, supplies both the occipital lobe and the splenium. Both regions are therefore subject to softening. However, which segment of the callosum, the forceps major connecting symmetrical portions of the cerebrum or the forceps tapetum of H. Sachs, must be disrupted in this case, is still in doubt.

The tapetum in the temporal lobe cannot be localized in the place designated by Von Monakow. In other ways his diagram is the same as Dejerine's—since that would be too close to the occipital lobe. In this regard refer to my discussion presented above. However, the possibility of involvement of both tracts has not been excluded. This would account for variations in the clinical picture, such as the patient's ability to copy.

One may also ascertain the approximate site of focal lesions in respect to the rare relatively pure cases of literal agraphia by a comparison with certain related cases. Such lesions are felt to be located at the site of crossing of the sensory fibers of the corona radiation related to the extremities with the deep lying portions of the arcuate fasciculus.

The complexity of the anatomic situation of the speech region reviewed thus far contributes to the fact that the pathologic findings of the rather infrequent cases which are reported by reliable observers and are adequately studied clinically are frequently deficient in description and thus subject to many objections. Therefore, a purely clinical viewpoint in utilizing the pathologic findings is not successful. On the contrary, the clinical observations, which are generally valid, may be challenged collectively on the basis of contradictory observations. The wealth of material presented, such as the distinguished and unbiased work of Bastian, which since the contribution of Kussmaul stands as the most exhaustive summary available, can well support this statement. I find it extremely satisfying that in spite of this, a universal lawfulness obtains in this area, as can be seen in the harmony of viewpoints of Pick, Von Monakow, and Dejerine, investigators whose unquestionable clinical objectivity established them as first-making are largely based on part of the words of these authors and in part on my own clinical experience and observations.

In regard to the actual areas of the motor and sensory speech center in a narrower sense, I refer to my discussion presented earlier. The anterior obliquely shaded area (Figure 27) reveals the common area of destruction in pure cases of motor aphasia. This syndrome, according to our nomenclature, also includes a verbal agraphia. Most of the cases of motor aphasia without agraphia appear to be cases of subcortical motor aphasia. In part, however, with respect to the demonstrated findings, we must also consider partial destruction of Broca's gyrus. In such cases it is damage only to the inferior lip of Broca's gyrus, facing the Sylvian fossa, which causes word-muteness. The preservation of the other portions, according to Monakow, is adequate to permit written language. Therefore, Figure 27 illustrates the seat of the lesions of cases of cortical motor aphasia which are not typically accompanied by agraphia.

The secondary degeneration which remains after cortical motor aphasia is localized to a specific place in the internal capsule in the accompanying illustration, Figure 28, is designated by the region (a-1). Unfortunately, confirmation of the exact site of the very small lesion responsible for causing subcortical sensory aphasia i.e., pure word-deafness, in my opinion can definitely be established in a single case. This is the case of Liepmann mentioned previously, whose autopsy findings have only recently been published. Certain unfavorable accompanying circumstances unfortunately permit it to be used only as proof by exclusion, in that destruction lies at the point of union between the corona radiata of the temporal lobe and the insula. Nevertheless, the evidence is most convincing since at the same time a secondary degeneration was found involving the lobe of the right hemisphere. This could only be explained on the basis of an old lesion in the white matter of the temporal lobe, since the cortex of the temporal lobe and entire occipital lobe was well preserved on the left side. The right hemisphere, however, revealed only the recent destructive lesion. Liepmann, in his interpretation of this case, very appropriately refers to H. Sachs, who on the basis of his observation of the tightly compact bundle of the corona radiata of the temporal lobe in its course between the posterior and inferior projection of the third branch of

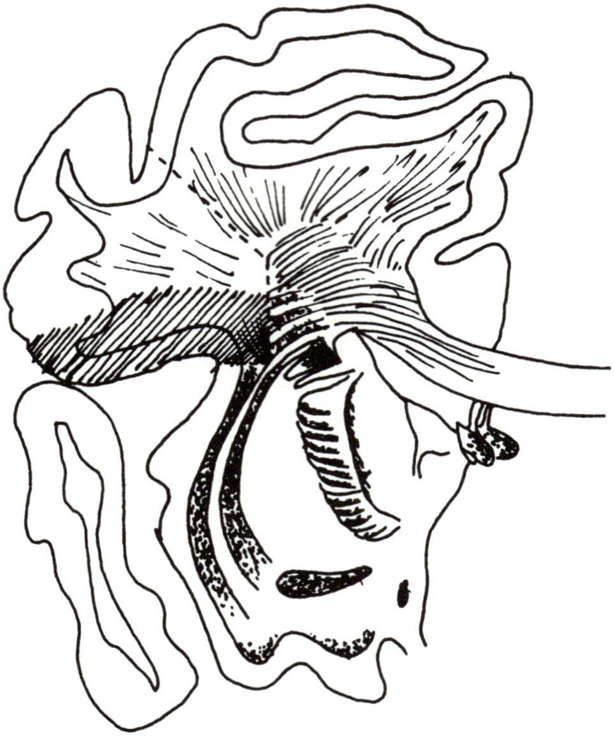

FIG. 28

Coronal Section of Left Hemisphere

the lenticular nucleus and the tail of the caudate nucleus located in the roof-of the inferior horn, predicted that a subcortical sensory aphasia could most readily be caused by damage to this area.

Many years ago I called attention to cases which demonstrated that a fiber tract must run inwardly from the posterior branches of the superior Burdach space, the destruction of which would cause motor aphasia. (Wernicke, 1882, *2*, pp., 173, 176, 179.) At that time I believed this tract coursed within the internal capsule and postulated the presence at that point of a special motor speech path, containing the projection fibers of Broca's gyrus to the bulbar nuclei. However, since that time numerous clinical cases have persuaded me that a sensory aphasia occurring with motor aphasia might be commonly overlooked. Moreover, it has been established that lesions of the internal capsule are not able to produce a cortical motor aphasia. There are other considerations regarding this matter which I shall report in the near future.

Therefore, I hold it ot be most probable that such observations must be attributed to instances of transcortical motor sensory aphasia. Von Monakow, who holds that the route of the impulse in spontaneous speech travels by way of the sensory speech center, designates with great certainty the archbundle (arcuate fasciculus) as the only association tract, apart from the island cortex, which connects the motor and sensory speech centers. Moreover, Heilbronner has recently stressed that the wealth of fiber connections between the temporal lobe and the third frontal gyrus compels one to regard the temporal lobe as the primary origin of the transcortical fiber tract for Broca's center. The decisive point in the question, however, I base on the case reported by Heubner, which permits no other interpretation than a transection of the major components of the arch-bundle or arcuate fasciculus. At least, there must be a disruption of the specific layer of white matter beneath the first temporal gyrus, which I have mentioned above. Clinically, this case unquestionably demonstrates features of a sensory as well as a motor transcortical aphasia. This case specifically demonstrates a cortical softening in essentially the form of a fissure by which the marginal gyrus appears to be isolated as it were from the surrounding cortical substance. Thus, just as this case demonstrates, nature may present us with focal lesions of the strongest and most fantastic form and extent in certain clinical cases which appear almost as planned experiments, offering for our study a wealth of varied combinations of lesions and symptoms and the most instructive clinical applications.

In respect to the area of diagnosis I refer the reader to the basic facts of general brain pathology in which we face the task of differentiating direct and indirect or transient signs in all focal symptom-pictures, to which the manifestations of aphasia belong in a broader sense. I shall not go into a definition of these here, since one may assume them to be generally known. It appears to me that only the transient symptoms have not always received the attention they have deserved. In this respect one may recall that the transient focal symptoms are caused by compensated arterial occlusions. Therefore, the involved cortical area is temporarily ischemic which does not progress to softening since the circulation is later re-established. One must always suspect this type of development in independent acute focal symptoms, which remit in the course of one to three weeks. In the individual case the occurrence of transient focal symptoms may indicate a specific diagnosis of embolism in contrast to hemorrhage, a diagnosis which cannot definitely be made in the majority of cases. Moreover, the diagnosis of subacute and chronic focal brain disease which are related to aphasia rests on the application of the same common principle, i.e., the presence of the accompanying general symptoms. The same holds for diagnosis of aphasic disturbances accompanying meningitis and paralytic dementia, in which motor as well as sensory aphasia may rather frequently be seen. Such cases as well as those presenting other focal symptoms related to this etiology hold a favorable prognosis. In all cases one must decide the question of the presence of a previous transient aphasia, the possession or lack of a disturbed control of written language before the attack. We may thank the contributions of A. Pick, who recently has demonstrated that this diagnosis may also apply to the process of a chronic progressive brain disease, namely, the simple cerebral atrophy most frequently of a senile or alcoholic etiology. He has indicated that, in addition to a generalized brain atrophy, a more strikingly localized atrophy may also be present, the site of which may be revealed by the accompanying focal symptoms. Thus, one or both temporal lobes, and specifically the first temporal gyrus may prove to be the seat of a marked focal-like atrophy. This betrays itself in a decrease in all parts of the gyrus, the cortex as well as the white matter. The resulting clinical-picture is that of a transcortical sensory aphasia, the occurrence of which can be explained also in unilateral focal-like atrophy in that the generalized atrophy, although mild, may limit compensation by the other hemisphere. Reliable description of cases have been presented by A. Pick and Dejerine. Because of the severe accompanying deafness, these were interpreted as cases of subcortical sensory aphasia or so-called pure word-deafness. Liepmann, however, has provided the evidence that the clinical picture belongs to that of transcortical sensory aphasia, even though a decided bilateral deafness obscures differential diagnosis. A more bilateral deafness, however, may develop in this kind of localized picture, particularly if the atrophy reduces the comparative size of the sensory speech centers bilaterally, as I have discussed above, which naturally masks the presence of an accompanying transcortical sensory aphasia. We must also consider the existence of such transcortical cases. A process involving a gyrus may involve all components to the same degree and yet cortical functions requiring transmission from the periphery may still be in evidence, although the transcortical connections have been damaged, since the gyral white matter contains subcortical as well as transcortical fibers. This may be readily explained on the basis of the firmness of once-developed sensory memory images and their ability to be completely reproduced even in the presence of very fragmentary and incomplete reports from the periphery. The best known example of this is the preservation of tactile ability of a hand in spite of a severe sensory disturbance of both pertinent nerve areas, the medianus and ulnaris, resulting in transmission of very imprecise sensory impressions from the periphery to the cortex. I must challenge Von Monakow's interpretation of the opposite view-point that impairment of sensory centers controlling these very specific cortical performances may occur on the basis of a mild functional disturbance.

In cases demonstrating good preservation of the motor capacity for speech, paraphasia of varying degrees may be the most striking symptom presented, while impairment in comprehension might easily be overlooked except by very experienced observers and is a symptom which must be carefully tested for and established in each case. It is the patient's well-preserved ability to gain cues through the situation at hand and the ability to adapt to it which is so—frequently responsible for overlokking a very gross disturbance in this area. This may readily occur when he in part is able to respond adequately to everyday questions or requests. If motor aphasia is present at the same time, it becomes more difficult to make a decision regarding comprehension of the spoken word, and in such cases one must examine even more carefully for presence of this particular symptom. In respect to disturbances of written language, I shall merely refer to my previous discussion. Whoever might be interested in a more exhaustive study of the finer points of diagnosis of speech disturbances as focal symptoms may find the same in A. Pick's (1898) work, which represents a substantial contribution in this area.

I shall make only a few comments in regard to aphasia therapy. This can only come into question if the focal symptom occurs in a brain which is otherwise healthy. The principle of management lies in speech practice, which in sensory aphasia involves a gradual remission of the disorder by itself. This spontaneous improvement does not occur if special circumstances are present, such as an accompanying generalized cerebral atrophy or a bilateral involvement of the temporal lobes. In regard to motor aphasia, as has already been emphasized, even systematically carried-out exercises may have small effects. Nevertheless, the success which Dejerine and Thomas have demonstrated in motor aphasia indicates that under certain circumstances or by use of certain teaching methods, such as the visual approach, speech movements may be accomplished by means of systematic practice. Therefore, it is recommended that it be used by individuals who are specialized in teaching this method. However, except for a few physicians who have become dedicated to this method, the teachers of deafmutes are best fitted for this task.

NOTES TO THE TRANSLATIONS

Notations followed by the symbol (r) [revised] indicate comments added to the original writings by the author in 1892, at which time they were reprinted together with a collection of other works. Notes not followed by (r) refer to footnotes included at the time of the initial publication.

1. Nothnagel's regression to the Flourens view in citations of experimental studies which consistently support localization, seems to me to reveal an inner conflict.

2r. I no longer support this interpretation, but on the contrary, feel that the cerebral cortex is the site of origin of such attacks.

3. Hitzig has recently stimulated motor response from the posterior regions of the central gyrus.

4r. So it was believed at that time. We now know that the posterior central convolution, the inferior, and a little of the upper portions of the parietal lobe are also regarded as part of the so-called motor area. However, the occipital and temporal lobes stand as sensory areas in sharp contrast to the anterior portions of the hemisphere.

5. Figures submitted in the Winter Semester, 1872-73 are as follows: Findings in the anterior area of the brain in cases of insanity: 46 males, 70 females: 41.5%, 41.90%. Findings in the anterior area of the brain in paralytics: 173 males, 30 females: 40.35%, 39.90%.

6. An additional motor area located in the frontal medullary substance, which Nothnagel has found in the posterior area of the hemisphere, according to his description, belongs to Ammonshorn, area which Meynert maintains, has motor functions.

Hitzig's recent experiment using monkey brains proves only that all fibers unite at certain points of the anterior area of the brain for specific, related movements. They do not therefore contradict the peculiar role of the entire frontal brain region as taught by Meynert.

7. Hitzig, in recent experiments with monkeys, found that stimulation of the left motor center of the mouth and tongue, located just behind the Broca gyrus, results in bilateral muscle movement.

8r. The olfactory nerve by means of its connections with the anterior commissure and the uncinate gyrus. The here specified, "portion of the posterior columns", was at that time regarded by Meynert, on the one hand, as a continuation of the so-called sensory pyramidal decussation, and on the other hand, as the external bundle of the cerebral peduncle, which may be traced to the temporo-occipital area.

9. On this assumption alone rests the reflex inhibitory action of the cerebral hemispheres, as has been emphasized recently by Goltz.

10. Should not mimicry, originating as a reflex process culminating in perfected performance by man, reflect the same innate, refined reflex capacity characteristic of all sensory areas? This feature differentiates us from all other animals, especially the closely-related ape. Actually many imitative movements of an involuntary nature are also present in adults. In how much greater measure would one expect to find this in adulthood, by which time the intellect has strongly developed its controlling effect on reflex activity.

11. Two such cases, demonstrating perforation have been reported by Dr. Grossmann, assistant in the Obstetric Clinic. The autopsy studies were carried out by Dr. Waldezer.

12. I am convinced that Meynert's error is justified, having reviewed his dissections. But many who reproach him for the error would not support him so openly.

13. This point shall be demonstrated later.

14r. That such partial forms of sensory aphasia exist, now seems to me completely improbable. At any event, such a type has not come to my attention, clinically.
15r. Incorrect. An indirect hemiplegia may accompany lesions of the temporal lobe.
16r. Likewise, incorrect. The uneducated as well as the educated are dependent on the same mechanism of spelling, as we have learned from Grashey.
17. See Meynert's ingenious interpretation of cerebral ciruclation in his, "*Bau der Grosshirnrinde.*"
18r. Refer to notation 16r, in which the stage of development is considered irrelevant.
19r. This applies, as Grashey teaches, only to words of such familiarity that they may be recognized without the intermediate step of spelling, such as the individual's signature. And yet, by way of exception, other words may be read in just such a manner. At least this appears to be the most natural explanation of the observations made in the case of Beckman.
20r. Refer to my work, "Recent Works on Aphasia," pp. 181-186.
21r. See below the cases of Beckmann and Kunschkel. Of all areas under consideration, the left optic tract lies closest to the island.
22r. If one accepts Grashey's explanation of the reading process, it appears that the pathway $\iota(\chi\text{-}\beta)$ is also involved in every instance in spontaneous writing, and thus there is the need to postulate a special pathway (χ=al - β).
23r. In regard to this idea see my work, "Recent Works on Aphasia," pp. 181-185
24r. At that time, under Meynert's influence, I had accepted the idea of interruption of the motor fibers in the ganglia of the corpus striatum, a theory which I myself later disproved. Refer to: "Proceedings of the Physiological Association of Berlin," 1879-80, No. 5.
25. One would need to be grounded in Meynert's anatomic theories to pursue this kind of construct. At that time, as is still held by some, the customary picture of hemiplegia was generally associated with destruction of the lenticular nucleus.
26r. Refer to my work, "The Motor Speech Pathway", which contains a discussion hypothesizing involvement of the corpus striatum in such cases.
27r. Refer to, "The Motor Speech Pathway," for a review of these same ideas.
28r. I am no longer able to recall the source of this fantastic tale.
29. In order that we may correctly utilize Finkelnburg's case-study, we assume the right of applying the term asymbolia also to the essential tactual and visual images.
30r. Refer to notation 8r.
31. All evidence supports the idea that most of the cranial nerves bilateral functions course to identical points of both hemispheres. Thus, the location of acoustic imagery must be the same on the right as on the left, for we hear with both ears throughout life. But only the left acoustic center is effectively connected with the motor speech center, and thereby perhaps the left acoustic center alone demonstrates pathways utilized in connection with the concept center. However, the right acoustic center can very quickly replace the left, as occurred in the case of Adam, which shall be reported later.
32. *Ein Beitrag zur Lehre der Aphasie,* Beslau, 1873.
33r. The case reported by Schmidt in *Allg. Zeitschrift f. Psychiatr. 27,* p. 304, first came to my attention later.
34. On necropsy study of a 73 year old man suffering from senile cataracts and senile cerebral atrophy, I found atrophy of the entire hippocampal gyrus and lingual-formation. At the same time, the fornix on the same side was grey in color, as was also the ipsilateral optic thalamus, which was very small. The opposite optic nerve showed a greyish degeneration.
35r. As is known, the semi-decussation of the optic nerve is now established beyond question, as is its exclusive connection with the occipital lobe.
36r. One may correctly state that the zone lying to the right of the fixation point showed diminution of perception. (See Foerster's article in Greaf-Saemisch, *Handbuch d. Augenheilkünde,* VII, 118).
37r. See reference 20r in regard to an explanation of this.

38r. See reference 16r.
39r. This is incorrect. The right hemianopsia itself does not abolish the ability to read. In regard to an explanation of this, I continue to hold the view stated in reference 19r.
40. The conclusion in regard to the left optic tract is not permitted if there is complete crossing in the chiasma. In that event the posterior angle of the chiasma would come under consideration.
41. If one accepts the postulate of complete crossing of fibers to the left.
42r. I have now presented and confirmed the localized findings in a different manner. The pathological studies were carried out by Foerster and are reported in my *Lehrbuch der Gehirnkrankheiten, II,* p. 193.
43r. Refer to the case discussed on page 201 of my "Recent Works on Aphasia," where the writing disturbance is described as a subcortical agraphia.
44r. A hypothesis which I now do not maintain.
45r. Refer to page 192 of my "Recent Works on Aphasia," where the opposite view is formulated with an interpretation of the occurrence of agraphia as a sequel to destruction of Broca's gyrus. This case, to be sure, does not represent a case of pure motor aphasia, but belongs to a special form of subcortical motor aphasia.
46r. Refer to page 201 of my "Recent Works on Aphasia," where to an even greater extent, the interruption of the pathway (b-χ) [Figure 22] comes into question.
47r. See references 24r and 25r.
48r. See reference 39r.
49r. I have changed my opinion of this. Refer to the introduction of my textbook, *Lehrbuch der Gehirnkrankheiten,* where the conditions for such localization are discussed in detail.
50. I have observed such a case which is described in the dissertation of Czarnowsky now in press.
51r. Only now after 18 years, am I approaching a realization of this long-harbored intention. With the support of the Royal Academy of Science, an atlas of the cerebral medullary tracts is now in preparation.
52r. It would seem to me that a patient who is unable to say the word "I" might fall into this category. (See: Guttmann, P., Ztschrf. f. Klin. Med. II, 1.)
53r. Refer to my textbook, *Lehrbuch der Gehirnkrankheiten,* I, 251.
54. One must add here that a positive feature of conduction aphasia, moreover, is present in the severe impairment in ability to mimic words. A very significant case of this type has recently been observed.
55r. I well appraciate the fact that the concept of the letter comprises more than this, including above all, the acoustic and motor images. However, it is evident that these cannot be invested with an independent significance. The oral production of letters, according to my view is one of the most complicated performances of centers (a) and (b), and has developed out of an established word-existence, just as the refined movements of the individual fingers have evolved from the gross, mass movements of the hand. The acoustic and motor images of the letters are contained with the word in centers (a) and (b).
56r. Paraphasia alone can follow any arbitrary disruption of the arc (a-B-b).
57r. Not exclusively visual, however, since specific motor processes participate in all form and spatial imagery, as discussed in regard to the concepts of concrete objects; nevertheless, to a great extent, visual, since we essentially read with the macula lutea, which can be readily demonstrated by experimentation, and the macula, as is known, is invested with the most refined spatial-sense.
58r. This passage requires some correction in the sense that the left sagittal medullary layer which contains the transmission of the left optic tract is disconnected secondary to the hemianopsia and thus cannot contribute to reading; the subcortical disruption also involves the end-terminals of the left optic tract, the center (χ), which is accessible to stimulation from the outside world by means of the right optic tract and its cortical endings. Subcortical here includes also a stretch between the same projection fields of the right and left hemispheres, which, no doubt is contained in the corpus callosum.

The term subcortical here has the same relative significance as it has in cases of subcortical verbal alexia and agraphia.

I am indebted to my colleague, Bruns, from Hanover, for calling my attention to this error.

59r. Thus, with the exception of letters of the alphabet, which alone of all visual impressions could not be identified, if in addition, the cortical terminals of the right optic tract were involved, a combination of subcortical alexia with psychic blindness, a condition similar to that of Lissauer's case, would result.

60r. In August, 1891, I again examined this patient. He was at that time again able to write with the right hand, although awkwardly. Tactual sense was still completely absent, and a minimal disturbance in position-sense of the fingers on the right could be detected. In the year 1886, the same defects in position-sense were present but masked by the gross disturbances which I had earlier described.

The minimal disturbance in position-sense is not responsible for the complete loss of tactual ability. This is demonstrated among others by cases of disturbance of position-sense related to spinal or peripheral causes. It is more likely due to an actual loss of tactual imagery.

REFERENCES

Amidon.
1885 On the pathological anatomy of sensory aphasia. *New York Med. Journ.*, January.

Bastian, C.
1869 On the various forms of loss of speech in cerebral disease. *British and Foreign Med. Chir. Review.* January.

Berger, O.
1885 Zur localization der cortical Sehsphäre beim Menschen. *Bräsl. Artzl. Ztschr.* 1.

Berlin Wanderversammlung sudwestdeutsch Irren ärzte u. Neurologen. *Arch f. Psych.* 15, 276

Bezold.
1895-6 Das Hörvermögen der Taubstummen und Nachträge dazu. *Z.f. Ohrenheilk. 36.*

Broadbent, W.
1883 Proc. of British Med. Association Meeting No. 53. *British Med. Journ.* August.

Charcot, J.
1883 Des différentes formes de l'aphasie - de la cecité verbale. Progr. Med., Paris, *11.*
Des variétés de l'aphasie. I. De la cécité des mots. II. Aphasie motrice. *Prog. Med.*, Paris III, 468-471; 487-488; 521-525; 859-861.

Dax
1836 Lesion de la moitié gauche de l'encéphale coincident avec l'oubli des signes de la pensée . *Gaz. Hebd. med. 2,*

Dejerine, J.
1884 De l'aphasie et de ses diffé́rentes formes. *Somain med.* 44, 423-449.

D'Heilly, E. et Chantemesse, A.
1883 Note sur un case de cécité et de surdité verbales. *Prog. med., 22.*

Freund, C.
1889 Ueber optische Aphasie und Seelenblindheit. *Arch. f. Psych. 20,* 276-297.

Grashey,
1885 Ueber Aphasie und ihre Beziehungen zur Wahrehmung. *Arch. f. Psych.* 16, 654-688.

Heilbronner.
1897 Aphasie und Geisteskrankheit. *Psych. Abhandl.* 1.
1901 Uber die transcorticale motorische Aphasie und die als Amnesie bezeichnete Sprachstörung. *Arch. f. Psych.* 34.

Jackson, H.
1883 Proc. of British Med. Assoc. Meeting No. 54. *British med. Journ.*, August.

Kahler
1885 Kasuistische Beitrage zur Lehre von der Aphasie *Prager med. Wchschrft.*, 16.

Körner
1885 Zwei Fälle von grossen erwerben Defekten im Schläfolappen. *Ber. Klin. Wchschrft.*, 16.

Kussmaul, A.
1877 *Die Störungen der Sprache.* Leipzig: Vogel.
Lichtheim, L.
1885 Ueber Aphasie. *Deut. Arch. f. Klin. Med.*, 36, 204, 608,
Liepmann, H.
1898 Ein Fall von reiner Sprachtaubheit, Pysch. Abhandl. *7, 8* Beslau.
Marie, P.
1883 De l'aphasie (cécité verbale, surdite verbale, aphasie motrice, agraphie). *Rev. de med.*, 693, 702.
Pick, A.
1892 *Arch. f. Psych. 23.*
Beitrage zur Pathologie u. pathologischen Anatomie des Centralnervensystems. Berlin.
Pitres, A.
1884 Considérations sur l'agraphie a propos d'une observation nouvelle d'agraphie motrice pure. *Revue de med.*, 855-873.
1898 L'Aphasie amnesique et ses variétés cliniques, *Progres Med.*
Prevost, J.
1882 Aphasie (cécité et surdite verbales) *Revüe med. de la Suisse romande.* No. 11, 12.
Redlich, E.
1895 Ueber die sogenannte subcorticale Alexie. *Jahrbuch f. Psych. u. Neuro. 13,* 243-302.
Rieger, C.
1888 Beschreibung der Intelligenz-störungen infolge einer Hirnverletzung Verhandl. der Phys. med. Gesellschaft zu Würzburg, *12.*
Rosenthal, A.
1885 Ein Fall von corticaler Hemiplegia mit Worttaubheit. *Central. f. Nervenheilk.*, 1.
Ross, J.
1883 *Treatise on the Diseases of the Nervous System.* London: Churchill.
Schmidt
1871 Gehör und Sprachstörungen in Folge von Apoplexie. *Allg. Zeitschrift. f. Psych.* 27.
Seppilli
1884 La sordite verbale ed afasiea sensoriale Studio clinico ed anatomo-pathologico. *Revist. sparimont. di fremiatria,* 10, 94-125.
Sommer
Zur Theorie der cerebralen Schreib u. Lesestörungen. *Z. f. Psych. u. Phys. der Sinnesorgane,* 5. p. 305.
1894 *Centralbl. fl Nervenheilk.* u. Psych.
Starr, A.
1884 Cortical lesions of the brain. A Collection and Analysis of the American Cases of Localized Cerebral Disease. *Amer. Journ. of the Med. Sc.*, July.
Storch, E.
1901 Versuch einer psycho-physiologischen Darstellung des Bewusstseins. Berlin
1903 Zwei Falle von reiner Alexie. *Monatschr. f. Psych. und Neurol., 13.*
Wernicke, C.
1881-83. *Lehrbuch der Gehirnkrankheiten.* 3 vols. Berlin: Fischer.
1886 Einige neure Arbeiten uber aphasie. *Fortschritte der Med.*, 3, 824, 1885; 377, 463.
1903 Ein Fall von isolierter Agraphie. *Monatschr. f. Psych. u. Neurol.* 13.
Westphal, A.
1884 Ueber einen Fall von Zerstörung des linken Schläfelappens durch Geschwulsbildung ohne aphasichen Störungen. Linkshändigkeit. *Berlin. klin. Wchschrft.* No. 49.
Wolff,
1897 Ueber krankhafte Dissociation der Vorstellungen. Habilitationsschrift., *Z.f. Psych. d. Sinnl 15.*

AUTHOR INDEX

SUBJECT INDEX

Bei Fragen zur Produktsicherheit wenden Sie sich bitte an:
If you have any questions regarding product safety,
please contact:

Walter de Gruyter GmbH
Genthiner Straße 13
10785 Berlin
productsafety@degruyterbrill.com